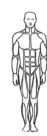

A Practical Approach to Strength Training

4th Edition

Matt Brzycki

Assistant Director of Campus Recreation, Fitness
Department of Athletics, Physical Education and Recreation
Princeton University

Coadjutant Faculty
Department of Exercise Science and Sport Studies
School of Arts and Sciences
Rutgers, The State University of New Jersey

First edition published in 1989.
Second edition published in 1991.
Third edition published in 1995.

ISBN: 9781935628132

Cover design by Mark Collins

Book design by Wish Publishing

Printed in the United States of America
10 9 8 7 6 5 4 3 2 1

Printed by
Versa Press, Inc.
1465 Spring Bay Road
East Peoria, Illinois 61611

Distributed by
Cardinal Publishers Group
2402 Shadeland Avenue, Suite A
Indianapolis, Indiana 46219

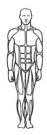

TABLE OF CONTENTS

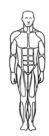

Acknowledgements

Sincere thanks to the following individuals, without whom this book wouldn't have been possible:

Mark Collins of Bright Ideas Graphics (Delran, New Jersey) who designed the front and back covers.

Holly Witten Kondras of Wish Publishing (Terre Haute, Indiana) who designed the interior of the book and coordinated the project with the printer.

Raymundo Abayon, Bobbi Augustyn, Tony Alexander, Dan Bennett, Ryan Bonfiglio, Jim Bryan, Brendan Brzycki, Ryan Brzycki, Anita Carley, Crista Collins, Nickolas Conte, Marguerite Cutchey, Roger Doobraj, David Durell, Patty Durell, Charity Fesler, Alexa Fornicola, Fred Fornicola, Jason Gallucci, Mark Harrison, Stevie Harrison, Troy Harrison, Dave Hauger, Dave Heebner, Kris Heebner, Sharon Henderson, Curt Hillegas, Jane Hunter, Vanessa Jones, Charles Kruger, Jake Marcin, Eliza Martinez, Tom O'Rourke Jr, John Quigley, Paul Quigley, Marty Riehm, Linda Salonek, Peter Silletti, Kurt Siudzinski, Michael Snaer, Illiana Stoilova-Rogers, Zach Turcotte, Shikha Uberoi and Lauren Woods whose photographs appear throughout the book.

Mark Asanovich, Ryan Bonfiglio, Michael Bradley, Margaret Bryan, Mark Brzycki, Luke Carlson, Patty Durell, Fred Fornicola, Lori Fornicola, Greg Fried, Greg Hammond, Mark Harrison, Stevie Harrison, Troy Harrison, Pilar Martinez, Tom Nowak, John Quigley, Melanie Silletti, Peter Silletti, Chris Stone, Ken Stone, Shikha Uberoi and Karl Wright who took or provided photographs that appear throughout the book.

Cybex International, Incorporated, for providing the artwork that appears on the first page of each chapter and in Figures 1.1 and 1.2.

The US Department of Agriculture for providing the MyPlate icon that appears in Chapter 19.

The U.S. Food and Drug Adminstration for providing the Nutrition Facts panel that appears in Chapter 19.

Except as noted here or elsewhere, all photographs were taken by or provided by Matt Brzycki.

v

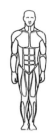

1 Basic Anatomy and Muscular Function

Before discussing any type of physical training, it's necessary for you to gain a basic understanding of your muscles and how they work. Essentially, any physical activity is a series of movements that are made by your muscles acting on your skeleton. (Their combined efforts are reflected in the term musculoskeletal system.)

More to the point, your body is basically a system of levers. Movement of these levers – your bones – is produced by your muscles which are anchored to your bones by tendons. (Tendons link muscle to bone; ligaments link bone to bone.) Perhaps the most well-known and noticeable tendon in your body is the Achilles tendon which fastens your calf muscles to your heel bone.

MUSCLE: TYPES AND STRUCTURE

There are three different types of muscle tissue: cardiac, smooth and skeletal. Cardiac muscle makes up most of your heart wall, smooth muscle is found in the walls of your blood vessels and skeletal muscle acts across your joints to produce movement.

Your muscles are made up of numerous muscle fibers (or cells) which, in turn, are made up of many myofibrils. (To get an idea of this arrangement, picture a telephone cable containing hundreds of wires.) Myofibrils contain two contractile protein filaments that run parallel to one another: the thinner actin and the thicker myosin. Muscular contraction occurs at this level.

TYPES OF MUSCULAR CONTRACTIONS

In normal dialogue, contraction means getting smaller or shorter. But with a muscular contraction, this definition doesn't always hold true. Here, contraction refers to the process in which a muscle generates force. (The force that's exerted by a muscle on the weight of an object is known as the tension; the force that's exerted by the weight of an object on a muscle is known as the load. So, tension and load are opposing forces.)

There are three types of muscular contractions: concentric, eccentric and isometric. Concentric and eccentric contractions are more common than isometric contractions in physical training. But isometric contractions do occur and, therefore, must be considered.

A concentric contraction is one in which a muscle shortens against a load. The resistance moves in a direction away from the earth or opposite the direction of gravity. Examples of concentric contractions are raising a weight, ascending from a squat position and running up a hill. In a concentric contraction, muscular tension is more than the external load. Since the mechanical work is positive, a concentric contraction is sometimes referred to as the positive phase of a movement or repetition.

An eccentric contraction occurs when a muscle lengthens against a load. The resistance moves in a direction toward the earth or in the direction of gravity. Examples of eccentric contractions are lowering a weight, descending into a squat position and running down a hill. In an eccentric contraction, muscular tension is less than the external load. Since the mechanical work is negative, an eccentric contraction is sometimes referred to as the negative phase of a movement or repetition.

Finally, an isometric (or static) contraction is one in which the contractile component of a muscle shortens while the elastic connective tissue lengthens by the same amount thereby producing no change in the overall muscle-tendon length.

1

Examples of isometric contractions are holding a weight in a static position, maintaining a squat position and doing an iron cross on the still rings. Because there's no joint movement during an isometric contraction, the mechanical work is zero. (Of course, energy must be provided in order to perform an isometric contraction. Although there's no mechanical work, there's metabolic work.)

THE SLIDING FILAMENT THEORY

As noted earlier, movement of your skeletal system is produced by contraction of your muscles. Though it was first met with some skepticism, the most widely accepted theory of explaining muscular contraction is the Sliding Filament Theory. In something that's worthy of Ripley's Believe It or Not, the theory was proposed simultaneously in 1954 – in the same journal, no less – by two pairs of researchers: Sir Andrew Huxley and Dr. Rolf Niedergerke at the University of Cambridge in Cambridge, England, and Drs. Hugh Huxley and Jean Hanson at the Massachusetts Institute of Technology in Cambridge, Massachusetts. (In case you're wondering, the two Huxleys weren't related.)

As the name of this theory implies, one set of protein filaments is thought to slide over the other and overlap (like pistons in a sleeve) thereby shortening the muscle. Here's how: The myosin filaments have tiny protein projections in the shape of globular heads that extend toward the actin filaments. During a concentric contraction, it's believed that these projections (or cross-bridges) bind to the actin filaments and then swivel in a ratchet-like fashion – much like oars in a boat – in such a way that it pulls the actin filaments over the myosin filaments. The cross-bridges then uncouple from the actin filaments, pivot, reattach and repeat the cycle. Thus, the process can be summed up as attach-rotate-detach-rotate.

This action occurs along the entire myofibril and among all the myofibrils of a muscle fiber. However, the cross-bridges don't attach-rotate-detach-rotate at the same time since this would result in a series of jerks rather than a smooth movement.

A myosin filament may attach to and detach from an actin filament thousands of times in the course of a single contraction (such as during one repetition of an exercise). Given that a muscle only shortens a small amount when it contracts, this means that one cycle of cross-bridging is virtually undetectable.

JOINT JARGON

Several terms are frequently used in the vernacular of physical training to describe the movement of joints. Familiarity with these terms will assist you in understanding the function of most muscles.

Flexion is a decrease in the angle between two bones and extension is an increase in the angle between two bones. Abduction is movement of a limb away from the mid-line of the body and adduction is movement of a limb toward the mid-line of the body. Finally, rotation is turning about the vertical axis of a bone.

THE MAJOR MUSCLES

Incredible as it may seem, there are more than 600 muscles in the human body (and about six billion muscle fibers). In fact, each one of your forearms has 19 separate muscles with such exotic-sounding names as extensor carpi radialis brevis and flexor digitorum superficialis. Don't worry, it's well beyond the scope and purpose of this book to discuss your muscles in such great detail; instead, the focus will be on your major muscles.

It's convenient to organize the major muscles into these nine areas: hips, upper legs, lower legs, torso, upper arms, lower arms, abdominals, lower back and neck. Brief notes on the location and primary functions of each muscle are given along with anatomical terminology that's generally accepted in discussions of physical training. (Anterior and posterior views of the muscles are illustrated in Figures 1.1 and 1.2, respectively.) Also provided are examples of how a particular muscle would be used.

HIPS

Your hip region is made up of three major muscle groups: the gluteals, adductors and iliopsoas.

Gluteals

Your gluteals (or "glutes") are located on the back of your hips. They're composed of three main muscles: the gluteus maximus, gluteus medius and gluteus minimus. The largest and strongest muscle in your body is the gluteus maximus (which forms your buttocks or "butt"). The primary function of this muscle is hip extension (driving your upper legs backward). Your gluteus medius and gluteus minimus cause hip abduction (spreading your legs apart). Your gluteal muscles are involved significantly in walking, jogging/running, jumping and stairclimbing.

Adductors

Your adductor group is composed of five muscles that are found throughout your inner thigh: the gracilis, pectineus, adductor longus, adductor brevis and adductor magnus (which is the largest of the five). The muscles of your inner thigh are used during hip adduction (bringing your legs together).

Iliopsoas

The iliopsoas is actually a collective term for three muscles on the front of your hips: the iliacus, psoas major and psoas minor. The main function of the iliopsoas is hip flexion (bringing your knees to your chest). Your iliopsoas has a major role in many activities such as lifting your knees when walking, jogging/running and stairclimbing. The iliopsoas is sometimes considered with the muscles of the abdomen.

UPPER LEGS

The two major muscle groups of your upper legs (or thighs) are the hamstrings and quadriceps.

Hamstrings

Your hamstrings (or "hams") are found on the back of your upper legs and actually include three muscles. From the medial (inner) side to the lateral (outer) side, the muscles are the semimembranosus, semitendinosus and biceps femoris. Together, these muscles are involved in knee flexion (bringing your heels toward your buttocks) and hip extension (driving your upper legs backward). Your hamstrings are used extensively during jogging/running and jumping. One of the best reasons to strengthen your hamstrings is that they're quite susceptible to pulls and tears. Clearly, strong muscles on the back of the upper legs are necessary to counterbalance the powerful muscles on the front of the upper legs.

Quadriceps

Your quadriceps (or "quads") are the most important muscles on the front of your upper legs. As its name suggests, your quadriceps are made up of four muscles. The vastus lateralis is located on the lateral side of your thigh; the vastus medialis resides on the medial side of your thigh above your patella (kneecap); between these two thigh muscles is the vastus intermedius; and, finally, laying on top of the vastus intermedius is the rectus femoris. The main function of your quadriceps is knee extension (straightening your legs). Your quadriceps are involved in jogging/running, kicking, jumping, biking and stairclimbing.

LOWER LEGS

The calves and dorsi flexors are the two major muscle groups in your lower legs.

Calves

Your calves are comprised of two important muscles that are located on the back of your lower legs: the gastrocnemius (or "gastroc") and soleus. The gastrocnemius is a superficial muscle that makes up the visible bulk of the calves; the soleus lies beneath the gastrocnemius. These two muscles have a common tendon of insertion – the Achilles tendon – and are jointly referred to as the triceps surae or, more simply, the gastroc-soleus. (The "triceps" designation counts the two heads of the gastrocnemius along with the soleus. Another perspective, though less popular, includes the gastrocnemius, soleus and plantaris as the triumvirate.)

The gastrocnemius and soleus are employed in plantar flexion (straightening your ankles as in pointing your foot downward or rising up on your toes). Normally, the gastrocnemius is involved more than the soleus in plantar flexion. However, when the angle between your upper and lower legs is about 90 degrees or less – such as in the seated position – the function of the gastrocnemius is diminished and the soleus makes a greater contribution to the movement. Your calves play a major role in jogging/running, jumping and stairclimbing.

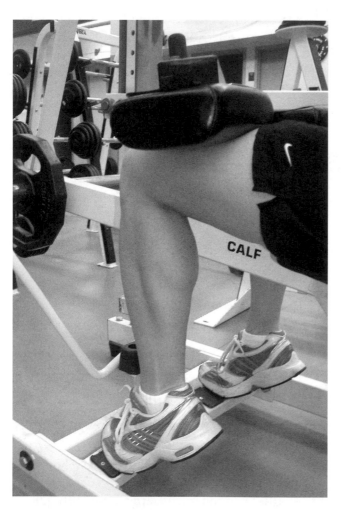

When the angle between your upper and lower legs is about 90 degrees or less, the function of the gastrocnemius is diminished and the soleus makes a greater contribution to the movement.

Dorsi Flexors

The front of your lower legs contains four muscles that are sometimes simply referred to as the dorsi flexors. The largest of these muscles is the tibialis anterior. The dorsi flexors are primarily used in dorsi flexion (bending your ankles as in bringing your foot upward). It's critical to strengthen your dorsi flexors as a safeguard against shin splints.

TORSO

The three major muscle groups in your torso are the chest, upper back and shoulders.

Chest

The main muscles that surround your chest area are the pectoralis major and pectoralis minor which are collectively known as the "pecs." The pectoralis major is thick, flat and fan-shaped and the most superficial muscle of your chest wall. The pectoralis minor is thin, flat and triangular and positioned beneath the pectoralis major. Together, these two muscles pull your upper arms across your torso. The chest is involved in pushing and throwing movements.

Upper Back

The latissimus dorsi is a long, broad muscle that comprises most of your upper back. As a matter of fact, the "lats" are the largest muscle in your upper body. Its primary function is to pull the upper arms backward and downward. Your lats are an essential muscle in assorted pulling movements and climbing skills. In addition, developing your upper back is necessary to provide muscular balance between the anterior (front) and posterior (back) segments of your torso.

Shoulders

Your shoulders are made up of numerous muscles. The primary muscles are the deltoids, trapezius, rhomboids and so-called rotator cuff.

Perhaps the most important muscles of your shoulders are the deltoids. Your "delts" are actually composed of three separate parts (or heads). The anterior deltoid is found on the front of your shoulder and is used to raise your upper arm forward; the middle deltoid is found on the side of your shoulder and is used to lift your upper arm sideways; and the posterior deltoid is found on the back of your shoulder and is used to draw your upper arm backward.

The trapezius is a kite-shaped (or trapezoid-shaped) muscle. Its upper portion resides at the base of your neck and across your shoulders; its middle portion covers much of your upper back. There are three primary functions of the "traps." The upper portion does shoulder elevation (shrugging your shoulders as if to say, "I don't know") and neck extension (bringing your head backward); the middle portion does scapulae adduction (pinching your shoulder blades together). The trapezius is sometimes considered with the muscles of the neck.

Lying beneath the middle portion of the trapezius are the rhomboid major and rhomboid minor. The main job of the rhomboids is scapulae adduction.

Your rotator cuff is comprised of several deep muscles that are sometimes referred to as the internal rotators (the subscapularis and teres major) and the external rotators (the infraspinatus and teres minor). In addition to performing rotation, these muscles are also largely responsible for maintaining the integrity of your shoulder joint and preventing shoulder impingement.

UPPER ARMS

The two major muscles of your upper arms are the biceps and triceps.

Biceps

The prominent muscle that's located on the front of your upper arm is technically known as the biceps brachii. As its name suggests, the muscle has two separate parts (or heads). When the biceps are fully contracted, this separation can be seen as a groove on a well-developed upper arm. The primary function of your biceps is elbow flexion (bending your arms). Your biceps assist your upper back in pulling and climbing movements.

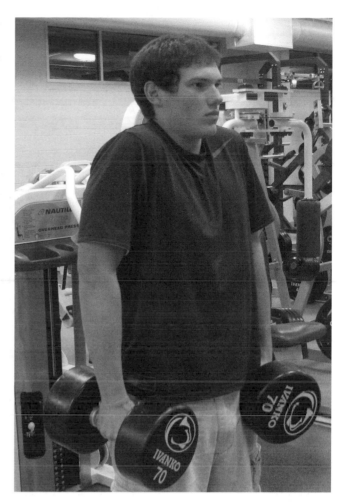

The upper portion of the trapezius is involved in shoulder elevation. (Photo by Mark Harrison.)

Triceps

The prominent muscle that's located on the back of your upper arm is technically known as the triceps brachii. As its name suggests, the muscle has three distinct heads: the long, lateral and medial. When the triceps are fully contracted, these three heads produce a horseshoe-shaped appearance on a well-developed upper arm. The primary function of your triceps is elbow extension (straightening your arms). Your triceps assist your chest and shoulders in pushing and throwing movements.

LOWER ARMS

The forearms are the major muscles in your lower arms.

5

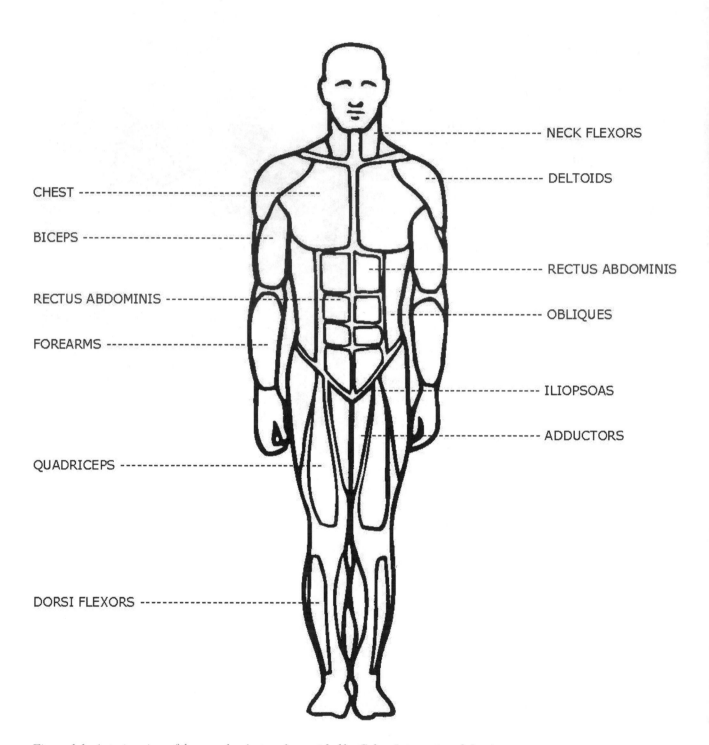

Figure 1.1: Anterior view of the muscles (artwork provided by Cybex International, Inc.)

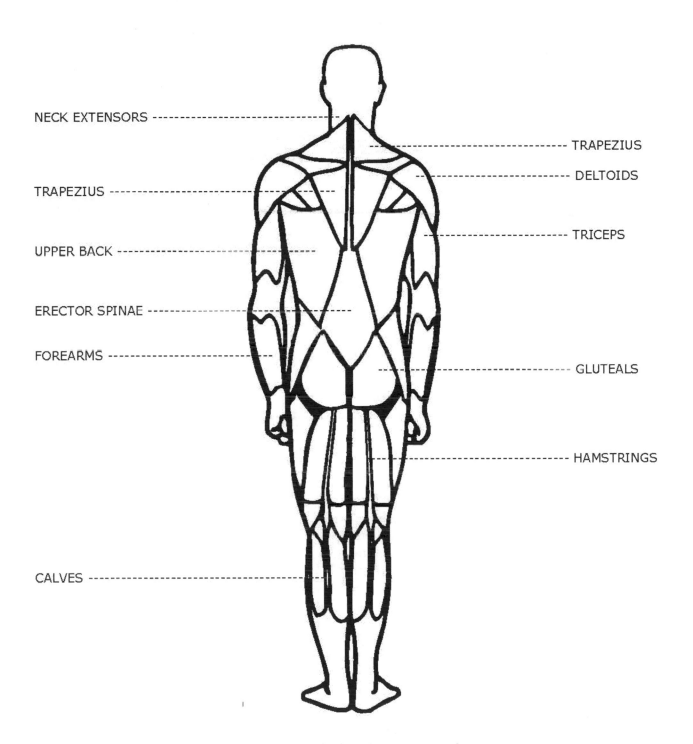

NECK EXTENSORS

TRAPEZIUS

DELTOIDS

TRAPEZIUS

TRICEPS

UPPER BACK

ERECTOR SPINAE

FOREARMS

GLUTEALS

HAMSTRINGS

CALVES

Figure 1.2: Posterior view of the muscles (artwork provided by Cybex International, Inc.)

Forearms

As mentioned previously, each one of your forearms has 19 different muscles. These muscles can be divided into two groups on the basis of their position and function. The anterior group on the front of your forearm causes wrist flexion (flexing your wrist) and pronation (turning your palm downward); the posterior group on the back of your forearm causes wrist extension (extending your wrist) and supination (turning your palm upward). Since the muscles of the forearms affect your wrists, hands and fingers, they're extremely important in pulling movements, climbing skills and tasks that involve gripping.

ABDOMINALS

The abdominal muscles are comprised of the rectus abdominis, obliques and transversus abdominis.

Rectus Abdominis

The rectus abdominis is a long, narrow muscle that extends vertically across the front of your abdomen from the lower rim of your rib cage to your pelvis. Its main function is torso flexion (pulling your torso toward your thighs). The fibers of this muscle are interrupted along their course by three horizontal fibrous bands which inspire the term washboard abs when describing an especially well-developed abdomen. This distinctive architecture has led to the popular but erroneous belief that there are upper abs and lower abs. Your rectus abdominis helps to control your breathing and plays a major role in forced expiration during intense activity.

Obliques

The external and internal obliques reside on both sides of your mid-section. The external oblique is a broad muscle; its fibers form a V across the front of your abdomen, extending diagonally downward from your lower ribs to your pubic bone. The external oblique has two main functions: torso lateral flexion (bending your torso to the same side) and torso rotation (turning your torso to the opposite side). The internal oblique is located immediately under the external oblique on both sides of your abdomen; its fibers form an inverted V along the front of your abdomen, extending diagonally upward from your pubic bone to your lower ribs. The internal oblique has two functions: torso lateral flexion (bending your torso to the same side) and torso rotation (turning your torso to the same side). In a nutshell, your obliques are used during movements in which your torso bends laterally or twists. The external and internal obliques are also active during expiration and inspiration, respectively.

Transversus Abdominis

The muscle that comprises the innermost layer of your abdominal wall is the transversus abdominis. The fibers of this muscle run horizontally across the abdomen. The primary function of the transversus abdominis is to constrict your abdomen. This muscle also helps to control your breathing and is involved in forced expiration during intense exercise.

LOWER BACK

The most important muscles in your lower back are the erector spinae (or spinal erectors).

Erector Spinae

Located on the posterior and lateral portion of your mid-section, the main function of your erector spinae is torso extension (straightening your torso from a bent-over position). However, the erector spinae also assist in torso lateral flexion (bending your torso to the side) and torso rotation (turning your torso).

NECK

The major muscles of your neck include the neck flexors and neck extensors.

Neck Flexors

The muscles on the front of your neck can be collectively referred to as the neck flexors. A major neck flexor is your sternocleidomastoideus. This muscle has two parts – one located on each side of your neck – that start behind your ears and run down to your sternum (breastbone) and clavicles (collarbones). When both sides of the sternocleidomastoideus contract at the same time, it results in neck flexion (bringing your head toward your chest); when one side acts alone, it results in neck lateral flexion (bending your neck to the side) or neck rotation (turning your head). Like the other muscles of the neck, your neck flexors help to stabilize your head. Your neck flexors are also used in several sports and activities, most notably soccer. It's critical for those who participate in combat sports –

including football, rugby, boxing, judo and wrestling – to strengthen all of the muscles that influence their neck.

Neck Extensors

The muscles on the back of your neck can be collectively referred to as the neck extensors. These muscles are mainly used in neck extension (bringing your head backward).

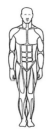

2 The Physiological Basis of Physical Training

It's beneficial for you to know how your body produces and utilizes energy during your physical training. Familiarity with these concepts will help you to understand how the physiological processes affect your physical performance. In addition, this knowledge will help you to structure your aerobic and anaerobic training in an effective manner. Also important is an understanding of the basic operations and functions of your circulatory and respiratory systems.

ADENOSINE TRIPHOSPHATE

The energy that's produced from the breakdown of food – carbohydrates, protein and fat – isn't used directly to perform mechanical work (physical activity). Instead, this energy is stored as adenosine triphosphate (ATP), a molecule that resides in most cells, particularly muscle cells, and has an extremely high energy yield.

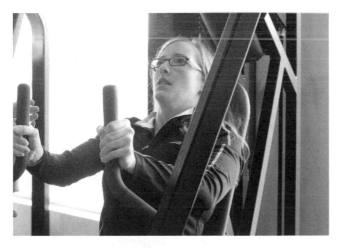

The energy that's liberated during the breakdown of ATP is your primary and immediate source of energy that's used to accomplish muscular work. (Photo provided by Luke Carlson.)

The structure of ATP consists of an adenosine component (made of adenine and ribose) that's bonded to three phosphate groups. The energy from ATP isn't necessarily in its chemical make-up but in the high-energy phosphate bonds that hold the molecule together. When the outermost phosphate bond is broken – meaning that one phosphate is separated from the rest of the molecule – energy is released. This process yields adenosine diphosphate (ADP) and inorganic phosphate as end-products. The energy that's liberated during the breakdown of ATP is your primary and immediate source of energy that's used to accomplish muscular work.

THE ENERGY SYSTEMS

In order for you to perform physically for prolonged periods of time, a steady supply of ATP must be made available to your muscle cells. Unfortunately, muscle cells can only store a limited amount of ATP. As such, your muscle cells must be able to rebuild – or rephosphorylate – ATP from ADP and inorganic phosphate.

A typical ATP molecule may exist for only a few seconds before its terminal bond is broken and energy is released. The ADP formed by this chemical event is remade rapidly back into ATP. Interestingly, energy is also required to reconstruct ATP. In fact, all of your energy systems have one common and primary purpose: to resynthesize ATP in order to furnish energy so that your muscles can perform mechanical work.

The process by which ATP is reassembled involves the interaction of three different series of chemical reactions. Two of these ATP-generating pathways can operate in the absence of oxygen and are labeled anaerobic; the other can only operate in the presence of oxygen and is labeled aerobic. The two anaerobic pathways are the ATP-PC System and Anaerobic Glycolysis; the aerobic pathway is the Aerobic System.

The ATP-PC System

In the ATP-PC (or Phosphagen) System, the energy that's used to rebuild ATP comes from the breakdown of a chemical compound that's known as phosphocreatine (PC) or, alternately, creatine phosphate (CP). Since ATP and PC both contain phosphate groups, they're collectively referred to as phosphagens.

Like ATP, PC is stored in your muscle cells. Also like ATP, PC releases a large amount of energy when its phosphate group is removed. This process yields creatine and inorganic phosphate as end-products. The phosphate is "donated" to ADP to convert it back into ATP. As quickly as ATP is broken down during brief, intense efforts, it's immediately and continuously remanufactured until your PC stores are depleted. Ironically, PC can only be rebuilt from the energy that's released by the breakdown of ATP. (This occurs during rest or a reduced level of intensity.)

Without being replenished, the ATP stores in a working muscle would be spent from an all-out exertion within a handful of seconds. If you're in reasonably good condition, this correlates to running about 40 meters at breakneck speed. When replenished by PC, the ATP stores in a working muscle would be spent from an all-out exertion within about 30 seconds.

So, the total amount of energy that's available from the ATP-PC System is very limited. Obviously, the usefulness of your stored phosphagens is in their rapid availability, not in their total quantity. Fast, powerful movements – such as sprinting and jumping – couldn't be performed without this energy system. It's no surprise, then, that your ATP-PC System is the predominant energy pathway for physical efforts of high intensity and brief duration, about 30 seconds or less.

Anaerobic Glycolysis

In your body, carbohydrates are converted into glucose (blood sugar) which can either be utilized instantly in that form or stored as glycogen in your liver and muscles for later use. The term glycolysis means to break down glycogen and, as noted earlier, anaerobic means in the absence of oxygen. Therefore, Anaerobic Glycolysis literally means to break down glycogen in the absence of oxygen.

When glycogen is broken down, energy is released and used to reassemble ATP. A complete breakdown of glycogen requires oxygen. Since the presence of oxygen isn't necessary during Anaerobic Glycolysis, the breakdown of glycogen is only partial and pyruvic acid is formed as a byproduct. Pyruvic acid is subsequently converted into a substance called lactic acid which is why Anaerobic Glycolysis is often referred to as the Lactic Acid System. (Note: Pyruvate and lactate are the salts of pyruvic acid and lactic acid, respectively.)

In burning a log, ash is left as a waste product. In this sense, lactic acid is the ashen remnant of Anaerobic Glycolysis. The point at which lactic acid first begins to appear in your blood is known as your anaerobic threshold or lactate threshold. When lactic acid enters your blood at a greater rate than it leaves, it builds up and becomes more concentrated. High concentrations of lactic acid can irritate your

The accumulation of lactic acid is also believed to cause heaviness in the muscles, labored breathing and fatigue. (Photo by Lori Fornicola.)

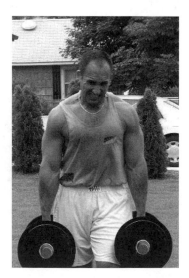

nerve endings and cause pain, discomfort and distress. The accumulation of lactic acid is also believed to cause heaviness in the muscles, labored breathing and fatigue. Because it's a fatiguing byproduct, lactic acid essentially acts as a performance inhibitor during Anaerobic Glycolysis. (A small amount of lactic acid is formed under resting conditions but doesn't accumulate since the rate at which it's produced equals the rate at which it's removed.)

Anaerobic Glycolysis – with a helping hand from your ATP-PC System – is responsible for supplying ATP for all maximum efforts that last between about 30 and 90 seconds. If you're in reasonably good condition, this correlates to sprinting a distance of about 200 to 400 meters. Therefore, the first minute or so of physical training depends on your ability to replenish ATP without the use of oxygen. The resynthesis of ATP is quite rapid but, in the absence of oxygen, is somewhat limited.

The Aerobic System

There's an infinite supply of oxygen available to meet your physiological needs. Think about it: Oxygen is literally everywhere around you. But the amount of energy that you can produce with oxygen is determined by the efficiency of your Aerobic System.

During prolonged physical efforts, your Aerobic System is the last process in your chemical chain-of-command for energy production. Like Anaerobic Glycolysis, the Aerobic System breaks down glycogen. Unlike Anaerobic Glycolysis, however, oxygen is used in the Aerobic System which means that the breakdown of glycogen is complete. (Since glycogen is broken down in the presence of oxygen, it's easy to see why the Aerobic System is sometimes referred to as Aerobic Glycolysis.)

Relative to your anaerobic pathways, your aerobic pathway can operate for a longer duration because no fatiguing byproducts – such as lactic acid – are produced in the presence of oxygen. Rather than form lactic acid from pyruvic acid, your Aerobic System converts pyruvic acid into two end-products: carbon dioxide and water. Carbon dioxide is continually removed by the blood and transported to the lungs where it's exhaled; water is either used in the cells or excreted in the urine. So although glycolytic reactions occur in both the anaerobic and aerobic domains, the difference is that lactic acid isn't formed when oxygen is available. Another feature of your aerobic pathway is that it can break down both carbohydrates and fat to liberate energy for the reconstruction of ATP while your anaerobic pathways can only use carbohydrates. (Energy can also be provided by protein. However, protein isn't normally used as a source of energy.)

The process of rebuilding ATP aerobically occurs in specialized areas of your muscle cells called mitochondria. Because such a large amount of energy is produced, the mitochondria are often referred to as the powerhouse of the cell. Muscle cells are usually very rich in mitochondria; in particular, an abundance of mitochondria is found in cardiac muscle (which makes up most of your heart wall) and slow-twitch muscle fibers.

Your Aerobic System becomes the predominant energy pathway once your anaerobic systems are unable to keep up with the metabolic demands of an activity and lactic acid begins to accumulate. Physical efforts that are between about 1.5 and 3.0 minutes in duration are the shared responsibility of Anaerobic Glycolysis and the Aerobic System. If you're in reasonably good condition, this correlates to running a distance of about 400 to 800 meters. For the most part, your Aerobic System becomes the predominant energy pathway after about three minutes of continuous exertion. If you're in reasonably good condition, this correlates to running a distance that's more than about 800 meters.

The longer the duration of an activity, the greater the importance of your Aerobic System. Interestingly, your Aerobic System is also the preferred energy pathway under resting conditions.

The major advantage of your Aerobic System is that it produces relatively large amounts of energy. But due to the transport and delivery of oxygen, it's a time-consuming process. As a

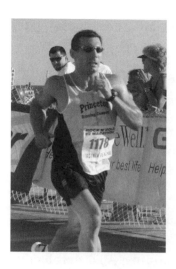

Your Aerobic System becomes the predominant energy pathway after about three minutes of continuous exertion. (Photo provided by Ryan Bonfiglio.)

result, the Aerobic System can't produce energy quickly enough to meet the demands of brief, intense movements such as jumping for a rebound or sprinting to first base.

THE "ENERGY CONTINUUM"

The need for a particular energy system is determined by the time and intensity requirements of a specific activity. At one end of the so-called energy continuum is the ATP-PC System which is the predominant energy pathway for immediate, high-intensity efforts; at the other end of the continuum is the Aerobic System which is the predominant energy pathway for long-term, low-intensity efforts. In between these two extremes is Anaerobic Glycolysis which partners with either the ATP-PC System or the Aerobic System to supply energy for short-term, high-intensity efforts that require a mixture of both your anaerobic and aerobic pathways. So, the production of ATP can be immediate (the ATP-PC System), short term (Anaerobic Glycolysis) or long term (the Aerobic System).

Your body doesn't exclusively choose one energy pathway over another; your exercising muscles simply use whatever energy pathway is readily available to meet the existing physiological challenge. Generally, your body selects the most efficient energy pathway to maximize the resynthesis of ATP and minimize the accumulation of lactic acid.

Blood lactate is an excellent indicator of which energy system you mainly relied on during your effort. A high level of blood lactate indicates that the primary energy system was Anaerobic Glycolysis; a low level of blood lactate means that the primary energy system was the Aerobic System.

Although one of your energy pathways may serve as the principal source of energy for a given activity, all three pathways contribute to the supply of ATP that's required to perform most activities. For example, playing full-court basketball is mainly anaerobic because it involves a series of brief, all-out efforts such as sprinting, jumping and so on. But it also has an aerobic component since the anaerobic efforts are required over an extended period of time. So, energy is needed from the anaerobic pathways as well as the aerobic pathway. In fact, a blend of all energy systems is the most likely scenario for the majority of physical activities that you might perform.

Remember that as the time of an activity increases, the continuum shifts away from anaerobic work toward aerobic work. It should also be noted that your energy systems operate in phases on a progressive scale. Moreover, your body doesn't shift abruptly from one energy system to another; the transition between the three systems is very subtle. In a sense, all three metabolic processes overlap each other. Clearly, if you can improve the efficiency of your energy systems through physical training, then you can also improve your performance potential.

To summarize: The ATP-PC System is used for efforts of about 30 seconds or less. The ATP-PC System and Anaerobic Glycolysis are used for efforts of about 30 to 90 seconds. Anaerobic Glycolysis and the Aerobic System are used for efforts of about 1.5 to 3.0 minutes. And the Aerobic System is used for efforts of about three minutes or more.

Blood Lactate

As indicated earlier, lactate threshold – which can be improved through training – is the point at which lactic acid first begins to appear in the blood. Being able to delay and/or tolerate the accumulation of blood lactate allows an individual to perform at a high level of effort for a sustained length of time with less fatigue. Everything else being equal, those who have a higher lactate threshold have a greater potential to resist fatigue during prolonged activities than those who have a lower lactate threshold.

Here's an illustration: Oxygen intake – discussed in detail in Chapter 14 – is an excellent indicator of aerobic fitness. Consider two male athletes with the same oxygen intake but different lactate thresholds. Suppose that Athlete A has a higher lactate threshold and, as a result, can sustain 75 to 85% of his maximum oxygen intake and Athlete B can sustain 50 to 60%. Since Athlete A can perform at a higher percentage of his maximum oxygen intake than Athlete B, everything else being equal, Athlete A would have a greater aerobic potential. Or look at it this way: For the same level of effort, lactic acid would appear much sooner in the blood of Athlete B than in the blood of Athlete A. This would put Athlete B at a huge disadvantage.

Underscoring this point further is an interesting anecdote about Lance Armstrong and lactic acid. Armstrong, of course, was a professional road-racing cyclist who won the Tour de France a record seven consecutive times; in those days, he was one of the top endurance athletes on the planet and underwent extensive physiological testing. When analyzed at the Human Performance Laboratory at the University of Texas at Austin in September 1993, Dr. Edward Coyle found that Armstrong had a high lactate threshold. This physiological characteristic enabled him to function at an intensity that was closer to his aerobic limits in comparison to most people. Dr. Coyle also found that Armstrong accumulated significantly less blood lactate during exhaustive exercise (stationary cycling) than other highly competitive cyclists.

A similar finding was reported on Paula Radcliffe, the world-record holder in the women's marathon with a time of 2:15:25. Dr. Andrew Jones found that Radcliffe – who has run four of the five fastest times ever in the

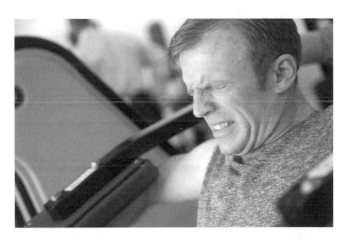

It's important for you to make your physical training progressively more challenging in order to provide an overload. (Photo provided by Luke Carlson.)

marathon – accumulated roughly half as much blood lactate during exhaustive exercise (treadmill running) than other highly competitive runners.

PHYSIOLOGICAL OVERLOAD

Any type of physical training – whether it's done for anaerobic, aerobic, strength, flexibility, metabolic, power or skill improvements must incorporate a well-known foundational concept in exercise science called the Overload Principle. The term overload means that a targeted physiological and/or neurological system is made to work harder than it's accustomed to working. This suggests that there's a minimum threshold that must be surpassed before a specific, long-term adaptation is produced.

Over a period of time, you'll likely find that the same activity – which was originally difficult – can be performed with less effort. As a result, it's important for you to make your physical training progressively more challenging in order to provide an overload and produce further physiological improvements in the target system (such as your musculoskeletal, respiratory and/or circulatory system).

Because of this, it's vital that you keep accurate records of your physical performances. Maintaining records permits you to track your progress thereby making your workouts more productive and more meaningful.

THE "ULTIMATE PUMP"

A thorough discussion about the physiological basis of physical training wouldn't be complete without mention of the most important muscle in your body and primary driving force behind the three energy systems: your heart. The heart is a large, hollow, cone-shaped organ that's located just behind your sternum (breastbone). It's about 5.0 inches long, 3.5 inches wide and 2.5 inches thick, roughly the size of a man's clenched fist. The average adult male heart weighs about 10 ounces while its female counterpart weighs about eight ounces.

Your heart is the ultimate endurance muscle or "pump." It contracts about 100,000 times each day, pausing only briefly after a contraction to fill with more blood for its next contraction. This muscular pump is comprised of left and right halves. Each half of your heart consists of two chambers: an atrium and a ventricle. The atria are the recovery chambers of your heart and the ventricles are the pumping chambers.

Your blood has two routes or circuits: the systemic circuit and the pulmonary circuit. In the systemic circuit, the powerful left ventricle of your heart pumps oxygen-enriched blood to your body tissues (such as your skeletal muscles). The blood collects carbon dioxide and other metabolic wastes and returns to the right atrium of your heart. In the pulmonary circuit, the right ventricle of your heart sends oxygen-depleted blood that's laden with carbon dioxide to your lungs. The blood drops off carbon dioxide, picks up oxygenated blood and returns to the left atrium of your heart.

Normally, the right half of your heart pumps the same amount of blood as the left half of your heart. However, the left half of your heart is much stronger and better developed than the right half. This is because the left half of your heart must pump blood throughout your entire body (the systemic circuit) while the right half only has to pump blood to your lungs (the pulmonary circuit).

Heart Rate

As the blood surges out of the ventricles, it pounds the arterial wall. This impact is transmitted along the length of the artery and can be felt as a throb or a "pulse" at those points where an artery is just under your skin. The beat of your pulse is synchronous with the beat of your heart. To a degree, the rate of the heartbeat is dependent on the size of the organism. A good rule of thumb is that the smaller the size of the organism, the faster the beat of the heart. A normal resting heart rate for humans is about 60 to 80 beats per minute (bpm). Women's hearts beat about six to eight times per minute faster than those of men. Children's hearts beat even more rapidly. At birth, a baby's heart rate could be as high as 130 bpm. Animals that are larger than humans have slower heart rates; an elephant's heart rate is about 30 bpm. Animals that are smaller than humans have faster heart rates; a shrew's heart rate is more than 800 bpm (and holds the distinction of having perhaps the highest heart rate ever recorded in any animal with 1,511 bpm).

Active individuals usually have lower resting heart rates than inactive individuals. It wouldn't be unusual for a person who's highly active to have a resting heart rate of 50 bpm or less. A lower resting heart rate would be especially important if the heart is limited to a certain number of beats over the course of a lifetime. For instance, suppose that the human heart can only beat about 2.5 billion times before it simply wears out from the labors of continual usage. In this scenario, an individual with an average resting heart rate of 70 bpm could expect to live a little less than 68 years; on the other hand, an individual with an average resting heart rate of 60 bpm could expect to live a little more than 79 years. If there's a limit to the number of times that a heart can beat in a lifetime, a decrease in the resting heart rate of just 10 bpm would translate into more than 11 additional years of life. While this notion has yet to be proven scientifically, it's still quite intriguing. And it does generate an added importance of having a lower resting heart rate.

Blood Pressure

When your heart forces blood through your circulatory system, the fluid is under pressure. Your blood pressure is a measure of the force that's exerted by your blood against the arterial walls. Blood pressure has two measures: systolic and diastolic. Your systolic blood pressure is the maximum pressure in your arteries when your ventricles contract; your diastolic blood pressure is the maximum pressure when your ventricles recover (refilling with blood).

Blood pressure is measured in milliliters of mercury (mmHg). An example of a blood-pressure reading would be 124/82 in which the upper number (124) is the systolic pressure and the lower number (82) is the diastolic pressure.

Of no small concern is high blood pressure (hypertension). The Seventh Joint National Committee on Prevention, Detection, Evaluation and Treatment of High Blood Pressure defined several categories of resting blood pressure for adults: Normal is a systolic pressure of less than 120 *and* a diastolic pressure of less than 80; pre-hypertension is a systolic pressure of 120 to 139 *or* a diastolic pressure of 80 to 89; and hypertension is a systolic pressure of at least 140 *or* a diastolic pressure of at least 90. Those who have chronic high blood pressure should consult with a physician. The same holds true for those who have chronic low blood pressure (aka hypotension). Note: If the systolic and diastolic pressures are in different categories, the classification is based on the higher category. For instance, if the systolic pressure is 119 (normal) and the diastolic pressure is 90 (hypertension), it would be classified as hypertension.

THE RESPIRATORY PROCESS

Respiration is a combination of inspiration and expiration. Inspiration (or inhalation) is an active process in which your lungs inflate and air enters your body. The primary muscle of respiration is your diaphragm. Located in your upper abdominal cavity, the diaphragm is a large, dome-shaped sheet of muscle. Expiration (or exhalation) is a passive process in which your lungs deflate and air is released into the environment. During intense activity, however, expiration is an active process – referred to as forced expiration – that's facilitated by your abdominals and internal intercostals (which reside between your ribs along with your external intercostals).

The respiratory process is accomplished without continuous conscious effort. Actually, respiration is a rhythmic action: Inflation of your lungs during inspiration causes expiration; deflation of your lungs during expiration causes inspiration.

Your respiratory system has two major functions: to exchange gases and maintain your acid-base balance.

The Gas Exchange

Your diaphragm – with assistance from your external intercostals in conjunction with the natural changes of pressures within your body – produces an open exchange of oxygen and carbon dioxide. The right ventricle pumps venous blood to your lungs that's low in oxygen and high in carbon dioxide. In the lungs, your blood unloads carbon dioxide and loads oxygen. The blood returns to the left atrium as arterial blood that's high in oxygen and low in carbon dioxide.

A second exchange of gases occurs between your blood and tissues. In this case, your left ventricle pumps arterial blood to your tissues that's high in oxygen and low in carbon dioxide. In the tissues, the blood unloads oxygen and loads carbon dioxide. Essentially, this gas exchange converts arterial blood into venous blood. The venous blood returns to your right atrium where the entire process of gas exchange and transport is repeated over and over again.

Acid-Base Balance

The respiratory process also regulates your acid-base balance, quantified as the pH of your body. Recall that lactic acid is a byproduct of anaerobic training and is the prime suspect in muscular fatigue. Without a system to remove or buffer the buildup of this metabolite, your body fluids would become more acidic and unsettle the delicate acid-base balance.

Your pH is a direct measure of acidity or alkalinity. The lower the pH, the greater the acidity. A pH that's less than 7.0 is considered to be acidic while a pH that's more than 7.0 is considered to be basic or alkaline. (A pH of 7.0 is neutral.) The lactic acid diffuses from your muscles into neighboring tissues and ultimately overflows into your blood. This decreases your blood pH. An environment that's too acidic may inhibit several chemical reactions that are needed for energy production. So in a sense, your acid-base system acts as an alarm mechanism that alerts you to reduce your level of effort because your acid levels have become too high.

BETTER FUNCTION = BETTER PERFORMANCE

As you improve the function of your energy systems through physical training, you'll be better suited to delay the accumulation of lactic acid, discard waste products and exchange gases thereby delaying muscular fatigue. Otherwise, you must abbreviate – or perhaps even terminate – your activities until you attain a more acceptable metabolic environment.

Being able to resist fatigue is an absolute requirement for training and competing at high levels. It's clear that your physical performance is linked to the development and improvement of your three energy systems.

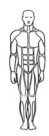

3 Genetics and Strength Potential

enetics is the study of heredity. It's well known that people inherit a variety of physical and behavioral traits from their parents. These traits are passed along from one generation to the next by the estimated 25,000 or so genes in the body which are made of deoxyribonucleic acid or DNA.

The potential for individual variation is simply enormous. These variations are most evident in physical appearance and include eye color, hair color and skeletal height.

Individual variation plays an extremely important role in a person's response to strength training. Because of their genetic (inherited) profile, some people make superior gains in strength (and size) while others make inferior ones, even when employing an identical strength program (doing the same exercises and using the same number of sets and repetitions). The fact of the matter is that with the exception of monozygotic (identical) twins, each individual is a unique genetic entity with a different potential for improving strength (and size).

GENETIC FACTORS

A number of genetic factors determine your response to strength training. These include the following:

Muscle Fiber Type

One of the most influential of all genetic factors is your muscle fiber type. Your muscle fibers can be broadly categorized as slow twitch (ST) or Type I and fast twitch (FT) or Type II. From a functional standpoint, muscle fibers differ in several ways, including speed of contraction, magnitude of force and degree of fatigability.

Relative to FT fibers, ST fibers contract slower, produce less force and have more endurance;

relative to ST fibers, FT fibers contract faster, produce more force and have less endurance. (This isn't to say that ST fibers contract slowly. ST fibers contract quickly but not as quickly as FT fibers. The contraction time of fibers is measured in thousandths of a second. The time to peak force is about 50 milliseconds in FT fibers and 100 milliseconds in ST fibers. To put this into perspective, a proverbial "blink of an eye" takes about 300 milliseconds.)

Because of their fatigue characteristics, ST fibers are often referred to as being oxidative, meaning that the fibers are highly aerobic and heavily dependent on oxygen for energy; FT fibers are often referred to as being glycolytic, meaning that the fibers are highly anaerobic and heavily dependent on glycogen for energy. (Research also recognizes one or more intermediate fiber types that possess characteristics of both FT and ST fibers.)

Most muscles have a blend of about 50% ST fibers and 50% FT fibers but some muscles have a higher proportion of one type or the other. For example, the soleus tends to have a greater percentage of ST fibers (as much as 85%) and the triceps a greater percentage of FT fibers (as much as 70%). Regardless of the distribution, the different fiber types are intermingled throughout each muscle, arranged in a mosaic pattern.

Some individuals inherit a higher-than-average proportion of one fiber type that influences their performance potential in sports and activities that require speed, strength, power and endurance. It has been noted that FT fibers produce more speed and force than ST fibers. (The greater force production is mainly because FT fibers have a larger diameter.) Everything else being equal, those who inherit a high percentage of FT fibers have a greater potential to exhibit speed, strength and power than those who inherit a low percentage of FT fibers. Examples are highly accomplished sprinters, competitive weightlifters and others whose success is predicated on speed, strength and power. Everything else being equal, those who inherit a high percentage of ST fibers have a greater potential to exhibit endurance than those who inherit a low percentage of ST fibers. Examples are highly accomplished long-distance runners, triathletes and others whose success is predicated on endurance.

It should be mentioned that an individual's fiber-type mixture can vary from one muscle to another. And the mixture may even vary from one side of the body to the other. In one study, for instance, there was a 26% difference in the proportion of ST fibers in the vastus lateralis of a volleyball player (73% in the right leg and 47% in the left).

Both FT and ST fibers have the potential to hypertrophy which is an increase in muscular size. (Atrophy is a decrease in muscular size.) However, FT fibers display a much greater potential for hypertrophy than ST fibers. This means that individuals who have a high percentage of FT fibers have a greater potential to increase the size of their muscles. It's interesting to note that FT fibers not only hypertrophy faster and to a greater degree than ST fibers but also atrophy faster and to a greater degree.

Incidentally, there's no scientific evidence that consistently and convincingly supports the notion that ST fibers can be converted into FT fibers or vice versa. It appears as if one type of muscle fiber may take on certain metabolic characteristics of another type but actual conversion doesn't occur. Stated differently, you can't convert one fiber type into another any more than you can convert lead into gold. Simply put, it's impossible to switch the twitch.

While on the subject, an increase in the number of muscle fibers – known as hyperplasia – is thought to take place by fiber splitting or budding. Although hyperplasia has been demonstrated experimentally in several avian and mammalian species – including quails, chickens, cats, rats and mice – there's no

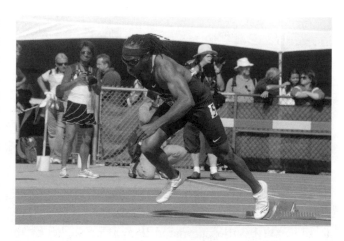

Those who inherit a high percentage of FT fibers include highly accomplished sprinters and others whose success is predicated on speed, strength and power. (Photo by Ken Stone.)

definitive proof that it occurs in humans. Most likely, strength training results in the addition of protein filaments – namely, actin and myosin – not in the addition of muscle fibers.

One last point in this regard pertains to charts that indicate how many repetitions individuals should strive to perform with a percentage their one-repetition maximum (or 1-RM). Because the proportion of FT and ST fibers has a major role in muscular endurance, the number of repetitions that can be done with the same percentage of a 1-RM won't be the same for everyone; individuals who have a high percentage of FT fibers aren't likely to do as many repetitions as individuals who have a high percentage of ST fibers. In effect, achieving the recommended number of repetitions could be too difficult (or outright impossible) for some and too easy for others. So, these charts are only useful for the segment of the population who happens to have inherited a mixture of fiber types that corresponds to the suggested repetitions.

Muscle-to-Tendon Ratio

The muscle organ consists of two parts: the belly (primarily muscle fibers) and the tendon (the fibrous connective tissue). The potential for a muscle to increase in size is related to the length of its belly and tendon. Everything else being equal, those who have long bellies and short tendons have a greater potential for achieving muscular size than those who have short bellies and long tendons.

Consider two individuals who have the same bone lengths but different muscle-to-tendon ratios. Suppose that Lifter A has a long bicep muscle and short bicep tendon and Lifter B has a short bicep muscle and a long bicep tendon. In this example, as depicted in Figure 3.1, Lifter A has a greater potential to increase the size of his bicep than Lifter B.

The dramatic impact of muscle-to-tendon ratios can be seen on the next page in the related photograph of two individuals who are contracting their calves. Note that the lengths of their lower legs are roughly the same. But the lengths of their muscle bellies and tendons are very different which dictates the size of their muscles. The individual on the right has a much longer muscle belly and shorter tendon than the individual on the left. At the time of the photograph, both individuals – female collegiate gymnasts in their freshman year – were training partners who had been doing the same strength program for nearly eight months, performing the same exercises and set/repetition scheme.

But how is the muscle-to-tendon ratio associated with strength potential? Well, a bigger muscle has a larger cross-sectional area. A larger cross-sectional area contains a greater number of protein filaments (actin and myosin) and cross-bridges thereby increasing the capacity to produce force. Therefore, a bigger muscle – in terms of its cross-sectional area – is also a stronger muscle. This means that individuals with long muscle bellies have the potential to be quite strong.

Understand, too, that a small difference in the length of a muscle makes a big difference in strength (and size) potential. In theory, the potential cross-sectional area of a muscle is equal to its length squared and the potential volume of a muscle is equal to its length cubed. To illustrate, a muscle that's three inches long would have a potential cross-sectional area of nine square inches [3 inches x 3 inches] and a potential volume of 27 cubic inches [3 inches x 3 inches x 3 inches]; a muscle that's four inches long would have a potential cross-sectional area of 16 square inches [4 inches x 4 inches] and a potential volume of 64 cubic inches [4 inches x 4 inches x 4 inches].

As with muscle fiber types, an individual's muscle-to-tendon ratio can vary from one muscle to another. It's difficult to determine the actual length of a muscle because it may be hidden by subcutaneous fat (located beneath the skin) or lie below other muscles. However, the length of the triceps, the forearms and especially the calves is usually easy to identify. The lengths of a muscle and its tendon aren't subject to change.

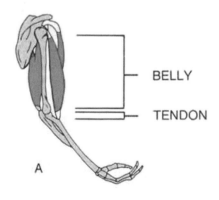

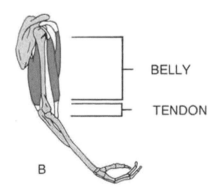

Figure 3.1: Muscle-to-tendon ratio

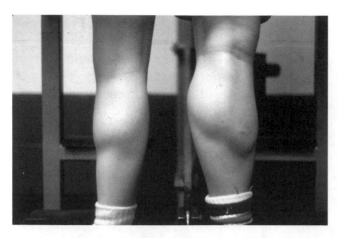

The dramatic impact of muscle-to-tendon ratios can be seen in this photograph of two individuals who are contracting their calves.

Testosterone Level

Although it's a male sex hormone, testosterone is also found in the blood of perfectly normal women. In men, testosterone is produced by the testes; in women, roughly 50% is produced by the ovaries and 50% by the adrenal glands. The secretion of testosterone is regulated by pituitary hormones.

Testosterone influences the secondary sexual characteristics. In men, for example, it lowers the voice and is associated with the growth of facial hair and, inexplicably, male pattern baldness. Additionally, testosterone stimulates increases in strength and muscle mass. In short, its major action is to promote growth. Everything else being equal, those who have high levels of testosterone have a greater potential to improve their strength (and size) than those who have low levels of testosterone.

Interestingly, a number of studies have also found a correlation between testosterone levels and aggressive behavior in both men and women. This isn't unique in the animal kingdom, by the way. Bull sharks are said to have the highest levels of testosterone found in any creature (land or sea) and their aggressive behavior is legendary. It is, perhaps, the most dangerous type of shark in the world.

Lever Lengths and Body Proportions

Archimedes, an ancient Greek mathematician, physicist and engineer, once said something along these lines: "Give me a place to stand and with a lever I will move the whole world." Considering the weight of the planet, that would involve quite a lever. His point, of course, was that levers can be used to lift heavy weights. And levers are a large part of genetics.

Some individuals have lever (bone) lengths and body proportions that give them greater leverage in lifting weights and a greater potential for increasing strength than other individuals. This can be readily seen in the sport of powerlifting. The three competitive powerlifts are the squat, bench press, and deadlift. Favorable lever lengths and body proportions in the bench press are short arms and a thick chest; favorable lever lengths and body proportions in the squat and deadlift are a short torso, wide hips and short legs. (Long arms also help in the deadlift.) Everything else being equal, those who have favorable lever lengths and body proportions have a greater strength potential in certain exercises because they don't have to move the weight as far as those who have less favorable lever lengths and body proportions. The end result is that the individuals can lift extraordinarily heavy weights. In fact, a study of 68 competitive powerlifters found that they were of average to below-average height and had relatively short limbs (which were attributed to their short stature).

Here's another way to look at it: Consider two individuals who are tasked with lifting 200 pounds in the bench press. Because of lever lengths and body proportions, suppose that Lifter A has to move the weight a distance of 20 inches and Lifter B has to move the weight 22 inches. Since work is defined as force (or weight) times distance, Lifter A must do 4,000 inch-pounds of work [20 inches x 200 pounds] and Lifter B must do 4,400 inch-pounds of work [22 inches x 200 pounds] to accomplish the identical task. In other words, Lifter A doesn't need to make anywhere near as much effort as Lifter B to lift the same weight. Lifter A would have greater leverage than Lifter B and, everything else being equal, would have a greater strength potential.

Short levers are highly favorable in most exercises. Ironically, however, long levers – the exact opposite – are highly favorable in most sports. Having long limbs, for example, is a valuable asset in baseball, basketball, boxing, rowing, swimming and volleyball. Much ado has been made about the wingspan – or arm span – of several highly successful athletes, including Michael Phelps, a swimmer who stands 6'4" with 6'7" wingspan and Brittney Griner, a basketball player who stands 6'8" with a 7'3.5" wingspan. But the most impressive measure among notable athletes might be the late Sonny Liston, a heavyweight boxer who stood 6'1" with a reported wingspan of 7'0" – nearly a one-foot difference between his wingspan and height. Liston won the world heavyweight championship in September 1962 and held the title until February 1964. In that fight, he lost to 22-year-old Cassius Clay who soon thereafter changed his name to Muhammad Ali. By the way, Ali stood 6'3" with a 6'8" wingspan. (Note: The average individual has a wingspan that's the same as his or her height.)

Body Type

Another genetic factor that plays a critical role in strength potential is your body type. In the 1940s, Dr. William Sheldon, a physician and

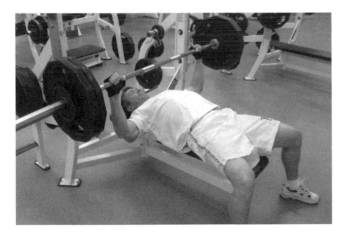

Favorable lever lengths and body proportions in the bench press are short arms and a thick chest.

psychologist, advanced the idea that there are three main physiques or body types: endomorph, mesomorph and ectomorph. These classifications are the ones that are most widely accepted in science and academia.

Endomorphs have a soft and round physique. They have a very high percentage of body fat without much muscle tone. An example of an endomorph is a sumo wrestler. Mesomorphs have a heavily muscled physique. They have an athletic build with broad shoulders, a large chest and a trim waist (giving them a V-shaped appearance). An example of a mesomorph is a competitive bodybuilder. Finally, ectomorphs have long limbs and a slender physique. They have a very low percentage of body fat but little in the way of muscular size. An example of an ectomorph is a long-distance runner.

Relatively few individuals can be classified as being purely one body type or another. Although people have a tendency toward one body type, most are a combination of two types. Many athletes, for instance, are mainly mesomorphs with some characteristics of endomorphs or ectomorphs. Thus, their body type would be that of a meso-endomorph or meso-ectomorph. A meso-endomorph has a high degree of muscular development (but not like that of a mesomorph) coupled with a round physique (but not like that of an endomorph); a meso-ectomorph has a high degree of muscular development (but not like that of a mesomorph) coupled with a slender physique (but not like that of an ectomorph).

A somatotype is a numerical descriptor of overall physique in terms of body shape and composition. Somatotypes are derived from various rating systems in which an individual is given a score for each of the main body types. There are three numbers used in a somatotype: a number for endomorphy, mesomorphy and ectomorphy (always in that order).

The system that was created by Dr. Sheldon employs a scale that ranges from 1 to 7 to designate the degree of each of the three components with 1 being the least amount and 7 being the greatest. In 1967, two researchers –

Barbara Heath and Dr. Lindsay Carter – published an article on the Heath-Carter Method that uses a 9-point scale. At the present time, this is the most common way of somatotyping.

With the Heath-Carter Method, ratings of 0.5 to 2.5 are considered low, 3.0 to 5.0 moderate, 5.5 to 7.0 high and 7.5 and above very high. In this system, a somatotype of 9-1-1 (read as "nine-one-one") indicates extreme endomorphy (fatness), 1-9-1 extreme mesomorphy (muscularity) and 1-1-9 extreme ectomorphy (leanness).

As mentioned earlier, some individuals have a propensity toward one body type but most are a combination of two. For instance, somatotypes of 5-5-1 and 4-4-2 would be indicative of a meso-endomorph and somatotypes of 1-5-5 and 2-4-4 would be indicative of a meso-ectomorph.

The three-number rating can be recorded on what's known as a somatochart. The chart can be used to plot groups of specific athletes – gymnasts, rowers, weightlifters or wrestlers, for example – where a cluster of ratings would indicate that a certain body type predominates

in a particular sport. Or it can be used to examine the body type of the same person over time. In Figure 3.2, for example, the somatochart shows an individual (the author) on two separate occasions: May 1982 (gray dot) and April 2005 (black dot). Note that there's no significant change over this 23-year period with somatotypes of 2.5-4.0-2.0 in 1982 at age 25 and 1.8-4.4-2.0 in 2005 at about age 48. After nearly a quarter of a century, the endormorphy rating is slightly lower and mesomorphy rating is slightly higher but the body type is still generally indicative of a mesomorph.

Having said all of this, how can you determine your somatotype? Well, it involves 10 anthropometric measurements: height, weight, four skinfolds (triceps, subscapular, suprailiac and calf), the circumferences of your flexed arm and calf and the widths between the epicondyles of your humerus and femur. A somatotype is then calculated from these measurements using various equations. Needless to say, the process can be complicated. Nonetheless, you can get a general idea of your body type by simply

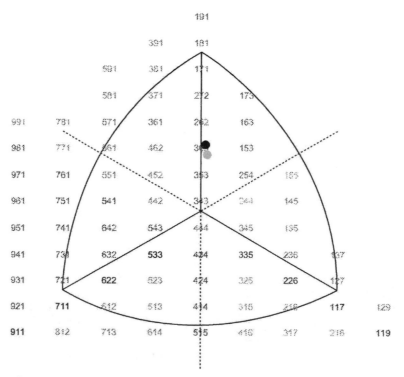

Figure 3.2: Sample somatochart

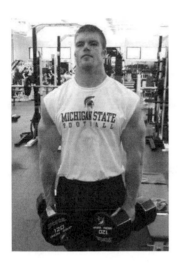

The body type that has the greatest potential to increase strength is the mesomorph. (Photo provided by Ken Mannie.)

considering your build. If you have a heavily muscled physique, your body type is mainly a mesomorph; if you have a slender physique, your body type is mainly an ectomorph. You get the picture.

A number of studies have related body type to physical performance. One study, for instance, found that meso-ectomorphs have a greater potential to improve their aerobic fitness than mesomorphs, endo-mesomorphs and ecto-morphs.

As you might suspect, the body type that has the greatest potential to increase strength is the mesomorph. In one study, the average somatotype of 54 male powerlifters was 4.3-8.8-0.5, showing that mesomorphy is dominant. Everything else being equal, those who have a high degree of mesomorphy have a greater potential to improve their strength than those who have a low degree of mesomorphy.

Body types can be modified a bit through an increase of muscle mass and/or decrease in body fat. However, certain aspects – such as bone structure – aren't subject to change.

Tendon Insertion

At one time or another, you've probably encountered individuals who were far stronger than they appeared. In fact, they may have been amazingly strong despite not having much in the way of size. If strength is directly related to size (in terms of the cross-sectional area of a muscle), how can this be? One possibility is that these individuals have favorable insertion points of their tendons.

The farther away that a tendon inserts from an axis of rotation, the greater the biomechanical advantage and strength potential. Consider two individuals who are tasked with holding 20 pounds in their hands a distance of 12.0 inches from their elbows while keeping their lower arms parallel to the ground and maintaining a 90-degree angle between their upper and lower arms. Suppose that Lifter A has a bicep tendon that inserts on his forearm 1.2 inches from his elbow and Lifter B has a bicep tendon that inserts on his forearm 1.0 inch from his elbow.

In this example, as depicted in Figure 3.3, the force necessary to maintain the weight (or resistance) in a static position can be calculated by using this equation: force times force arm equals resistance times resistance arm or, more simply, F x FA = R x RA. The force arm is defined as the distance from the axis of rotation – in this case, the elbow   to the point where the force is applied (the insertion point of the tendon); the resistance arm is defined as the distance from the axis of rotation to the point where the resistance is applied. Inserting the previously given values into the equation reveals that Lifter A must produce 200 pounds of force to hold the 20-pound weight in a static position while Lifter B must produce 240 pounds of force to accomplish the identical task. In other words, Lifter A doesn't need to make anywhere near as much effort as Lifter B to hold the same weight. Lifter A would have greater leverage than Lifter B and, everything else being equal, would have a greater strength potential.

This depiction of static forces is somewhat simplified. However, it still illustrates the fact that a very small difference in the insertion point of a tendon can produce a considerable amount of variation in leverage. Magnetic resonance imaging (MRI) and X-rays can be used to accurately determine the insertion point of tendons.

The effect that the insertion point of a tendon has on a bone can be likened to the position of a knob on a door. Placing the knob (tendon) away

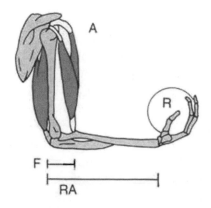
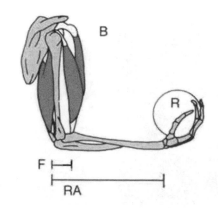
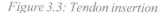
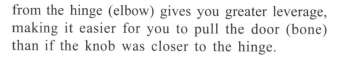

Figure 3.3: Tendon insertion

from the hinge (elbow) gives you greater leverage, making it easier for you to pull the door (bone) than if the knob was closer to the hinge.

Neurological Efficiency

One more genetic factor that has a significant role in determining strength potential deals with the nervous system; it has been dubbed neurological efficiency (or neuromuscular efficiency). This refers to an individual's inherited ability to innervate (or recruit) muscle fibers and is another reason why some individuals are far stronger than they appear.

It has been suggested that some individuals can recruit higher percentages of their muscle fibers than others which gives them a greater potential to improve their strength. Consider two individuals who have the same amount of muscle mass. Suppose that Lifter A can innervate 40% of his muscle fibers and Lifter B can innervate 30%. Lifter A would be able to access a higher percentage of muscle fibers than Lifter B and, everything else being equal, would have a greater strength potential.

HERITABILITY DICTATES TRAINABILITY

With all due respect to Abraham Lincoln, all men (and women) aren't created equal. If two individuals perform the same strength program, it's highly unlikely that they'll end up having the same level of strength (and size). Each individual responds in a different manner because – other

than monozygotic twins – everyone has a different potential for improving their strength (and size). Simply, some people are predisposed toward developing high levels of strength (and size) while others are not. And that's why the same strength program can result in one person who looks like Arnold Schwarzenegger and another who looks like Arnold Palmer.

So, your response to strength training isn't necessarily due to a particular program or workout. Indeed, following the routines of successful weightlifters doesn't mean that you'll attain their same level of strength; following the routines of successful bodybuilders doesn't mean that you'll attain their same level of size.

Train a chimpanzee like a gorilla and you might get a slightly stronger chimpanzee . . . but you'll never get a gorilla. The next time that you're in the fitness center (or weight room), take a look at different pairs of training partners. You'll see that individuals who work out together usually have different levels of strength (and size), despite doing the same exercises while using the same number of sets and repetitions.

The truth is that heritability dictates trainability. Your response to training is largely determined by your genetic profile. The cumulative effect of your inherited muscular, mechanical, hormonal and neural qualities is what determines your strength potential. An individual who has a high percentage of FT fibers, long muscle bellies coupled with short tendons, a high level of testosterone, desirable lever lengths

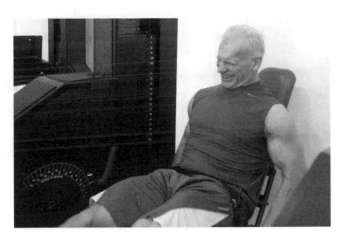

Your response to training is largely determined by your genetic profile. (Photo provided by Luke Carlson.)

and body proportions, a high degree of mesomorphy, favorable insertion points of tendons and an efficient neurological system would be incredibly strong (as well as physically impressive). Compared to the average person, this genetic marvel would be capable of almost unbelievable feats of strength. There are some individuals like that but most aren't as fortunate.

For all intents and purposes, you can't change the characteristics that you've inherited from your ancestors. And you can't travel back in time to pick your parents. However, this doesn't mean that there isn't any hope for you to get stronger; just be realistic about it. In terms of your response to strength training, the three letters in the English language that are of utmost importance are DNA. Regardless of your genetic destiny, your goal should be to achieve your strength potential.

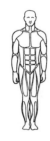

4 Strength Training

Strength can be defined as the ability of a muscle to produce force. It follows, then, that strength training is a means to improve this ability.

BENEFITS

There are many benefits of strength training. First of all, increasing your strength will improve your capacity to perform everyday tasks more easily. Strength training will also increase your muscle mass and decrease your body fat which will improve your body composition and physical appearance.

In addition, strength training can increase your bone mineral density thereby combating the destructive effects of osteoporosis. There are psychological benefits as well. This includes increased mental alertness, self-confidence and self-esteem.

For athletes, strength training can reduce the frequency and severity of injuries. If you can increase the strength of your muscles, connective tissues and bones to tolerate more stress, you'll reduce the likelihood of incurring an injury. By increasing their functional strength, athletes will also take an important step toward realizing their physical potential. Having greater strength allows them to perform their activities more easily and be more resistant to fatigue.

WHAT APPROACH?

Most fitness authorities agree that strength training can be extremely beneficial. Many, however, disagree over which approach is best for increasing strength (and size). The different approaches – and the enormous amount of conflicting advice – often leave people utterly confused.

A common practice is to adopt the strength programs of successful individuals or teams, a practice that frequently adds to the confusion. If you were to compare the strength programs of individuals who are very strong, you might be in for quite a surprise: Not only is it likely that their programs are vastly different but also that, in many cases, they offer contradictory information. Some strength programs use fast repetition speeds, others slow repetition speeds; some use mostly multiple sets of each exercise, others mostly single sets of each exercise; some use split routines, others total-body workouts; some use mainly free weights, others mainly machines; and so on.

Yet, despite these and other differences, many strength programs are highly effective. How, then, do you choose which program to follow if you're looking to improve your strength (and size)?

CHOOSING A PROGRAM

When deciding on what strength program to use, it's important to consider scientific research. Interestingly, research has been unable

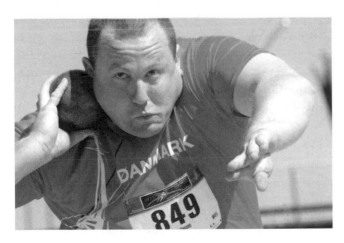

By increasing their functional strength, athletes will take an important step toward realizing their physical potential. (Photo by Chris Stone.)

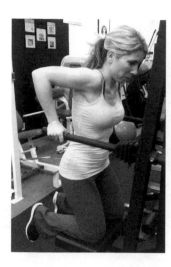

Research has shown that a variety of methods can be used to increase strength. (Photo by Fred Fornicola.)

to determine that one method of strength training is superior to another. If anything, research has shown that a variety of methods can be used to increase strength. In one study, significant improvements in strength were made by nine groups that did different combinations of one, two and three sets and two, six and ten repetitions. Moreover, research has shown that a variety of equipment can be used to increase strength. In several studies, significant improvements in strength were made by groups that used free weights and groups that used machines.

When choosing a strength program, it's also important to consider anecdotal evidence. Though anecdotal reports lack the same scientific scrutiny as research studies, their sheer volume is so overwhelming in this case that they can't be discounted. The inescapable fact is that countless individuals have attained significant improvements in their strength (and size) with a wide variety of programs.

So, it's possible for many types of strength programs to yield favorable results. In determining which program to implement, you should ask the following five questions:

Is It Productive?

The program must be productive. It makes little sense for you to invest time in a strength program if it doesn't produce meaningful results.

A program will be productive as long as it's based on scientific research, common sense and deductive reasoning not unfounded advice, wild speculation and wishful thinking.

Is It Comprehensive?

The program must be comprehensive. A strength program should address all of the major muscles in your body, not just the "showy" or "cosmetic" ones. Frequently, muscles that are often injured get ignored (such as those surrounding the knee, ankle, neck and lower back) while muscles that are often flaunted get emphasized (such as the chest, biceps, triceps and abdominals). If you happen to be a competitive athlete, a comprehensive strength program is one that's performed year-round, including throughout the off-season and in-season. Training during the season is especially critical since this is when athletes need to be at their best in terms of strength and conditioning.

Is It Practical?

The program must be practical. In other words, it must be relatively easy to understand. In some instances, strength programs are grossly overcomplicated and correspondingly confusing. The use of pseudoscientific terminology adds to the confusion. Strength training needn't be complex.

Is It Efficient?

The program must be efficient. It should produce the maximum possible results in the minimum amount of time. A strength program that requires you to lift weights for lengthy periods of time and/or more than several workouts per week isn't an efficient use of your time . . . nor is it necessary. By utilizing a program that's time-efficient, you'll have a greater opportunity to pursue other activities such as preparing for academic endeavors and, if you're an athlete, performing sport-specific skills and conditioning. And don't forget about the extra time that you could dedicate toward your personal activities and interests. You should *invest* time in the fitness center, not *spend* time.

Is It Safe?

The program must be safe. At first glance, many strength programs can look quite appealing. Closer inspection, however, may reveal that the programs are highly questionable in terms of safety. There's no need whatsoever to perform potentially dangerous activities or exercises in the fitness center (or weight room). It's certainly true that physical activities have inherent participatory risks. But this doesn't mean that you should do activities that present risks to your orthopedic health.

In short, the program that you choose should be productive, comprehensive, practical, efficient and safe. It's these criteria that form the underlying theme for the ensuing information.

CONSIDERATIONS FOR STRENGTH TRAINING

Unless you happen to be a competitive weightlifter or bodybuilder, there's absolutely no need for you to train like one. These athletes have different goals than most of the population. Essentially, the main goal of a competitive weightlifter (a powerlifter or an Olympic-style lifter) is to do one repetition with as much weight as possible; the main goal of a bodybuilder is to achieve the best physique possible. With no disrespect intended, neither of these goals has much relevance to the average person or the average athlete, for that matter.

You can increase your strength (and size) in a manner that's productive, comprehensive, practical, efficient and safe by considering and incorporating these 10 concepts:

1. Level of Intensity

The most important factor that determines your results from strength training is your genetic (inherited) profile (which includes your predominant muscle fiber type, lever lengths, insertion points of tendons and so on). However, you can't control the genetic cards that you were dealt. The most important factor that you can control is your level of intensity. (In strength training, intensity shouldn't be confused with a

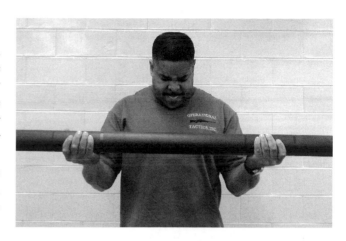

A high level of intensity is necessary for maximizing your response to strength training. (Photo by Peter Silletti.)

percentage of a maximum weight. Rather, intensity is another word for effort.)

A high level of intensity is necessary for maximizing your response to strength training. Here, a high level of intensity is characterized by performing a set to the point of muscular fatigue or "failure." In simple terms, this means that you've exhausted your muscles to the extent that you literally can't do any additional repetitions with proper technique.

The Overload Principle

If you fail to reach an appropriate level of intensity – or muscular fatigue – your increases in strength (and size) will be less than optimal. Evidence for this notion is found in the Overload Principle. Coined by Dr. Arthur Steinhaus in 1933, it has become perhaps the most widely referenced principle in exercise science. According to Dr. Roger Enoka – a renowned biomechanist and author – the Overload Principle states, "To increase their size or functional ability, muscle fibers must be taxed toward their present capacity to respond." He adds: "This principle implies that there is a threshold point that must be exceeded before an adaptive response will occur."

Stated otherwise, a minimum level of muscular fatigue must be produced in order to provide a stimulus for adaptation. Your effort must be great enough to surpass this threshold so that a sufficient amount of muscular fatigue is created to trigger an adaptive response. Given proper nourishment and an adequate amount of recovery between workouts, your muscles will adapt to these demands by increasing in strength (and size). The extent to which this compensatory adaptation occurs then becomes a function of your genetics.

The General Adaptation Syndrome

Make no mistake about it: In order for you to achieve optimal improvements in strength (and size), you must produce an appropriate level of muscular fatigue. So if you produce too little muscular fatigue, you may not have stimulated any compensatory adaptation. But if you produce too much muscular fatigue, you may not have permitted any compensatory adaptation; it may even cause a loss of strength (and size).

In the 1930s, Dr. Hans Selye proposed the General Adaptation Syndrome (GAS) to explain the physical effects of stress. This three-stage process can be applied to the physiological stress that's encountered by the muscles during strength training. In the Alarm Stage, the stress causes damage to the muscles (or micro-trauma). This is followed by the Resistance Stage during which the body defends itself against the stress-induced damage through compensatory adaptation (by increasing in strength and size). Stress that's too severe induces the Exhaustion Stage in which the demands that are placed on the muscles exceed their ability to recover and adapt.

Therefore, your level of intensity should be high . . . but it should also be appropriate. Consider this analogy: If you used a hammer on a regular basis for short periods of time you'd form calluses on your palm. Basically, the calluses are a compensatory (and protective) adaptation to frictional heat. If you hammered for a long enough period of time, however, you'd develop blisters instead. Here, the excessive demands have surpassed the adaptive ability of your tissue because the stress was too much and too frequent. In brief, you should train with a high level of intensity without overdoing it.

How do you know if the demands on your muscles are too little or too much? You should monitor your performance in terms of the resistance that you use and the repetitions that you do. If you continue to make progress in your performance, then the demands are appropriate.

Favorable Results

The main reason why most people fail to realize their strength (and size) potential is simply because they don't train with a high enough level of intensity. Simply, a sub-maximum effort yields sub-maximum results. Athletes should also keep in mind that "you play like you practice." If you're an athlete and do your strength training with a low level of effort, will you be able to ratchet up your intensity when needed in competition?

That being said, you must also use your judgment in deciding what level of intensity is appropriate for you. Intensity is a relative term that depends on your level of fitness. Exercise of low intensity for an active individual may be of high intensity for an inactive individual. So if you haven't been training on a regular basis or aren't in the best of shape, then you should adjust your effort accordingly. Also, some individuals may not be comfortable exercising to the point of muscular fatigue. Those who feel uneasy about training with a high level of intensity should terminate the set a few repetitions short of muscular fatigue. Remember, you can control your level of intensity when you train; your efforts can be as easy or as hard as you desire.

The fact that your results from strength training are directly related to your level of effort shouldn't come as much of a surprise. It's like anything else in life: How hard you work at your other physical training, your job and even your relationships largely determines your success at those endeavors.

2. Progressive Overload

In the late 1940s, Dr. Thomas DeLorme, a physician, coined the term progressive-resistance exercise. In fact, he's often referred to as the father of progressive-resistance exercise. Dr. DeLorme began lifting weights in 1932 at the age of 16 in an attempt to increase his size and strength. During World War II, he applied the lessons that he had learned from his own experience to the rehabilitation of large numbers of wounded soldiers at the Gardiner Army General Hospital in Chicago.

Unfortunately, little of what's done in most fitness centers and weight rooms can be characterized as progressive. It's not uncommon to hear of someone who performs the same number of repetitions with the same amount of resistance over and over again, workout after workout. Suppose that today you did 10 repetitions with 150 pounds on the seated row and a month later you're still doing 10 repetitions with 150 pounds. Did you increase your strength? Probably not. On the other hand, what if you were able to do 12 repetitions with 165 pounds in that exercise a month from now? In this case, you performed 20% more repetitions with 10% more resistance; excellent progress over the course of one month.

The Overload Principle, Revisited

Changes in the functional and structural abilities of your muscles depend on the continued application of the Overload Principle. This means that your muscles must be overloaded with progressively greater demands. For this reason, your muscles must experience a workload that's increased steadily and systematically throughout the course of your strength program. This is often referred to as progressive overload.

Legend has it that Milo of Croton – a renowned warrior and athlete who won numerous prizes as a wrestler in the Olympic and Pythian Games in ancient Greece – periodically lifted a baby bull on his shoulders. As the bull increased in size and weight, so did Milo's strength. This crude method of progressive overload has been credited with the improvement of his legendary strength.

In order to overload your muscles, every time you train you must attempt to increase the resistance that you use and/or the repetitions that you do in comparison to your previous workout. This can be viewed as a double-progressive technique ("double" referring to resistance and repetitions). Stated otherwise, you must impose demands on your muscles that they haven't previously encountered by using more resistance

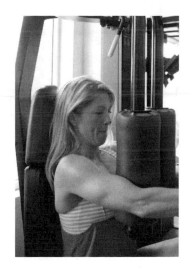

Your muscles must experience a workload that's increased steadily and systematically throughout the course of your strength program. (Photo provided by Luke Carlson.)

and/or doing more repetitions. Exposing your muscles to progressively greater demands stimulates compensatory adaptation in response to the unaccustomed workload. Specifically, your muscles adapt to such demands by increasing in strength (and size). The extent to which this occurs then becomes a function of your genetic profile.

In a nutshell, the double-progressive technique would be implemented in this manner: If you reach muscular fatigue within your prescribed repetition range – say you did 14 repetitions and your range is 10 to 15 – you should repeat the weight for your next workout and try to increase the number of repetitions that you did; if you attain or surpass the maximum number of prescribed repetitions in an exercise – say you did 15 repetitions and your range is 10 to 15 – you should increase the weight for your next workout.

Appropriate Progressions

Your progressions in resistance need not be in Herculean leaps and bounds. You should increase the resistance in an amount with which you're comfortable . . . but the resistance that you use must always be challenging. Fortunately, this may be accomplished much more systematically than the method that was used by Milo and his growing bull.

Progressions should be thought of in *relative* terms, not *absolute*. Always increasing the resistance by a set value of, say, five pounds can be problematic. Think about it: Making a five-pound progression from 100 to 105 pounds is an increase of 5%; making a five-pound progression from 10 to 15 pounds is an increase of 50%.

Your muscles will respond better if the progressions in resistance are about 5% or less, depending on the degree to which the set was challenging. Suppose, for example, that an exercise has a repetition range of 15 to 20. If it was fairly hard for you to do 20 repetitions, then you should make a slightly smaller progression in resistance; if it was fairly easy for you to do 20 repetitions, then you should make a slightly larger progression in resistance.

The idea behind making smaller progressions – known as micro-loading – is the fact that you'll hardly notice a slightly heavier resistance and your repetitions won't decline much if at all. In other words, it's much easier for your muscles to adapt to subtle increases in resistance. Consider this example: Imagine that an exercise has a repetition range of 15 to 20 and you did 200/20 (200 pounds/20 repetitions). If you increased the resistance by 10% (by 20 pounds) the next time you do that exercise, it's likely that you'd notice the significantly heavier weight and might do 220/15 or 220/16. Doing 16 repetitions means that you must improve the number of repetitions by 25% (from 16 to 20) before you can make your next progression in resistance which may prove to be a very daunting task. If, instead, you increased the resistance by 1.25% (by 2.5 pounds), it's not likely that you'd notice the slightly heavier weight and might do 202.5/20. Another 2.5-pound increase the next time you do that exercise may result in 205/20. Eventually, you might progress to the point where you were doing 220 pounds for at least 18 or 19 repetitions. So, you made the 20-pound increase in a number of small progressions instead of a large progression and, as a result, you allowed your muscles to adapt gradually to the resistance. And now, you'd only need to increase your repetitions by one or two in order to make your next progression in resistance. This scenario is hypothetical, of course, but it wouldn't be unusual for this to actually happen. The point is that your muscles will respond better to smaller increases in resistance than larger ones.

To make smaller progressions in resistance, you can use fractional plates or lighter Olympic plates for exercises that are done with free weights and plate-loaded machines. Fractional plates weigh as little as 0.25 pounds; Olympic plates weigh as little as 1.25 pounds. If lighter plates aren't available, you can simply hang something from the bar (or the movement arm of the machine) such as a small ankle weight.

Selectorized machines have weight stacks with plates that are usually 10, 12.5, 15, 20 or 25 pounds. Many of these machines offer a self-contained system of making smaller progressions in resistance such as the use of a drop-down weight. With some selectorized machines, a saddle plate (or add-on weight) must be placed on the top plate of the weight stack. (Standard weights for saddle plates are 2.5 and 5.0 pounds.) Another option is to secure a fractional plate or light Olympic plate to the weight stack of the machine by first inserting a selector pin through the hole in the plate and then into the weight stack. (This is often referred to as "pinning" a plate.) You can also place any object that weighs about one or two pounds on top of a weight stack as long as it won't fall off while you're using the equipment.

With dumbbells, you can use magnetic add-on weights. These weights – which can be round or hex to match the shape of the dumbbells – can be secured to the ends of the dumbbells and allow you to make increases in resistance that are much more desirable. So instead of having to jump from 25- to 30-pounders – a 20% increase in resistance – the use of 1.25-pound magnetic add-on weights can produce a pair of dumbbells that weigh 26.25 pounds. (Magnetic add-on weights can also be secured to the weight stacks of selectorized machines.) Another option for making smaller progressions with dumbbells is to employ ankle weights. Using 20-pound dumbbells with 1.25-pound ankle weights around your wrists produces 21.25 pounds of resistance.

Again, the resistance that you use must always be challenging. If you recently began a strength program or changed the exercises in your routine, it may take several workouts before you find a challenging weight. That's understandable; simply continue to make progressions in the resistance as needed.

For those who want to achieve their physical potential, progressive overload has always been – and will always be – of utmost importance. To summarize: You must place a demand on your muscles that's beyond what they're accustomed. If you lifted 200 pounds today for 12 repetitions, then in a subsequent workout you must attempt to increase the resistance and/or do more repetitions.

3. Number of Sets

For many years, most individuals have done multiple-set training simply because that's what they've heard, read or been told to do. The roots of multiple-set training can be traced back to the time when virtually every authority in strength training came from the ranks of the professional strongmen, competitive weightlifters and, to a lesser degree, bodybuilders. In the early 1970s, the notion was advanced that strength (and size) could be improved with far fewer sets – and, thus, less volume of training – than had been traditionally thought. The debate concerning the ideal number of sets has been raging ever since.

Research and Utilization

Research has been unable to determine how many sets of each exercise are necessary to produce optimal increases in strength (and size). But the overwhelming majority of scientific evidence indicates that single-set training is at least as effective as multiple-set training. An exhaustive review of the literature in 1998 by Drs. Ralph Carpinelli and Robert Otto of Adelphi University (NY) and later reviews by Dr. Carpinelli examined dozens of studies that compared different numbers of sets (dating back to 1956). Collectively, their research found five studies that showed multiple-set training was superior to single-set training and 57 that did not.

For instance, researchers at the University of Florida randomly assigned 42 subjects to groups that did either one set of nine exercises or three sets of the same nine exercises. Prior to the study, the subjects had done strength training for an average of 6.2 years. After 13 weeks of training, both groups had significant improvements in strength, endurance and body composition. And there were no significant differences between the groups in the improvements that were made in any of those measures.

So, the basis for performing single-set training – or a relatively low number of sets – has powerful and compelling support in the scientific literature. But is single-set training actually done in the "real world"? More importantly, can experienced or "trained" individuals obtain the same results from single-set training as they can from multiple-set training? The answer to both questions is an emphatic yes. The fact of the matter is that single-set training has been popular since the idea was first promoted in the early 1970s. And to quote Drs. Carpinelli and Otto: "There is no evidence to suggest that the response to single or multiple sets in trained athletes would differ from that in untrained individuals." Indeed, numerous authorities advocate single-set training including the strength coaches for many collegiate and professional teams. Dan Riley – who logged 27 years as a strength coach in the National Football League (with the Washington Redskins and Houston Texans) and another 8 at the collegiate level (with the US Military Academy and Penn State) – notes, "Your goal must be to perform as few sets as possible while stimulating maximum gains. If performed properly, only one set is needed to generate maximum gains. In our standard routines, one set of each exercise is performed."

Recall that in order for your muscles to increase in strength (and size), they must experience an adequate level of fatigue. It's just that simple. It really doesn't matter whether your muscles are fatigued in one set or several sets as long as you produce an adequate level of muscular fatigue.

Efficient Applications

If doing one set of an exercise produces virtually the same results as doing multiple sets, then single-set training represents a more efficient means of strength training. After all, why perform multiple sets when you can obtain similar results from one set in a fraction of the time?

This isn't to say that multiple-set training can't be done. If performed properly, multiple-set training can certainly be effective in overloading your muscles. Multiple-set training has been used successfully by an enormous number of individuals for decades.

If you have a preference for multiple-set training, you should be aware of several things. First of all, simply doing multiple sets doesn't guarantee that you've overloaded your muscles. If the weights you use aren't demanding enough then you won't produce sufficient muscular fatigue and your workout won't be as effective as possible. Remember, a large amount of low-intensity work doesn't necessarily produce an overload. So if you'd rather do multiple sets, make sure that you're challenging your muscles with appropriate demands. In addition, keep in mind that performing too many sets (or too many exercises) can create a situation in which the demands that are placed on your muscles have surpassed your ability to recover. If this happens, your muscle tissue will be broken down in such an extreme manner that your body is unable to regenerate muscle tissue (essentially the resynthesis of protein filaments). Also, doing too many sets (or too many exercises) can significantly increase your risk of incurring an overuse injury such as tendinitis and bursitis. And as was indicated earlier, multiple-set training is relatively inefficient in terms of time so it's undesirable for time-conscious individuals. If you're like most people, time is a precious commodity; most people simply don't have much free time. The point is this: Keep your sets to the minimum amount that's needed to produce an adequate level of muscular fatigue.

Clearly, single-set training can be just as effective as multiple-set training. There's one caveat, however: If a single set of an exercise is to be productive, it must be done with an appropriate level of intensity (to the point of muscular fatigue). Your muscles should be thoroughly exhausted at the end of each set.

You should emphasize the *quality* of work that's done in a strength program, not the *quantity* of work. Don't perform meaningless sets; make every set count. The most efficient program is one that produces the maximum possible results in the minimum amount of time.

4. Number of Repetitions

Determining an appropriate repetition range depends on a number of factors and, even then, has some degree of variability. Understand first that strength training isn't an aerobic activity that's characterized by long-term, low-intensity efforts; rather, it's an anaerobic activity that's characterized by short-term, high-intensity efforts. Therefore, the duration of a series of repetitions – a set – should be in the anaerobic domain. Efforts that last from a split second to several minutes are considered to be anaerobic (assuming, of course, that the level of effort is great enough to justify an anaerobic response). Intense efforts at the lower end of this time frame carry a higher risk of injury and those at the upper end have an increasingly greater reliance on the aerobic pathway. Narrowing the window of time to roughly 30 to 120 seconds represents a safe and effective range for strength training with lower durations assigned to smaller muscles and higher durations to larger ones. (Larger muscles – those in your hips and legs – should be trained for a slightly longer duration because of their greater size and work capacity.) Thus, time frames might be 90 to 120 seconds for a hip exercise, 60 to 90 seconds for a leg exercise and 30 to 60 seconds for a torso exercise.

Be that as it may, doing sets for a specified amount of time under load (TUL) can be tricky and tedious. But you can use the aforementioned time frames to formulate repetition ranges. Suppose that you prefer to use a speed of movement that's six seconds per repetition. Dividing six seconds into the time frames that have been noted yields repetition ranges of 15 to

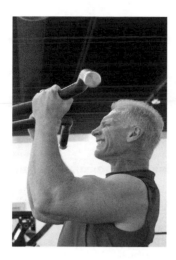

Strength training is an anaerobic activity that's characterized by short-term, high intensity efforts. (Photo provided by Luke Carlson.)

20 for your hips, 10 to 15 for your legs and 5 to 10 for your torso. (A repetition range of 8 to 10 is recommended for torso exercises that have an abbreviated range of motion.) Remember, these ranges are based on six-second repetitions. Different repetition speeds require different repetition ranges. Suppose that you prefer to use a speed of movement that's 10 seconds per repetition. Dividing 10 seconds into the time frames that have been noted yields repetition ranges of 9 to 12 for your hips, 6 to 9 for your legs and 3 to 6 for your torso. (You're encouraged to experiment with different repetition speeds and vary them based on your personal preferences and performance objectives.)

Genetic Considerations

Due to certain aspects of their genetic profile – most notably their predominant muscle fiber type some individuals may require repetition ranges that are either a bit higher or lower than that prescribed for the general population. For example, individuals who have a high percentage of slow-twitch (ST) fibers would probably benefit more from doing slightly higher repetitions because their predominant fiber type is more suited for muscular endurance. Here, repetition ranges might be 20 to 25 for the hips, 15 to 20 for the legs and 10 to 15 for the torso. Individuals who have a high percentage of fast-twitch (FT) fibers would probably benefit more from doing slightly lower repetitions because their predominant fiber type is less suited for muscular

endurance. Here, repetition ranges might be 12 to 15 for the hips, 9 to 12 for the legs and 4 to 8 for the torso.

In one study, sprinters trained with low repetitions, middle-distance runners with medium repetitions and long-distance runners with high repetitions. All three groups experienced excellent and equal gains in strength. (In all likelihood, successful sprinters have a high percentage of FT fibers and successful long-distance runners have a high percentage of ST fibers.)

Muscle fiber types can be identified in a laboratory by doing a biopsy in which a small plug of muscle tissue is removed and later analyzed under a microscope. A muscle biopsy isn't for everyone, though, since it results in the destruction of tissue and most people are understandably reluctant to give away free samples. Moreover, the accuracy of muscle biopsies has also been questioned. For one thing, fiber "headcounts" are subject to different interpretations. And since the distribution of fibers varies throughout a muscle, the site from which the biopsy is taken may not be indicative of the overall fiber-type mixture.

One way to guesstimate your fiber types is to assess their fatigue characteristics during a test of muscular endurance. To do this, you'd determine the most weight that you could lift one time (which is your one-repetition maximum or 1-RM). Then, you'd take 75% of your 1-RM and perform as many repetitions as possible using good technique. For instance, if you find that your 1-RM is 80 pounds on the bicep curl, you'd use 60 pounds for the endurance test [80 lb x 0.75 = 60 lb]. It would be expected that 10 repetitions could be done with 75% of a 1-RM. If you do a relatively high number of repetitions with 60 pounds (more than about 10), it's likely that your biceps have a high percentage of ST fibers; if you do a relatively low number of repetitions with 60 pounds (less than about 5), it's likely that your biceps have a high percentage of FT fibers. But remember, since the composition and distribution of fibers can vary from muscle to muscle, the results of an endurance test aren't necessarily reflective of your entire muscular system; you'd have to perform different tests for different muscles.

How much do individuals really vary in terms of their muscular endurance? Dr. Wayne Westcott reported data on 141 subjects who did an endurance test with 75% of their 1-RMs on a 10-degree chest machine. Again, it would be expected that 10 repetitions could be done with this workload. And according to the data, the subjects completed an average of 10.5 repetitions. However, only 16 of the 141 subjects (11.35%) did exactly 10 repetitions. Many of the subjects were in the neighborhood of 10 repetitions. In fact, 66 of the 141 subjects (46.81%) did between 8 and 13 repetitions. But 75 of the 141 subjects (53.19%) did either less than 8 repetitions or more than 13. At the extremes, two subjects did 5 repetitions (a sprinter and a thrower) and one managed 24 (a triathlete). Researchers at the University of North Dakota also found wide variations in muscular endurance among 98 football players. In this study, four of the athletes had the same 1-RM in the bench press (300 pounds). But when tested with 75% of this weight (225 pounds), they completed 9, 10, 11 and 16 repetitions. So while other factors may certainly come into play, the influence that fiber types have on muscular endurance can't be overlooked or underemphasized.

You can also make a logical guesstimate of your fiber type based on your performance in certain activities. If you're successful in activities that require muscular endurance, you probably have a high percentage of ST fibers and should perform slightly higher repetitions; if you're successful in activities that require strength, speed and/or power, you probably have a high percentage of FT fibers and should perform slightly lower repetitions.

Another way of making a reasonable guesstimate of your fiber types is to consider your muscular development. FT fibers have a much greater potential to increase in size than ST fibers. Therefore, if you have a significant amount of muscular development, you probably have a high percentage of FT fibers; if you have an insignificant amount of muscular development,

you probably have a high percentage of ST fibers (assuming, of course, that your lack of muscular development isn't the result of inactivity).

A final point about FT and ST fibers: The use of lower repetitions isn't suggested as a way to convert ST fibers to FT fibers. Nor is the use of higher repetitions suggested as a way to convert FT fibers to ST fibers. As noted in Chapter 3, there's no scientific evidence that consistently and convincingly supports the belief that one fiber type can be converted into another type. In other words, you can't convert one fiber type into another any more than you can convert a draft horse into a racehorse. So if you were to take a draft horse and train it like a racehorse, you might get a slightly faster draft horse . . . but you'll never get a racehorse. Performing different repetition ranges is done to maximize your response to training based on your already-established predominant fiber type.

Another genetic factor that influences repetition ranges is lever length. In many exercises, those who have long limbs (levers) must move the weight over a greater distance and, therefore, must maintain muscular tension over a greater distance than those who have short limbs. Everything else being equal, a long-limbed individual would probably be more fatigued after doing the same number of repetitions than a short-limbed individual. Here, then, using a lower repetition range would prevent muscular fatigue from occurring beyond the recommended anaerobic window of time. As a result, someone with long limbs would benefit more from doing slightly lower repetitions, especially in multiple-joint exercises (such as the bench press, lat pulldown and leg press) and free-weight exercises (such as the bicep curl) where limb length is a factor.

Special Considerations

Repetition ranges of 15 to 20 for the hips, 10 to 15 for the legs and 5 to 10 for the torso will be safe and effective for most of the population. However, slightly higher repetition ranges are suggested for certain individuals. This includes younger teens and older adults along with anyone who has orthopedic issues. In addition, women who are pregnant should do slightly higher repetitions because of the increased laxity in their ligaments and joints during gestation. Slightly higher repetition ranges would also be recommended for those who have hypertension or are doing rehabilitative training.

In these cases, repetition ranges might be 20 to 25 for the hips, 15 to 20 for the legs and 10 to 15 for the torso. These higher repetition ranges necessitate using lighter weights which reduces the orthopedic stress that's placed on the bones, connective tissues (including tendons and ligaments) and joints.

5. Proper Technique

Most people have no understanding of – or pay no attention to – how they perform their repetitions. Regardless of the type of strength program that you utilize, a productive program begins with a productive repetition. Remember, the repetition is the most basic and integral aspect of your strength program. If your repetitions aren't productive, your sets won't be productive; if your sets aren't productive, your workouts won't be productive; and if your workouts aren't productive, your program won't be productive.

A repetition has four checkpoints: the positive (or raising) phase, the mid-range position, the negative (or lowering) phase and the range of motion.

Checkpoint #1: The Positive Phase

A repetition starts with raising the weight. To minimize the use of momentum, you should raise the weight in a smooth, controlled manner without any explosive or jerking movements.

Raising a weight with high speeds isn't recommended for two main reasons. First of all, high-speed repetitions are less productive than low-speed repetitions. Here's why: When weights are lifted too quickly, the muscles produce tension during the initial part of the movement . . . but not for the last part. In simple terms, the weight is practically moving by itself. In effect, the load on the muscles is decreased – or eliminated – and so are the potential gains in strength (and size).

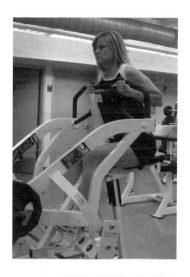

You should raise the weight in a smooth, controlled manner without any explosive or jerking movements.

Unfortunately, the use of excessive momentum is demonstrated in fitness centers and weight rooms across the world on a daily basis (albeit, in most cases, unknowingly). Imagine that you raised the weight so quickly during the leg extension that the pad left your lower legs partway through the repetition. Think about it: The pad is attached to the movement arm of the machine which, in turn, is connected to the resistance by some means (such as a chain, cable or belt). If the pad is no longer in contact with your lower legs, there's no load on your muscles. If there's no load on your muscles, there's no stimulus – or reason – for them to adapt. Sure, you will obtain some benefit when your muscles were loaded during the first part of the repetition (when the pad was against your shins). However, you will not obtain any benefit when your muscles were unloaded during the last part of the repetition (when the pad wasn't against your shins). There's no question that the more momentum is used to raise a weight, the less productive will be the repetitions.

Secondly – and more importantly – high-speed repetitions also carry a greater risk of injury than low-speed repetitions. Using an excessive amount of momentum to raise a weight increases the shear force that's encountered by a given joint; the faster a weight is raised, the higher this force is amplified, especially at the point of explosion. (Note: Shear force acts parallel to a joint; compressive force acts perpendicular to a joint.) In one study, a subject squatting with 80%

of his four-repetition maximum incurred a 225-pound peak shear force during a repetition that took 4.5 seconds to complete and a 270-pound peak shear force during a repetition that took 2.1 seconds to complete. This is clear evidence that a slower speed of movement reduces the shear force on joints. When the shear force exceeds the structural limits of a joint, an injury occurs to the muscles, connective tissues or bones. In addition, it's also possible that some injuries that occur outside the fitness center actually had their genesis inside the fitness center from employing certain techniques – such as high-speed repetitions – that weakened the joint structures. To ensure that your repetitions are safe and productive, it should take at least one to two seconds to raise the weight.

Checkpoint #2: The Mid-Range Position

After raising the weight, you should pause briefly in the mid-range position where the muscle is fully contracted. Where's the mid-range position of a repetition? These two examples should help to make it clear: When performing a tricep extension, the mid-range position is where your arms are almost completely straight (extended); when performing a bicep curl, the mid-range position is where your arms are completely bent (flexed).

Most people are very weak in the mid-range position of a repetition because they rarely, if ever, emphasize it. Pausing momentarily in the mid-range position allows you to focus your attention on your muscles when they're fully contracted.

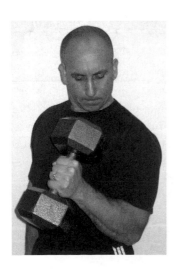

Pausing momentarily in the mid-range position of a repetition allows you to focus your attention on your muscles when they're fully contracted. (Photo by Lori Fornicola.)

Furthermore, a brief pause in the mid-range position permits a smooth transition between the raising and lowering of the weight and helps to decrease the influence of momentum. If you can't pause momentarily in the mid-range position, it's likely that you're raising the weight too quickly and literally throwing it into position.

Checkpoint #3: The Negative Phase

A repetition ends with lowering the weight. The importance of emphasizing the negative phase of a repetition can't be overstated. Numerous studies have shown that repetitions involving both concentric and eccentric contractions produce greater increases in strength (and size) than those involving just concentric contractions.

Why? Because the same muscles that you use to raise a weight are also used to lower it. In a bicep curl, for example, your biceps are used in raising and lowering the weight. The only difference is that when you raise the weight, your biceps are shortening against the load and when you lower the weight, your biceps are lengthening against the load. So by emphasizing the lowering of the weight, each repetition becomes more efficient and each set becomes more productive. Because a "loaded" muscle lengthens as you lower the weight, emphasizing the negative phase of a repetition also guarantees that the muscle is being stretched properly and safely.

You have three levels of strength: concentric, isometric and eccentric. Your eccentric strength is always greater than your concentric strength in the same exercise (with your isometric strength ranked approximately midway between the two). Stated differently, you can always lower more weight than you can raise (again, in the same exercise).

One theory is that the differences in the levels of strength are due to the effects of internal muscular friction; friction that's produced when a muscle contracts. During a concentric contraction, friction is produced by the contact between the myosin cross-bridges and the actin surfaces as these two filaments slide past each other. Friction is also produced during an eccentric contraction as the two filaments slide past each other, this time in the opposite direction. When you raise a weight, the friction works against you; you're lifting the weight plus internal muscular friction. When you lower a weight, the friction works for you; you're lowering the weight minus internal muscular friction.

Regardless of the reason why eccentric strength is greater than concentric strength, the fact is that it takes less effort to lower a weight than it does to raise a weight. Indeed, walking down stairs is much easier than walking up stairs. It makes sense, then, that lowering the weight should take more time to complete than raising the weight. To ensure that your repetitions are safe and productive, it should take at least three to four seconds to lower the weight back to the start/finish position.

Effectively, then, it should take at least four to six seconds to perform a repetition. A 16-week study reported a 50% increase in upper-body strength and a 33% increase in lower-body strength in a group that did each repetition by raising the weight in two seconds and lowering it in four seconds. Using the same six-second guideline for raising and lowering the weight, two different eight-week studies reported increases in strength of 55% and 58%.

Another thing to remember here is that all exercises don't have the same range of motion (ROM). And that affects repetition speed. For instance, the elbow joint normally has a ROM that's about 135 degrees during the bicep curl and tricep extension. In order to raise the weight in two seconds, you'd need to move at about 67.5 degrees per second. In comparison, the wrist joint normally has a ROM that's about 90 degrees during wrist flexion and wrist extension. In order to do raise the weight in two seconds, you'd need to move at about 45 degrees per second.

Checkpoint #4: The Range of Motion

A repetition should be done throughout the greatest possible ROM that safety allows: from a full stretch to a full contraction and back to a full stretch. Performing your repetitions throughout a full ROM allows you to maintain – or perhaps increase – your flexibility. In one study, 25

exercise science majors at the University of North Dakota were randomly assigned to groups that did either strength training or flexibility training for the same muscles and joints. (A third group acted as a control and didn't train.) After five weeks, both groups significantly increased their ROM in three of four measures of flexibility and there were no significant differences between the groups. (The two groups made a small but non-significant improvement in the fourth measure of flexibility.)

Moreover, it ensures that you're stimulating your entire muscle – not just a portion of it – thereby making the repetitions more productive. Research has shown that strength training is very angular-specific. When a muscle is trained at a specific angle, increases in strength are limited to about 15 to 20 degrees on either side of that point. In other words, full-range exercise is necessary for a full-range effect.

This doesn't imply that you should avoid limited-range repetitions altogether. During rehabilitative training, for example, you can exercise throughout a pain-free ROM and still manage to stimulate some gains in strength (and size). However, full-range repetitions are more productive and should be performed whenever possible.

Safe and Productive Repetitions

It's much safer and more productive to raise and lower the weight in a smooth, controlled manner without any explosive or jerking movements. Raising the weight in at least one to two seconds and lowering it in at least three to four seconds is a good indication that momentum didn't play a significant role in the performance of the repetition.

Remember, *how well* you lift is more critical than *how much* you lift. Your strength program will be safer and more productive when you perform each repetition with proper technique.

6. Duration of a Workout

When it comes to strength training, more isn't necessarily better. An inverse relationship exists between time and intensity: As the time of an activity increases, the level of intensity decreases.

Stated otherwise, you can't train with a high level of intensity for a long period of time. Consider this analogy: With respect to anaerobic training, compare the time (length) and intensity of a workout that consists of four 400-meter sprints to a workout that consists of eight 400-meter sprints. In doing four sprints, the time of the workout would be relatively low but the level of intensity would be relatively high; in doing eight sprints, the time of the workout would be relatively high but the level of intensity would be relatively low. So as the time of an activity goes up, the level of intensity goes down.

The fact is that you can train for a short period of time with a high level of intensity or a long period of time with a low level of intensity. But you can't train with a high level of intensity for a long period of time. In order to train with a high level of intensity, you must train for a brief period of time. If you lengthen the duration of your workout – by increasing either the number of exercises or sets that you normally perform – you must reduce your level of intensity. And, of course, using a lower level of intensity isn't desirable.

It's important to note that carbohydrates are your preferred source of energy during intense activity. Carbohydrates circulate in your bloodstream as glucose and are stored in your liver and muscles as glycogen. The liver and muscles can only stockpile a limited amount of glycogen. For the average individual, estimates vary but seem to be around 375 to 500 grams or about 1,500 to 2,000 calories. (A negligible amount of glucose circulates in the blood.) The rate at which you use calories is a function of your level of intensity; as your level of intensity increases, your rate of caloric expenditure increases. Now, suppose that you did strength training with a high level of intensity which required an average of 16 calories per minute. If you had 1,500 to 2,000 calories of glycogen available, this means that you could conceivably work out for about 90 to 120 minutes or so before draining the reservoir. The amount of glycogen that's available can vary considerably among individuals. But even if you have enough glycogen to provide energy for as much as two

hours, it doesn't mean that your workout has to be that long. An intense and comprehensive workout can be completed in approximately one hour or less.

Be advised that the duration of a workout is a critical factor in program adherence, especially among those who are new to training. Studies have shown that individuals tend to discontinue their programs when given lengthy workouts to complete.

The exact duration of your workout depends on several factors such as the size of the facility, the amount of equipment, the preparation for each exercise/set (such as adjusting seats, setting weights and so on), the number of people using the facility, the transition time between each exercise/set and the availability of a training partner. Generally speaking, however, you should be able to complete a comprehensive workout in no more than about one hour.

You can make your workouts more efficient – and more intense – by taking as little recovery as possible between exercises/sets. The length of your recovery interval depends on your level of fitness. Initially, you may require several minutes of recovery between exercises/sets to catch your breath or feel that you can produce a maximum level of effort. With improved fitness, your pace between exercises/sets can be quickened. (The speed with which you do your repetitions shouldn't be quickened, just the pace between

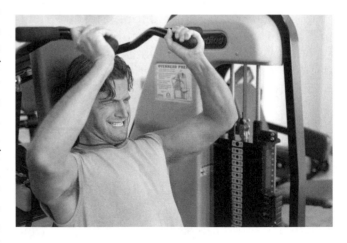

You can make your workouts more efficient – and more intense – by taking as little recovery as possible between exercises/sets. (Photo provided by Luke Carlson.)

exercises/sets.) Doing your strength training with a minimum amount of recovery between exercises/sets will elicit improvements in your metabolic fitness that can't be approached by multiple-set training.

7. Volume of Exercises

Most individuals can accomplish a total-body workout with 14 exercises or less. The focal point for the majority of these exercises should be your major muscles: your hips, legs and torso. Include one exercise for your hips, hamstrings, quadriceps, calves/dorsi flexors, biceps, triceps, abdominals and lower back. Because your shoulder joint allows movement at many different angles, you should perform two exercises for your chest, upper back and shoulders. You can choose any exercises that you prefer to address those body parts.

Some individuals may need to do slightly more than 14 exercises. For instance, those who participate in combat sports – such as football, rugby, boxing, judo and wrestling – should also include an additional two to four exercises for their neck to strengthen and protect their cervical area against catastrophic injury. Those who participate in sports or activities that require grip strength – such as baseball, golf and tennis – should include one exercise for their lower arms (forearms).

Once again, more isn't necessarily better when it comes to strength training. Performing too many exercises can produce too much stress which will impede compensatory adaptation. A total-body workout that contains 20 exercises could be metabolically devastating for someone who has a low tolerance for strength training. And the more exercises that you perform, the more difficult it will be for you to maintain an appropriate level of intensity.

This isn't to say that you can't do an extra exercise or two in order to emphasize a particular body part. As long as you continue to make improvements in your strength, you're not performing too many exercises. So if your workout consists of 20 exercises and you're making progress, then you're not overtraining. But if you plateau in one or more exercises, it's

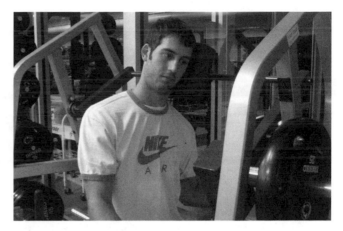

Those who participate in combat sports should include two to four exercises for their neck to strengthen and protect their cervical area against catastrophic injury. (Photo by Troy Harrison.)

probably because the volume of your training has compromised your ability to recover.

8. Order of Exercise

The order in which you perform your exercises is essential in producing optimal improvements in strength (and size). The order of your exercises also determines which muscles you emphasize or target.

Researchers randomly assigned 48 men from the Brazilian Navy Academy into two experimental groups: One group trained their muscles from largest to smallest, doing the bench press, lat pulldown, shoulder press, bicep curl and tricep extension; the other group trained their muscles from smallest to largest, doing the same five exercises but in the reverse order. (A third group acted as a control and didn't train.) The two experimental groups did three sets of each exercise three times per week for eight weeks.

The order in which the exercises were completed was critical in the improvements that were made. For example, gains in the bench press were 39.8% when the exercise was done first and 18.6% when it was done last; gains in the tricep extension were 74.3% when the exercise was done first and 50.0% when it was done last. In other words, doing an exercise earlier in the workout led to the greatest improvements.

As a rule of thumb, the idea is to train your most important muscles as early as possible in your workout. It stands to reason that you'd want to address those muscles while you're fresh, both mentally as well as physically. Larger muscles are generally more important than smaller muscles. In effect, then, your workout should begin with exercises that involve your largest muscles and proceed to those that involve your smallest ones.

The Lower Body

The largest and most powerful muscles are found in your lower body specifically, your hips and legs. What's the best order of exercise for training your lower body? Consider this: Multiple-joint movements that are done for your lower body – such as the leg press and deadlift – require the use of your upper legs for assistance. Your upper legs – your hamstrings and quadriceps – are the "weak link" in those exercises because they have a smaller amount of muscle mass. So if you fatigue your upper legs first, you'll weaken an already weak link thereby limiting the workload placed on the muscles of your hips. As a result, it's usually best to train your hips before your upper legs.

What would happen if you did train your upper legs immediately prior to your hips? In other words, what if you did the leg extension and then the leg press? This sequence of exercises would be very effective in fatiguing your quadriceps but not so much for your hips.

After training your upper legs, you should proceed to your lower legs, either your calves or dorsi flexors. If you train your calves and your dorsi flexors in the same workout, the order in which you do so really doesn't matter.

So in general, you should start with your hips and literally work down your legs. In other words, the best sequence would be hips, upper legs (hamstrings and quadriceps) and lower legs (calves or dorsi flexors).

The Upper Body

Once you've exercised your lower body, you can now direct your attention to your upper body. What's the best order of exercise for training your upper body? Not to be redundant but from a conceptual standpoint, it sounds quite similar to that which has been discussed for your lower body. Multiple-joint movements that are done for your upper body – such as the bench press, seated row and shoulder press – require the use of your arms for assistance. Your arms – your biceps, triceps and forearms – are the weak link in those exercises because they have a smaller amount of muscle mass. So if you fatigue your arms first, you'll weaken an already weak link thereby limiting the workload placed on the muscles of your torso. As a result, it's usually best to train your upper back before your biceps; your biceps before your forearms; and your chest and/or shoulders before your triceps.

What would happen if you did train your triceps immediately prior to your chest and/or shoulders or your biceps immediately prior to your upper back? In other words, what if you did the tricep extension and then the bench press or the bicep curl and then the seated row? This sequence of exercises would be very effective in fatiguing your arms but not so much for the major muscles of your torso.

You have at least two options for the order in which you train your chest, upper back and shoulders. One way is to do all of the exercises for a given muscle – your chest, for example – and then proceed to the next muscle. Another way is to alternate "pushing" movements with "pulling" movements. (To avoid confusion, it's important to note that all muscles pull when they contract; however, muscular contractions cause joints to extend and flex which produce movements that can be described as either pushing or pulling.) Your chest, anterior portion of your shoulders and triceps are used in pushing movements while your upper back, posterior portion of your shoulders and biceps are used in pulling movements. In a push-pull application, you might do the following sequence for your torso: bench press (push), seated row (pull), incline press (push), underhand lat pulldown (pull), front raise (push), bent-over raise (pull), tricep extension (push) and bicep curl (pull).

Performing all of the exercises for a given muscle before moving to another muscle produces a large amount of fatigue since the muscle being exercised gets little relief (assuming, of course, that the time taken between exercises/sets is minimal); alternating exercises in a push-pull fashion allows one muscle to recover while another muscle is being trained. (You're encouraged to experiment with these two applications and vary them based on your personal preferences and performance objectives.)

So in general, you should start with your chest, upper back and shoulders and literally work down your arms. In other words, the best order of exercise would be torso (chest, upper back and shoulders) and upper arms (biceps and triceps). If you include an exercise for your lower arms (forearms) in your workout, it's best to do it after you complete your upper-arm exercises.

The Mid-Section

Many people begin their workouts by training their mid-section (their abdominals and lower back). But early fatigue of the mid-section isn't advisable.

During intense activity, your abdominals force expiration. Therefore, fatiguing your abdominals early in your workout would detract from your performance in other exercises that involve larger, more powerful muscles.

In one study, 12 subjects ran as far as possible in 12 minutes on an outdoor track under two conditions: one with prior fatigue of the abdominals and one without. To produce fatigue, the subjects inhaled freely through their nose and exhaled through a mouthpiece that offered resistance to breathing. (An earlier study found that this type of resistive breathing elicits abdominal fatigue.) In 12 minutes, the subjects ran about 2,872 meters when their abdominals were fatigued and about 2,957 meters when they weren't. So, prior fatigue of the abdominals resulted in a significant decrease in maximal running distance.

Take-home message: Exercise your abdominals at the *end* of a workout, not at the *beginning*.

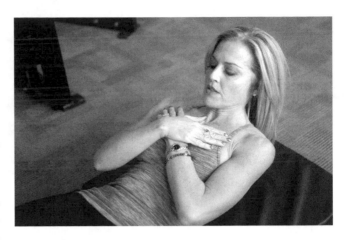

Exercise your abdominals at the end of a workout, not at the beginning. (Photo provided by Luke Carlson.)

The very last muscle that you train should be your lower back. Fatiguing your lower back early in your workout will also detract from your performance in other exercises.

So, the last area that you should train in your workout is your mid-section. And the best order of exercise would be abdominals and lower back.

The Neck

As mentioned earlier, individuals who participate in combat sports should train their neck muscles. If you include exercises for your neck in your workout, it makes the most sense to do them at the beginning of your workout or just after you complete your lower-body exercises (prior to beginning your upper-body exercises). This violates the largest-to-smallest rule but at the end of your workout, you will be – and should be – physically and mentally drained. If you wait until this point to train your neck, you'll be less likely to address this all-important area with a desirable level of effort or enthusiasm. Training your neck earlier in your workout when you're less fatigued will yield a more favorable response.

In summary, the best order of exercise in a total-body workout would usually look like this: hips, upper legs (hamstrings and quadriceps), lower legs (calves or dorsi flexors), torso (chest, upper back and shoulders), upper arms (biceps and triceps), abdominals and lower back. If included, exercises for your neck should be done at the beginning of your workout or just after your lower body (prior to the exercises for your torso); exercises for your lower arms (forearms) should be done just after your upper arms.

If you prefer to do a split routine – in which the body is divided or split into parts that are trained over the course of several workouts instead of one total-body workout – the aforementioned order of exercise would still apply. In a workout that targeted your chest, shoulders and triceps, for example, you should still address those body parts from largest to smallest.

9. Frequency of Training

Intense strength training places great demands on your muscles. In order to adapt to this stress, your muscles must receive an adequate amount of recovery between your workouts.

Compensatory adaptation to the demands occurs during the recovery process. Believe it or not, your muscles don't get stronger during your workout . . . your muscles get stronger *after* your workout. If the demands are of sufficient magnitude, a muscle is literally torn. Although these "tears" are quite small – microscopic, in fact – the recovery process is essential in that it allows the damaged muscle enough time to repair itself. Think of this as allowing a wound to heal. If you had a scab and picked at it every day, you'd delay the healing process. But if you left it alone, you'd permit the damaged tissue time to heal. So in a sense, the recovery that follows a workout is a process in which damaged tissue – in this case, muscle tissue – is healed.

There are individual variations in recovery ability; everyone has a different tolerance for exercise. However, a period of at least 48 hours is usually necessary for muscle tissue to recover sufficiently from intense strength training. Keep in mind, too, that intense strength training relies heavily on carbohydrates as the primary source of energy. When glycogen (carbohydrate) stores are depleted as a result of intense strength training, it appears as if about 48 hours are needed to refill those stores. The process for replenishing glycogen is actually biphasic. When adequate carbohydrates are consumed after a workout, glycogen is reestablished rapidly; within

24 hours, glycogen is almost at the pre-training level. Thereafter, however, glycogen is reestablished slowly. One study found that almost 46 hours were needed to reach pre-training glycogen levels; this, despite consuming a carbohydrate-enriched diet and without doing physical activity for as long as possible.

As such, it's suggested that you do strength training two or three times per week on non-consecutive days (such as on Monday, Wednesday and Friday). This advice is consistent with the recommendation of the American College of Sports Medicine. (Note that this assumes total-body workouts.)

An appropriate frequency (and volume) of strength training can be likened to doses of medication. In order for medicine to improve a condition, it must be taken at specific intervals and in certain amounts. Taking medicine at a greater frequency or in a larger quantity beyond what's needed can have harmful effects. Similarly, an overdose of strength training – in which workouts are done too often or have too much volume – can also be detrimental.

Most individuals respond well from three total-body workouts per week. But because of a low tolerance for strength training, others respond more favorably from two total-body workouts per week. In rare circumstances, an individual may respond better from one total-body workout per week. Performing any more than three doses of total-body workouts per week will gradually become counterproductive if the demands placed on your muscles exceed your recovery ability.

Many authorities believe that a muscle begins to lose strength (and size) if it's not adequately stimulated within about 96 hours of a previous workout. Anecdotal reports suggest that it may be more than 96 hours, at least for some individuals. Clearly, however, a loss of strength (and size) will occur after some period of extended inactivity. If you're an athlete, then, it's important for you to continue strength training even while in-season or while competing. However, the workouts should be reduced to twice a week due to the increased level of activity from practices and competitions. One workout should be done as soon as possible following a competition and another not within 48 hours of the next competition. So, an athlete who competes on Tuesdays and Saturdays should do strength training on Wednesdays and Sundays (or Thursdays, providing that it's not within 48 hours of the next competition). From time to time, an athlete may only be able to do strength training once per week because of a particularly heavy schedule such as competing three times in one week or several days in a row.

In general, it appears as if training three days per week is better than training two days per week. But you can still make significant improvements in strength from two weekly workouts. In one study, 117 subjects were randomly assigned to four groups that trained either two or three times a week for either 10 weeks or 18 weeks. (A fifth group acted as a control and didn't train.) The two groups that trained three days per week increased their strength by 21.2% (10 weeks) and 28.4% (18 weeks); the two groups that trained two days per week increased their strength by 13.5% (10 weeks) and 20.9% (18 weeks). So overall, doing two weekly workouts achieved about 80% of the gains in strength as doing three weekly workouts.

How do you know if your muscles have had an adequate amount of recovery? You should see a gradual improvement in the amount of resistance and/or number of repetitions that you're able to do over the course of several weeks. If not, then you're probably not getting enough recovery between your workouts which, again, could be the result of performing too many sets, too many repetitions or too many exercises. Remember, strength training will be effective if it provides an overload, not an overdose.

The Split Routine

A method that has been popularized by bodybuilders and competitive weightlifters is known as the split routine. When using a split routine, the body is split into different parts that are trained on different days.

There are many possibilities for a split routine. One example is to split the muscles such that the

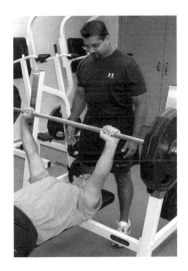

In order to adapt, your muscles must receive an adequate amount of recovery between your workouts. (Photo by Peter Silletti.)

hips, legs and mid-section are trained on Monday and Thursday; the chest, shoulders and triceps on Tuesday and Friday; and the upper back, biceps and forearms on Wednesday and Saturday. So in this split routine, each muscle would be trained twice per week during six workouts.

Despite the popularity of split routines, they're no more effective than total-body workouts. In one study, 30 female kinesiology students were assigned to groups that did either a split routine consisting of four workouts per week (two for the upper body and two for the lower body) or total-body workouts twice per week. (A third group acted as a control and didn't train.) After 20 weeks of training, it was found that both protocols were equally effective in improving maximum strength, increasing lean-body mass and decreasing body fat.

Split routines can be productive as long as they encourage progressive overload and provide adequate recovery. It's the latter area in which split routines often fall short. If a split routine is designed correctly, a person won't train the same muscles two days in a row. Recall, however, that it takes about 48 hours for your body to replenish its stockpile of glycogen following an intense workout. So if you trained your lower body on Monday with a desirable level of intensity, you exhausted much of your glycogen stores. Even if you train different muscles on Tuesday, your body wouldn't have enough time to return your glycogen stores to pre-training levels. Keep in

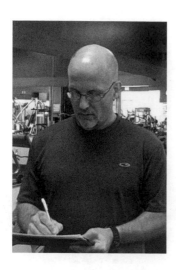

Records are an extremely valuable tool to monitor your progress and make your workouts more productive and more meaningful. (Photo by Patty Durell.)

mind, too, that even though you train part of your body in a workout, you still stress your entire anaerobic pathways (which provide metabolic support for your efforts). Your energy systems don't recover in parts; they recover as a whole. The researchers in the aforementioned study that compared split routines to total-body workouts noted that doing fewer workouts per week "would free more days for recovery or other types of training." This is an important consideration for competitive athletes who must invest significant amounts of their time in aerobic, anaerobic and skill training.

If you prefer to use a split routine, make sure that you group your muscles based on their functions and relations with other muscles. For instance, your triceps and shoulders are used to train your chest. So, these muscles should be included in the same workout. Likewise, your biceps and forearms are used to train your upper back. So, these muscles should be included in the same workout.

One final point: From a performance perspective, split routines don't make sense because they're not specific to the muscular involvement in most physical activities. When you use a split routine, you train different muscles on different days. However, a selective use of muscles almost never happens during a physical activity. Rather, you're required to integrate all of your muscles at once. Therefore, it makes little sense for you to prepare for physical activities by training your muscles separately on different days.

10. Record Keeping

Many people believe that they don't need to track their performance because they can remember their resistance and repetitions. In all likelihood, they've probably been using the same resistance and doing the same repetitions for so long that the numbers have become firmly entrenched in their long-term memories. If strength training is to be as productive as possible, it's absolutely critical for you to keep written records that are accurate and detailed.

Why? For one thing, records are the history of what you accomplished during each and every exercise of each and every workout. Moreover, records are an extremely valuable tool to monitor your progress and make your workouts more productive and more meaningful. Records can also be used to identify exercises in which you've reached a plateau. In the unfortunate event of an injury, you can also gauge the effectiveness of your rehabilitative training if you have a record of your pre-injury levels of strength.

Regardless of the means that you choose to employ for record keeping, you should be able to track your bodyweight, the date of each workout, the resistance used for each exercise, the number of repetitions performed for each set, the order in which the exercises were completed and any necessary seat adjustments.

The bottom line: Don't underestimate the importance of keeping records as a way to make your strength training more productive and more meaningful.

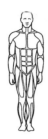

5 Strength Training for Females

Strength training isn't just for males. Many physical, physiological and psychological benefits of strength training have been noted in Chapter 4 but one that's especially important for females is worth mentioning again: an increase in bone mineral density.

Osteoporosis – literally, porous bones – is a condition that's characterized by decreased bone mineral density. According to the National Center for Health Statistics, 2% of American men aged 50 and older have osteoporosis of the hip while 10% of their female counterparts have the same condition. Osteoporosis impacts the quality of life in many ways but perhaps the biggest concern is a greater risk of fractures (mainly to the vertebrae, wrist and hip). Obviously, this could lead to permanent disability. Strength training can increase bone density thereby reducing the risk of osteoporosis (and bone fracture).

DISPELLING MISCONCEPTIONS

It wasn't until the early 1980s or so before it became socially acceptable for females to lift weights. Prior to that time, there were many worries that strength training would produce masculinizing effects.

Gradually, most of these fears have subsided. But even to this day, some concerns continue to linger. The two biggest misconceptions about females who lift weights are that they'll end up losing flexibility and developing large muscles.

Losing Flexibility

When conducted properly, strength training doesn't reduce flexibility. If anything, doing repetitions throughout a full range of motion against a resistance will maintain or even improve flexibility.

Females who have residual fears about becoming less flexible can do a series of stretches both before and after their strength training. As an added measure, they can also stretch the muscles that were involved in an exercise immediately after it's completed. Following the leg extension, for example, an individual can do a stretch for her quadriceps.

Developing Large Muscles

Increases in strength are often accompanied by increases in size (although the increases in size don't match the increases in strength). While this is true for both genders, the fact of the matter is that increases in size are much less pronounced in females. (An increase in strength without an attendant increase in size is thought to be the result of neural adaptation.)

Since the early 1960s, research has shown that most females can achieve increases in their strength without increases in their size. In a classic study that was conducted by Dr. Jack Wilmore at the University of California, Davis, a group of 47 women significantly improved their

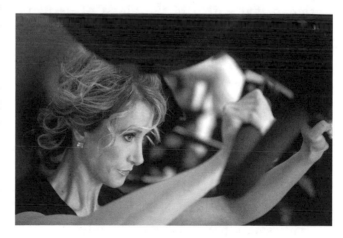

Females who life weights can make substantial gains in strength without developing large muscles. (Photo provided by Luke Carlson.)

49

strength in the leg press by 29.5% and bench press by 28.6% after eight weeks of training (in which they did two sets of eight exercises). Yet, the largest increase in size that was experienced by the women in any one of the 17 areas that were assessed was *less than one-quarter inch*. (This was a 10-week study but initial testing didn't take place until after the second week of training.)

It's very evident that females who lift weights can make substantial gains in strength without developing large muscles. From a physiological standpoint, there are at least three reasons why this is true.

Muscle Fiber Type

One reason why most females can't get large muscles has to do with their proportion of fast-twitch (FT) and slow-twitch (ST) fibers. Research has shown that females possess a slightly higher percentage of ST fibers than males. For example, a study that involved 418 subjects reported that females had 51% ST fibers in their vastus lateralis and males had 46%.

As noted in Chapter 3, FT and ST fibers have the potential to increase in size but FT fibers have a much greater potential. Since females have a higher percentage of ST fibers, their potential to increase the size of their muscles is lower.

Testosterone

Another reason why most females can't get large muscles pertains to testosterone, a male sex hormone that's also in the blood of perfectly normal women. Testosterone prompts muscles to increase in size. Everything else being equal, those who have high levels of testosterone have a greater potential to improve their size than those who have low levels of testosterone. Compared to males, most females have low levels of this hormone. In fact, the average female has about one tenth of the testosterone as the average male. This small amount restricts the degree to which females can increase the size of their muscles.

The small percentage of females who do develop relatively large muscles might have slightly higher levels of testosterone than the average female. In one study, researchers suggested that testosterone may play a role in a female's trainability (the degree to which she responds to strength training). In another study, 10 women participated in a brief but intense strength program. The researchers found a high correlation between their level of testosterone and the size of their muscles.

By the way, this doesn't mean that a female who has a high level of testosterone is any less of a woman. It simply means that she has a greater potential for increasing her size (and strength) than the average woman.

Body Fat

One more reason why most females can't get large muscles has to do with body fat. Females tend to inherit higher percentages of body fat than males. For example, the average 18- to 22-year-old female has about 22 to 26% body fat, whereas the average male of similar age has about 12 to 16%. A higher percentage of body fat corresponds to a lower percentage of lean-body (or fat-free) mass. This extra body fat tends to soften or mask the effects of strength training. Females who have very little body fat look more muscular than they actually are because their muscles are more visible. Along these lines, what appears to be an increase in muscle mass from strength training may be the result of a decrease in body fat which makes the same amount of muscle look more noticeable.

Interestingly, the distribution of fat is gender-specific. Even though there are individual differences, males tend to store fat in their abdominal area (aka an android pattern) which produces an apple-shaped look; females tend to store fat in their hips and thighs (aka a gynoid pattern) which produces a pear-shaped look. Moreover, the body type of the average female tends more toward endomorphy (fatness) while the body type of the average male tends more toward ectomorphy (leanness) and mesomorphy (muscularity).

Female Bodybuilders

In case you're wondering about female bodybuilders, they've inherited a greater potential to increase the size of their muscles than the average woman. In other words, female bodybuilders have developed large muscles because of their genetic profile, not simply because they lifted weights. Also, it's well within the realm of possibility that at least some female bodybuilders have used anabolic steroids or other pharmacological substances to enhance their muscular development.

Keep in mind, too, that female bodybuilders look much more muscular than normal while posing on stage. When training for a competition, female bodybuilders restrict their caloric intake – often severely – thereby reducing their body fat and body fluids. Immediately prior to posing on stage, they've also "pumped" their muscles. This engorges their muscles with blood and makes them temporarily bigger, a condition known as transient muscular hypertrophy. Finally, the stage lighting as well as their tans and clothing – and even the oil that's rubbed on their bodies – all contribute to making female bodybuilders appear as if they have much larger muscles than they actually do.

A relatively small number of females have inherited the ingredients that are necessary to attain significant increases in their size. But the overwhelming majority of females can gain considerable strength while experiencing little change in their size. In short, it's physiologically improbable for the average female to develop large muscles that are unsightly or unfeminine.

CONSIDERATIONS FOR STRENGTH TRAINING

It must be understood that there's no such thing as gender-specific training (or gender-specific exercises). Even with the use of an electron microscope, it's literally impossible for a scientist to differentiate between the muscle tissue of females and the muscle tissue of males. So in general, females can do the same strength program – and utilize the same exercises – as males.

Females can improve their strength in a manner that's productive, comprehensive,

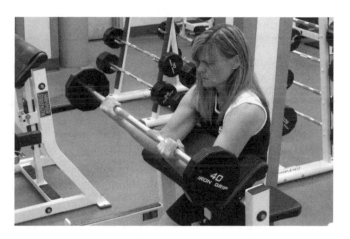

There's no such thing as gender-specific training or gender-specific exercises.

practical, efficient and safe by incorporating the concepts that have been detailed in Chapter 4.

GENDER DIFFERENCES IN STRENGTH

Researchers have investigated gender differences in strength since the early 1900s. This is often done as a measure of absolute strength: the amount of weight that can be lifted without considering any other factors. But it's also important to examine relative strength: the amount of weight that can be lifted in relation to bodyweight, body composition and muscular size.

Absolute Strength

In terms of absolute strength, the average male tends to be far stronger than the average female. An early review of the literature found that the absolute total-body strength of females is roughly 67% that of males. Since that time, numerous studies have compared the absolute strength levels of males and females and have reported varying degrees of differences. However, research has consistently shown that males tend to be stronger than females in absolute terms.

The differences in absolute strength between males and females vary according to the areas of the body that are being compared. As an example, a review of nine studies revealed that the absolute lower-body strength of females is about 57 to 86%

(averaging 71.9%) that of males while the absolute upper-body strength is about 35 to 79% (averaging 55.8%). The reason for this is probably related to the fact that both genders have had an equal opportunity to use their lower bodies to a similar degree (such as while standing, walking and running). But females have had less opportunity than males to use their upper bodies due to continued societal constraints. Another reason that has been cited is that males have wider shoulders than females, giving them a biomechanical advantage in upper-body strength.

Relative Strength

So in absolute terms, males are significantly stronger than females. However, males are significantly larger and heavier than females. In terms of absolute strength, the greater body size of males gives them a decided advantage over females. When assessing gender differences in strength, then, comparisons should be made relative to some measure of size.

As mentioned earlier, the average female has more body fat than the average male. And there's a direct correlation between a high percentage of body fat and a low percentage of lean-body mass which is, of course, functional tissue. For instance, the average college-aged male who weighs 154 pounds (lb) with 14% body fat has 21.56 pounds of body fat and 132.44 pounds of functional tissue [154 lb x 14% = 21.56 lb; 154 lb - 21.56 lb = 132.44 lb]. On the other hand, the average college-aged female who weighs 121 pounds with 24% body fat has 29.04 pounds of body fat and 91.96 pounds of functional tissue [121 lb x 24% = 29.04 lb; 121 lb - 29.04 lb = 91.96 lb]. So in this illustration, the average college-aged male has 27.27% more bodyweight [154 lb compared to 121 lb] and 44.02% more functional tissue [132.44 lb compared to 91.96 lb] than the average college-aged female. Clearly, strength must be expressed relative to bodyweight and/or body composition in order to make valid comparisons of males and females.

Strength Relative to Bodyweight and Body Composition

When the disparities in bodyweight and body composition are taken into consideration, the differences in strength between males and females are less substantial. The Wilmore study that was noted earlier also involved 26 men who did the same strength program as the 47 women. After eight weeks of training, when expressed relative to bodyweight, the leg strength of females was nearly identical to that of males. And when expressed relative to lean-body mass, the leg strength of females was actually slightly higher than males. (In this study, the upper-body strength of men was significantly greater than women regardless of how the values were compared.) Another study reported that the upper-body strength of females averaged 60 to 70% of males relative to bodyweight and 80 to 90% of males relative to lean-body mass. In a study involving 55 women and 48 men, the researchers concluded that gender differences in strength are a function of lean-body mass and body composition. So, it's quite clear that making comparisons relative to body composition essentially eliminates any gender difference in strength.

With respect to gender differences in strength relative to bodyweight, it's also interesting to examine highly experienced athletes. This can be done easily by looking at the performances of elite powerlifters. Their accomplishments are a measure of strength − essentially one-repetition maximums − and they compete in weight classes. Of course, the calculations aren't totally precise since someone who "makes weight" in the 60-kilogram class, for example, will likely weigh somewhat more or less than this when actually competing. Nevertheless, it's still a convenient way to obtain a rough estimate of gender differences in strength relative to bodyweight.

In powerlifting, males and females compete in three different lifts: the squat, bench press and deadlift. The upcoming data were gleaned from the world records of men and women that were officially recognized by the International Powerlifting Federation (IPF) as of June 2011 in seven mutual weight classes: 52.0, 56.0, 60.0, 67.5, 75.0, 82.5 and 90.0 kilograms. (The IPF has since changed the weight classes such that none are the same for men and women.) Relative to bodyweight, performances by women in the squat and deadlift ranged from 68 to 77% (averaging 72.8%) and 70 to 79% (averaging 75.2%) of their male counterparts, respectively, compared to the reported range of 57 to 86% (averaging 71.9%) for gender differences in absolute lower-body strength. And relative to bodyweight, performances by women in the bench press ranged from 64 to 75% (averaging 71.2%) of men compared to the reported range of 35 to 79% (averaging 55.8%) for gender differences in absolute upper-body strength. So again, it's clear that the differences in strength between males and females are less significant when bodyweight is considered.

On a related note, something else to ponder is that although the average male is stronger than the average female in terms of absolute strength, many females are much stronger than the average male. A number of women, for instance, have lifted more than 3½ times their bodyweight in the squat and deadlift with two women having squatted more than four times their bodyweight and one of those women having deadlifted more than four times her bodyweight. Also, many women have exceeded twice their bodyweight in the bench press with at least five women having bench pressed more than 400 pounds (Topping the list at this time is Natalia Zotova of Russia with a bench press of 451 pounds.) Needless to say, the vast majority of the male population will never be able to attain such remarkable performances in those three exercises.

Strength Relative to Muscular Size

There's a direct correlation between strength and muscular size (here, the cross-sectional area of a muscle). As an example, one study examined the strength per unit of cross-sectional area of muscle tissue of 18 physical education students (7 females and 11 males) and 5 male bodybuilders. The researchers found no significant differences between males and females when strength was expressed in relation to muscle cross-sectional area. As such, the differences in strength between males and females appear to be in the *volume* of muscle

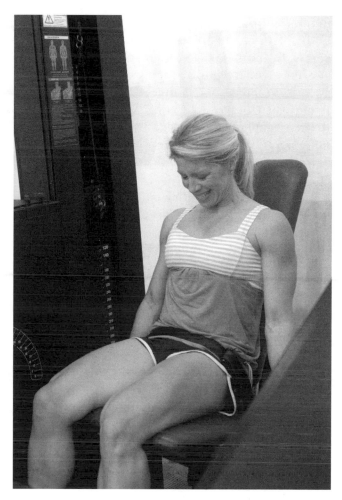

When the disparities in bodyweight and body composition are taken into consideration, the differences in strength between males and females are less substantial. (Photo provided by Luke Carlson.)

fibers, not in the *makeup* of muscle fibers. In other words, gender differences in strength are *quantitative* rather than *qualitative*. This means that although males usually have larger muscles than females, the force exerted by equal-sized muscles is the same in both genders. This isn't surprising since muscle tissue is essentially the same regardless of gender.

In short, the ability of muscle fibers to generate force is independent of gender.

ISSUE: EXERCISE AND PREGNANCY

The fundamental purpose of exercise during pregnancy – including strength training – is to maintain fitness and prepare a woman for labor and delivery. There doesn't appear to be any scientific evidence to suggest that women who exercise during their pregnancy will shorten or ease their labor and delivery. According to the American College of Sports Medicine, however, it's reasonable to expect that exercise will facilitate labor and the recovery from labor.

Potential Benefits

Many other potential benefits are associated with exercising during pregnancy. First of all, women who exercise can better meet the progressive physical demands of pregnancy. By strengthening the muscles of their torso and abdominals, women can compensate for the postural adjustments that typically occur during pregnancy as a result of the forward pull of the growing baby's weight. Women who have stronger muscles can counter fatigue and reduce the severity and frequency of common pregnancy-related discomforts such as low-back pain. In addition, women who do strength training experience minimal biomechanical changes and are better able to maintain their normal activities during pregnancy. Exercising also helps to control the amount of weight that women gain during pregnancy. Finally, improving strength can be good preparation for carrying a baby that may weigh 6 to 10 pounds at birth.

Concerns and Precautions

With regards to a fitness program, the most important consideration for a pregnant woman and her developing fetus is safety. Proper exercise poses little risk to the mother or her fetus. Nonetheless, women who have never participated in a fitness program shouldn't initiate one during their pregnancy. Additionally, women should consult with their physician before starting any fitness program.

Although exercise has little risk during pregnancy, the potential exists for adverse effects to both the mother and the fetus. As such, there are a few areas of concern that must be addressed.

With several precautionary measures for added safety, a pregnant woman can perform the same type of program that's recommended for the general population. If a pregnant woman shows signs of exertional intolerance and/or chronic fatigue, she should reduce her intensity, frequency, volume and/or duration of training. The American College of Obstetricians and Gynecologists advises women to terminate exercise if they experience any of the following conditions: vaginal bleeding; dyspnea (shortness of breath) prior to exercise; dizziness; headache; chest pain; muscle weakness; calf pain or swelling; or decreased fetal movement.

Competing Needs

During exercise, there may be competition for various maternal and fetal physiological needs such as blood flow, oxygen delivery and heat dissipation. The prospect of this biological struggle is greatest during exercise that's performed in the third trimester.

When a person exercises, there's an increased blood flow to the working muscles. In fact, the working muscles may receive 70% or more of the blood flow. During pregnancy, the diversion of oxygen-rich blood to the exercising muscles of the mother leads to a transient reduction in the flow of oxygen-rich blood to the fetus. This threatens the fetus with the possibility of an inadequate supply of blood and oxygen. Exercising with a low to moderate level of intensity for 30 minutes or less doesn't seem to disturb uterine blood flow.

A potential threat to the safety of the developing fetus – especially during the first trimester – is exercise-induced hyperthermia (an increased core temperature). Exercise is associated with a rise in both maternal and fetal core temperatures. The fetus usually maintains a core temperature slightly above that of the mother. In order to dissipate heat, the fetus must depend entirely on the mother's thermo-regulatory abilities. To avoid heat complications, an exercising mother must be adequately hydrated, use a level of intensity that's lower than her pre-pregnancy state and wear light clothing that permits heat loss. In addition, she must be aware of the existing environmental temperature and humidity. Pregnant women must avoid high ambient temperature and humidity during exercise due to potential problems in thermoregulation. During pregnancy, women shouldn't exercise when the ambient temperature is greater than 90 degrees Fahrenheit and the relative humidity exceeds 50%. Finally, workouts shouldn't be more than about 30 minutes in duration so that the fetus isn't exposed to prolonged thermal stress.

Increased Laxity

After contraception, the levels of relaxin increase significantly. Relaxin is a hormone that helps to loosen or, as you might suspect, "relax" the joints and connective tissues. This allows the ribs and pelvic cavity to expand in order to encompass the growing baby and make delivery easier. However, connective tissues soften throughout the entire body and the joints become less stable. The increased laxity of the joints during pregnancy can make women more susceptible to back, hip, knee and ankle injuries. Pregnant women shouldn't overstretch since extreme flexion or extension may be harmful to the joints and connective tissues. (During pregnancy, the aim of flexibility training should be to relieve muscle cramping and alleviate any pain in the low-back area.)

As a countermeasure against the increased laxity of the joints, pregnant women should use slightly higher repetition ranges than suggested for the general population. The higher repetition ranges require the use of lighter weights which reduces the orthopedic stress that's placed on their vulnerable joints and connective tissues. In this case, they should do about 20 to 25 repetitions for exercises involving their hips, 15 to 20 repetitions for their legs and 10 to 15 repetitions for their torso.

Exercise Caution

The American College of Obstetricians and Gynecologists recommends that women should avoid exercising in the supine (laying face-up) position after the first trimester. When in the supine position, the excess weight of the enlarging fetus may obstruct the flow of blood back to the mother's heart.

Also during pregnancy, high-impact activities and movements should be minimized and eventually eliminated. This includes jumping, hopping, bouncing and running. In addition, caution is advised for activities and movements that involve twisting.

Caloric Consumption

The intake of calories must be sufficient to meet the extra energy needs of pregnancy and any exercise that's done. During pregnancy, a woman should consume about 300 additional calories per day.

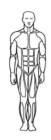

6 Strength Training for Youths

Strength training can be quite beneficial for youths. First and foremost is the fact that it can significantly improve their strength. As youths age, they'll increase their strength from normal growth and maturation. However, these processes may very well be expedited by strength training.

Like all other types of physical training, strength training produces an expenditure of calories that can help to establish a favorable percentage of body fat and improve appearance. Having greater strength can also reduce the frequency and severity of injuries and enhance athletic potential/performance. Moreover, youths can increase their self-confidence and self-esteem during the all-important identity-forming years.

One thing that shouldn't be expected in children and younger adolescents, though, is a noticeable increase in their muscular size. This is because they have low levels of androgens which are growth promoting hormones. (At younger ages, any improvements in strength are likely due to neural adaptation.)

DISPELLING MISCONCEPTIONS

A generation ago, the prevailing thought was that youths shouldn't do strength training prior to the development of their secondary sexual characteristics (such as a deeper voice and facial/ body hair in boys and breasts and wider hips in girls). These changes usually coincide with the onset of the so-called adolescent growth spurt. It had been believed that doing any strength training prior to this developmental stage would impair or stunt their growth.

Specifically, the worry was that strength training would damage the epiphyseal (or growth) plates which are cartilaginous discs that

reside at each end of a long bone (such as the femur and ulna). Injury to the epiphyseal plates can result in pre-mature closure of these structures which could impede the longitudinal growth of a bone.

As a result of this fear, it was recommended that youths should wait until the age of about 13 or 14 before they began strength training. While these concerns were certainly well intended, it turns out that they were unfounded. Attitudes have changed, largely due to a growing body of scientific research that has proven otherwise. Nowadays, participation by youths in strength training has gained much greater acceptance and is endorsed by many organizations including the American Academy of Pediatrics, the American College of Sports Medicine and the American Orthopaedic Society for Sports Medicine.

When to Begin?

Although there's no clear-cut borderline for determining an appropriate age to begin, research has shown that children as young as 10 can do strength training without risk of injury provided that certain guidelines are followed. Be advised, too, that a youth must be able to stay focused

Research has shown that children as young as 10 can do strength training without risk of injury provided that certain guidelines are followed.

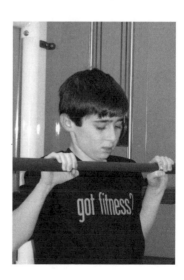

and follow directions before strength training is permitted.

Note: It's helpful to become familiar with several terms that are used frequently in this chapter. Children are boys and girls who haven't developed their secondary sexual characteristics which is about the age of 11 in girls and 13 in boys. Adolescents are girls aged 12 to 18 and boys aged 14 to 18. Youths encompass children and adolescents.

CONSIDERATIONS FOR STRENGTH TRAINING

Youths can improve their strength in a manner that's productive, comprehensive, practical, efficient and safe by incorporating these 10 concepts:

1. Level of Intensity

A high level of intensity (or effort) is needed to produce optimal gains in strength. Normally, this is one that reaches muscular fatigue (the point where no additional repetitions can be done with proper technique).

Because of their physical and mental immaturity, however, children shouldn't train to muscular fatigue. Instead, an appropriate level of intensity for children is to terminate a set a few repetitions short of muscular fatigue or when they feel that they've given a decent effort. As children get older and more mature, they should gradually increase their level of exertion.

2. Progressive Overload

In order for a muscle to get stronger, it must be "asked" to do progressively harder work. To accomplish this, an attempt must be made to increase either the resistance used or the repetitions performed in comparison to a previous workout.

Once the recommended number of repetitions is attained, the progressions in resistance should be made in small increments. Preferably, progressions should be no more than about 5%.

3. Number of Sets

There's no agreement as to how many sets of an exercise should be done by youths. Most of the recommendations, though, are between one and three sets. Doing one set of each exercise represents an efficient way of training and is highly recommended. An emphasis should be placed on the *quality* of work that's done in a strength program, not the *quantity* of work.

4. Number of Repetitions

It's generally agreed that youths need to perform a higher number of repetitions than most adults. Doing higher repetitions necessitates using lighter weights; this, in turn, reduces the stress that's placed on their bones, connective tissues and joints. Children should do about 20 to 25 repetitions for exercises involving their hips,

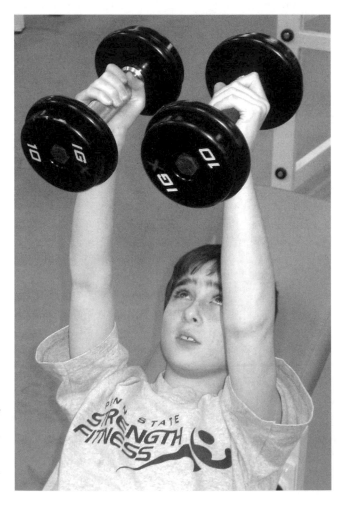

Youths need to perform a higher number of repetitions than most adults.

58

15 to 20 repetitions for their legs and 10 to 15 repetitions for their torso. As they get older and more mature, those ranges can be reduced over time to about 15 to 20 repetitions for their hips, 10 to 15 repetitions for their legs and 5 to 10 repetitions for their torso.

Youths shouldn't try to "max out" or do low-repetition sets. This increases the potential for injury and, therefore, should be discouraged.

5. Proper Technique

To make each exercise safer and more productive, it's important for youths to employ proper technique. The resistance should be raised in a smooth, controlled manner without any explosive or jerking movements. After raising the resistance, there should be a brief pause in the mid-range position. Then, the resistance should be lowered in a smooth, controlled manner. A repetition should be done throughout the greatest possible range of motion that safety allows. Emphasis should be placed on *how well* the weight is lifted, not *how much* weight is lifted.

6. Duration of a Workout

As noted in Chapter 4, more isn't necessarily better when it comes to strength training. The workouts of children should be limited to about 20 to 30 minutes; the workouts of adolescents should be limited to about 30 to 40 minutes.

There's no reason for them to spend much more time than that engaged in strength training. Lengthy workouts can lead to disinterest and dissatisfaction which will decrease adherence to the strength program. Furthermore, lengthy workouts can increase the risk of overuse injuries.

7. Volume of Exercises

Children should perform about nine exercises (one set each) per workout. A workout can consist of one exercise for their hips, hamstrings, quadriceps, calves/dorsi flexors, chest, upper back, shoulders, abdominals and lower back. This lower volume of exercises decreases the potential for overuse injuries and increases the potential for adherence to the strength program. As they get older and more mature, the volume can be increased to about 14 exercises (one set each) per

workout. In this case, a workout can consist of one exercise for their hips, hamstrings, quadriceps, calves/dorsi flexors, biceps, triceps, abdominals and lower back; two exercises (one set each) should be done for their chest, upper back and shoulders. If multiple sets of an exercise are performed, the total number of exercises should be reduced accordingly so as to stay within the aforementioned parameters for the duration and volume of training.

Youths who are involved in combat sports – such as football, judo and wrestling – should also include one or two exercises for their necks; youths who participate in sports or activities that require grip strength – such as baseball, field hockey and tennis – should also include one exercise for their lower arms (forearms).

8. Order of Exercise

A workout should begin with exercises that involve the largest muscles and proceed to those that involve the smallest ones. In general, the order of exercise would be hips, upper legs (hamstrings and quadriceps), lower legs (calves or dorsi flexors), torso (chest, upper back and shoulders), upper arms (biceps and triceps), abdominals and lower back.

If included, exercises for the neck should be done at the beginning of the workout or just after the lower body (prior to exercises for the upper body); exercises for the lower arms should be done after the upper arms.

Incidentally, exercises can be performed with a wide assortment of equipment including barbells, dumbbells, machines and resistance bands. Youths can also benefit from doing exercises that involve their own bodyweight (such as push-ups, dips, chin-ups, pull-ups and abdominal crunches).

9. Frequency of Training

Care must be taken to ensure that youths get an adequate amount of recovery between workouts. Children should do strength training once or twice per week on non-consecutive days. As they get older and more mature, strength training can be increased to two or three times

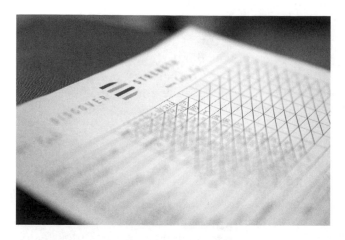

The value of keeping accurate records can't be overemphasized. (Photo provided by Luke Carlson.)

per week on non-consecutive days. (This assumes total-body workouts.)

10. Records

The value of keeping accurate records can't be overemphasized. A record is a log of what youths have accomplished in their strength program. This is an extremely useful tool to monitor their progress and make their workouts more productive and more meaningful. It can also be used to identify exercises in which they've reached a plateau.

SUPERVISION

It's of utmost importance that youths are monitored closely during their strength training. Competent and qualified individuals should provide adequate instruction in the proper performance of all exercises and direct supervision of all workouts. Simply put, an emphasis must be placed on safety.

ISSUE: PRACTICAL PROGRESSIONS

As mentioned earlier, an important aspect of strength training is progressive overload. It's well worth looking at how this can be incorporated in a practical manner.

Recall that with strength training, progression can be achieved by doing more repetitions or using more resistance in comparison to a previous workout. A practical progression that works well with children (and beginners) is to have them start with a resistance that allows them to easily reach the low end of the repetition range. Then, have them try to do one more repetition every workout or two. When they reach the high end of the repetition range, increase the resistance in their next workout by the smallest amount available and have them aim for the low end of the repetition range.

Example: In today's workout, Ryan did 10 repetitions with 30 pounds in the lat pulldown. In his next five workouts, he lifted the same weight for 11, 12, 13, 14 and 15 repetitions. In his next workout, the weight was increased to 31.25 pounds and he dropped back to 10 repetitions. In his next five workouts with that weight, he did 11, 12, 13, 14 and 15 repetitions. At this point, the weight was increased to 32.5 pounds and the aforementioned cycle repeated (dropping back to 10 repetitions).

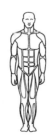

7 Strength Training for Older Adults

A slow but steady increase in life expectancy has resulted in the progressive aging of the American population. In 1990, for example, the median age was 32.9; in 2010, it was 37.2. Even more revealing is that between 2000 and 2010, the number of people aged 45 to 64 increased by 31.5% to 81.5 million which was 26.4% of the US population. And during that same 10-year span, the number of people aged 65 and over increased by 15.1% to 40.3 million which was 13.0% of the US population.

Older adults who do strength training stand to reap numerous rewards. For one thing, strength training can thwart the ravaging effects of osteoporosis. As people age, they have an increased risk of osteoporosis which means that they have a decreased bone mineral density. Although there are individual differences, bone density declines by about 0.5% or more per year after the age of 40. The result of a decrease in bone density is bones that are more porous and more prone to fracture. Also of importance is that with older adults, fractured bones take a longer time to heal. The good news is that strength training can increase bone density which decreases the risk of bone fractures.

With aging comes an increase in body fat; the rate is about 1.5 pounds per year. However, the *amount* of fat might be of less concern than the *distribution* of fat. In general, there are two types of body fat: subcutaneous (located beneath the skin) and visceral (located around the internal organs or viscera). Younger adults store about half of their fat as subcutaneous fat and half of their fat as visceral fat; older adults store a higher percentage of their fat as visceral fat. It's well known that visceral fat is associated with an increased risk of cardiovascular and metabolic diseases including diabetes, heart disease and hypertension. Similar to other types of physical training, strength training can produce a loss of body fat (visceral as well as subcutaneous).

Through strength training, older adults can also improve their overall mental health and well-being. This includes a reduced risk of depression and anxiety. In addition, they'll enhance various aspects of their cognitive function such as memory and attention.

Note: There's no clear guideline as to what age defines an older adult. This is partly due to the fact that everyone ages at different rates. The fact of the matter is that chronological age has nothing to do with physiological age. The recommendations that appear in this chapter are intended for those who are 65 and older but could be applicable for individuals who are much younger, depending on their level of fitness and function.

DISPELLING MISCONCEPTIONS

Perhaps the biggest misconception about older adults is that because of their advanced age, they'll experience little or no response to strength training in terms of the strength and size of their muscles. However, research tells another story.

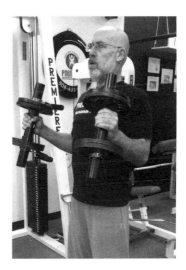

Older adults who do strength training stand to reap numerous rewards. (Photo by Fred Fornicola.)

Muscular Strength

As people age, they gradually lose muscular strength. In fact, strength usually peaks between the ages of 20 and 30 and then remains relatively stable until the age of about 45. But by the age of 50, strength declines progressively and precipitously with increasing age. Between the ages of 50 and 60, strength drops by about 1.5% per year and 3.0% per year thereafter. The loss of strength may actually be significant enough to hinder daily activities that nearly everyone else takes for granted such as rising from a chair or even walking.

The decline in strength is likely due to a loss of muscle mass. (The term for an age-related loss of muscle mass and strength is sarcopenia.) Indeed, studies show that much of the loss of strength is due to *quantitative* changes in the muscle, not *qualitative* changes. In other words, the muscles of older adults still function basically the same way as when they were younger; it's just that they have less muscle mass. (On a related note, research has found that a selective atrophy of fast-twitch fibers occurs with aging.)

While a loss of strength is inevitable, strength training can slow the rate of decline. A meta-analysis is a scientific way to combine the results of separate studies that examine the same topic. One meta-analysis pooled data from 47 studies that looked at the effects of strength training on older adults. The studies involved a total of 1,079 men and women who ranged in age from 50 to 83. The meta-analysis found that, on average, older adults who did strength training had significant improvements in strength in their lower body (29% in the leg press and 33% in the leg extension) and upper body (24% in the chest press and 25% in the lat pulldown).

Muscular Size

As people age, they gradually lose muscular size. Between the ages of 25 and 55, individuals lose muscle mass at the rate of about one-half pound per year. So, the average 55-year-old has 15 less pounds of muscle than at age 25. The loss of lean-body mass intensifies after the mid-50s.

Early studies that investigated the effects of strength training in older adults found marked gains in strength but little evidence of any gains in size. Because of the absence of significant hypertrophy, researchers speculated that the increases in strength achieved by older adults were due to neural adaptation. But in 1988, researchers at Tufts University reported significant increases in strength and size. In this landmark study, 12 older men (aged 60 to 72) trained three times per week for 12 weeks. They increased their quadriceps strength by 112% and their hamstring strength by 227%. This was accompanied by an increase in the cross-sectional area of their quadriceps by 10.6%.

And get this: Gains in size can be made by older adults even into their 90s. In one study, 10 men and women (aged 86 to 96) trained three times per week for eight weeks. The nine subjects who completed the study increased their quadriceps strength by 174% and the muscle area of their mid-thigh by 9%. (One subject stopped after four weeks due to a previous injury.) Of no small importance is that at the end of the study, two subjects no longer needed canes for assistance in walking.

More recently, a meta-analysis pooled data from 49 studies that looked at the effects of strength training on older adults. The studies involved a total of 1,328 men and women who ranged in age from 50 to 83. The meta-analysis found that, on average, older adults who did strength training 2.8 times per week for 20.5 weeks increased their lean-body mass by about 2.4 pounds. This might seem small but remember that after the age of 25, people lose about one-half pound of lean-body mass per year.

CONSIDERATIONS FOR STRENGTH TRAINING

Older adults can improve their strength in a manner that's productive, comprehensive, practical, efficient and safe by incorporating these 10 concepts:

1. Level of Intensity

A high level of intensity (or effort) is needed to produce optimal gains in strength. Normally, this is one that reaches muscular fatigue (the point where no additional repetitions can be done with proper technique).

Some older adults might not tolerate training to muscular fatigue, however. Those who aren't comfortable with this level of intensity can terminate a set a few repetitions short of muscular fatigue or when they feel that they've given a decent effort. As they become more accustomed to strength training, they should gradually increase their level of exertion.

2. Progressive Overload

In order for a muscle to get stronger, an attempt must be made to increase either the resistance used or the repetitions performed in comparison to a previous workout.

Once the recommended number of repetitions is attained, the progressions in resistance should be made in small increments. Preferably, progressions should be no more than about 5%.

3. Number of Sets

The American College of Sports Medicine recommends that older adults do one set of each exercise. This represents an efficient way of training. An emphasis should be placed on the *quality* of work that's done in a strength program, not the *quantity* of work.

4. Number of Repetitions

Older adults should perform a higher number of repetitions than their younger counterparts. Doing higher repetitions necessitates using lighter weights; this, in turn, reduces the stress that's placed on their bones, connective tissues and joints. Older adults should do about 20 to 25 repetitions for exercises involving their hips, 15 to 20 repetitions for their legs and 10 to 15 repetitions for their torso.

5. Proper Technique

To make each exercise safer and more productive, older adults must use proper technique. The resistance should be raised in a smooth, controlled manner without any explosive or jerking movements. After raising the resistance, there should be a brief pause in the mid-range position. Then, the resistance should be lowered in a smooth, controlled manner. A repetition should be done throughout the greatest possible range of motion that safety allows.

Older adults who suffer from arthritis should use a range of motion that's pain-free. Note that their pain-free range could change from one day to the next.

6. Duration of a Workout

More isn't necessarily better when it comes to strength training. The workouts of older adults should be limited to about 30 to 40 minutes. If more recovery is needed, the workouts should be limited to about 20 to 30 minutes.

Lengthy workouts can lead to disinterest and dissatisfaction which will decrease adherence to the strength program. Furthermore, lengthy workouts can increase the risk of overuse injuries and joint pain.

7. Volume of Exercises

Older adults can accomplish a total-body workout with 14 exercises or less. The focal point for the majority of these exercises should be their major muscles: their hips, legs and torso. A workout can consist of one exercise (one set each) for their hips, hamstrings, quadriceps, calves/dorsi flexors, biceps, triceps, abdominals and lower back; two exercises (one set each) should be done for their chest, upper back and shoulders.

If more recovery is needed, older adults can perform about nine exercises (one set each) per workout. In this case, a workout can consist of one exercise (one set each) for their hips, hamstrings, quadriceps, calves/dorsi flexors, chest, upper back, shoulders, abdominals and lower back. This lower volume of exercises decreases the potential for overuse injuries and increases the potential for adherence to the strength program.

8. Order of Exercise

A workout should begin with exercises that involve the largest muscles and proceed to those that involve the smallest ones. In general, the order of exercise would be hips, upper legs (hamstrings and quadriceps), lower legs (calves or dorsi flexors), torso (chest, upper back and shoulders), upper arms (biceps and triceps), abdominals and lower back.

9. Frequency of Training

Older adults must get an adequate amount of recovery between workouts. It's recommended that they do strength training two or three times per week on non-consecutive days. If more recovery is needed, the frequency should be reduced to once or twice per week on non-consecutive days.

10. Records

It's important for older adults to keep accurate records of what they've accomplished in their strength program. It's an extremely useful tool to monitor progress and make their workouts more productive and more meaningful. Records can also be used to identify exercises in which a plateau has been reached. In the event of an injury, the effectiveness of rehabilitative training can be gauged if there's a record of their pre-injury levels of strength.

ISSUE: WEIGHT GAIN WITH AGING

It has been noted that between the ages of 25 and 55, people lose about one-half pound of muscle mass per year. And as people age, they also gain body fat at a rate of about 1.5 pounds per year. So the net gain in weight is one pound per year but it's really a two-pound change in body composition.

Suppose that at the age of 25, a man weighed 170 pounds and his body fat was 15%. This means that he had 25.5 pounds of fat mass and

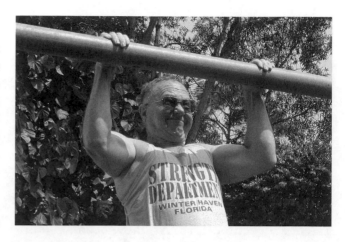

By engaging in a strength program on a regular basis, older adults will be able to slow down the weight gain that's associated with aging. (Photo by Margaret Bryan.)

144.5 pounds of fat-free (lean-body) mass. And now, 30 years later at the age of 55, his weight has increased by 30 pounds – one pound per year – to 200 pounds. But it's really a 60-pound swing in body composition as his fat mass has increased by 45 pounds (to 70.5 pounds) and his fat-free mass has decreased by 15 pounds (to 129.5 pounds). So in 30 years, his body fat has more than doubled, rising from 15% to 35.25%.

As people get older, it's natural for them to lose muscle mass and gain body fat. But by engaging in a strength program on a regular basis, they'll be able to slow down the weight gain that's associated with aging.

Note: According to the American College of Sports Medicine and the American Heart Association, men over the age of 45 and women over the age of 55 should consult with their physician before initiating a fitness program if one or more cardiovascular risk factors are present. This includes smoking (or having quit in the previous six months); high blood pressure (greater than 140/90); high cholesterol (greater than 200); family history of heart attack or heart surgery; physical inactivity; or overweight (by more than 20 pounds).

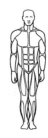

8 Free-Weight Exercises

Most fitness centers (and weight rooms) have at least some free weights (namely, barbells and dumbbells). And with good reason since free weights are perhaps the most popular pieces of equipment for strength training.

Josef Markl of Germany is credited with developing the plate-loading barbell in 1889 but a case could be made for Samuel Stockburger of Ohio who filed a patent for an "exercising bar" with removable weights that same year. In 1902, the Milo Bar-Bell Company of Philadelphia – which was founded by Alan Calvert – manufactured and sold the first adjustable barbell in the United States. The barbell had canister-like bells on each end that were loaded with lead shot or a similar substance. For the first time in this country, a barbell could be loaded with a different weight (though not very quickly). Previously, a different barbell was necessary for a different weight. By 1909, the company would sell plate-loading barbells. Largely because of Calvert, the American public was given access to equipment for strength training that for the most part had only been available to professional strongmen.

A dumbbell is essentially a shorter version of a barbell that's intended for use with one hand. People have been using dumbbells – or dumbbell-like objects – to improve their strength (and size) since at least the fifth century BC. But it took more than two millennia before the dumbbell got its name. In the middle of the 18th century, church-like bells – minus the clappers – were secured to the ends of a short handle. At the time, anyone who couldn't speak was referred to as dumb. Some researchers think that because the bell made no sound, it was christened a dumb bell.

ADVANTAGES OF FREE WEIGHTS

In comparison to machines, free weights offer the following advantages:

1. Free weights are generally less costly than machines.

In trying to furnish a fitness center with a limited or tight budget, the most important consideration in choosing equipment may very well be the price. It could easily cost $40,000 for a complete "line" of state-of-the-art selectorized equipment (10 to 12 machines). And larger fitness centers require far more than one line of machines. A considerable amount of free weights could be purchased for much less of an investment.

Note: Plate-loaded machines tend to be less expensive than selectorized machines. Not to be overlooked, however, is a hidden cost: A few thousand pounds or more of Olympic plates may need to be purchased to serve as the resistance.

2. Free weights give you more variety per dollar.

Most machines that are geared toward commercial use are designed to perform only one or two functions. An abdominal machine, for example, can only be used to train the abdominals. On the other hand, a bar and several hundred pounds of plates can allow you to perform exercises for just about every major muscle in your body.

3. Free weights can accommodate everyone regardless of their size from the tallest individual to the shortest.

When it comes to free weights, it's safe to say that one size fits all. Those who are at an extreme in terms of skeletal height and/or limb length may not be able to fit properly on some machines. This could make it difficult – or outright impossible – for some individuals to include certain machines in their strength program.

4. Having to balance free weights requires a greater involvement of synergistic muscles.

The degree to which this is considered as an advantage is debatable, though, since the significance of using synergistic muscles remains unclear. (A muscle is said to act as a synergist if it's used to prevent an undesired movement of a joint.)

ADVANTAGES OF DUMBBELLS

In this discussion, mention must be made of some benefits that are specific to dumbbells. In comparison to machines, dumbbells offer the following advantages:

1. Dumbbells can provide variety to your workout.

Remember, every exercise that can be performed with a barbell can also be performed with dumbbells. This means that every barbell exercise has a dumbbell counterpart that can be used as an alternative exercise.

2. With dumbbells, you have unrestricted freedom to change the position of your hands to best suit your natural biomechanics and level of comfort.

For instance, you can do a bicep curl with dumbbells using a traditional grip (palms facing up), a parallel grip (palms facing each other), a reverse grip (palms facing down) or even a grip that's somewhere in between.

3. Dumbbells force your limbs to work independently.

Most people are often stronger (and more flexible) on one side of their body than the other. Usually, this isn't a significant difference. But when there's a significant difference in the strength between limbs, the use of dumbbells is highly recommended. This is an important consideration for rehabilitative training, too. In this case, an individual may need to work one limb at a time while using a lighter weight for the injured limb. It should be noted that machines with independent movement arms allow you to work your limbs in an independent fashion.

THE EXERCISES

This chapter describes and illustrates the safest and most productive exercises that can be performed with free weights and your bodyweight. Included in the discussions of each exercise are the muscle(s) strengthened (if two or more muscles are involved, the first one listed is the prime mover), suggested repetitions (the time that the targeted muscles should be loaded is shown in parentheses), start/finish position, performance description and training tips for making the exercise safer and more productive.

These 36 exercises are described in this chapter: deadlift, ball squat, lunge, step-up, seated calf raise, standing calf raise, dorsi flexion, bench press, incline press, decline press, dip, bent-arm fly, bench row, bent-over row, chin-up, pull-up, pullover, shoulder press, lateral raise, front raise, bent-over raise, internal rotation, external rotation, upright row, shoulder shrug, scapulae adduction, bicep curl, tricep extension, wrist flexion, wrist extension, finger flexion, abdominal crunch, knee-up, side bend, back extension and stiff-leg deadlift.

DEADLIFT

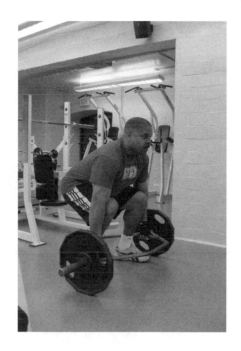 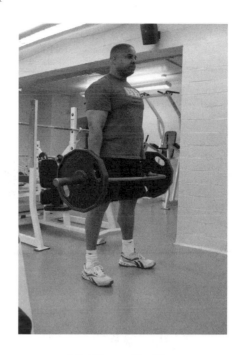

Start/Finish Position   *Mid-Range Position*

Muscles Strengthened: gluteus maximus, hamstrings, quadriceps and erector spinae

Suggested Repetitions: 15 to 20 (or 90 to 120 seconds)

Start/Finish Position: Step inside the opening of a trap bar and spread your feet slightly wider than shoulder-width apart. Reach down and grasp the bar on the outside of your legs with a parallel grip (your palms facing each other). Lower your hips until your upper legs are almost parallel to the floor. Flatten your back and look up slightly. Place most of your bodyweight on your heels. Straighten yor arms.

Performance Description: Stand upright by straightening your legs and torso. Pause briefly in this mid-range position (your legs and torso straight) and then lower the bar under control to the start/finish position (your legs and torso bent).

Training Tips:

- Avoid raising your hips too early. This negates their effectiveness and causes you to do the exercise almost entirely with your lower back. Ideally, your hips, legs and lower back should work together. However, your hips and legs should do most of the work.

- Exert force through your heels, not the balls of your feet.

- Avoid "locking" or "snapping" your knees in the mid-range position. Also, avoid hyperextending your torso (leaning backward excessively) in the mid-range position.

- Keep your arms straight, head up and back flat.

- Refrain from bouncing the weight off the floor between repetitions.

- You can also perform this exercise with a barbell and dumbbells. When doing this exercise with a barbell, use an alternating grip (your dominant palm facing forward and non-dominant palm facing backward); when doing this exercise with dumbbells, use a parallel grip and keep the weights at your sides.

- Use wrist straps if you have difficulty in maintaining your grip on the bar.

- This exercise may be contraindicated if you have low-back pain, hyperextended elbows or an exceptionally long torso and/or legs.

BALL SQUAT

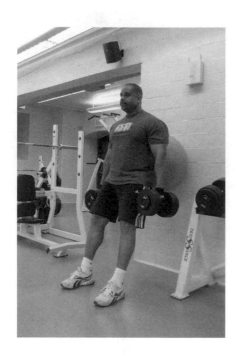

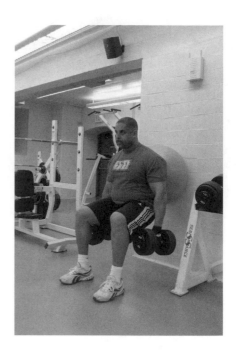

Start/Finish Position

Mid-Range Position

Muscles Strengthened: gluteus maximus, hamstrings and quadriceps

Suggested Repetitions: 15 to 20 (or 90 to 120 seconds)

Start/Finish Position: Grasp a dumbbell with each hand. Stand with your back toward a wall and have a spotter or training partner place a stability ball between your lower back and the wall. Position your feet so that your upper legs will be parallel to the floor and lower legs will be perpendicular to the floor in the mid-range position. Spread your feet slightly wider than shoulder-width apart and point them straight ahead. Keep your legs almost completely straight. Place most of your bodyweight on your heels. Straighten your arms and point your palms toward each other.

Performance Description: Lower your body under control to the mid-range position (your upper legs parallel to the floor). Without bouncing, return to the start/finish position (your legs almost completely straight).

Training Tips:

- Exert force through your heels, not the balls of your feet.

- Avoid "locking" or "snapping" your knees in the start/finish position.

- If you can't do 15 repetitions, perform this exercise without the dumbbells.

- Use wrist straps if you have difficulty in maintaining your grip on the dumbbells.

LUNGE

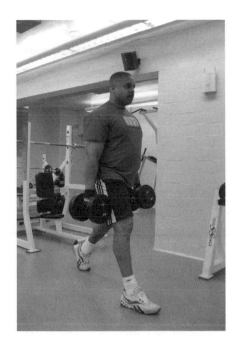

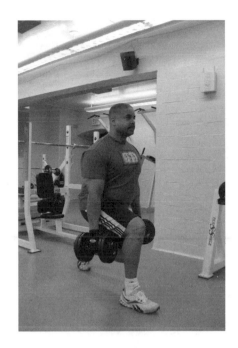

Start/Finish Position   *Mid-Range Position*

Muscles Strengthened: gluteus maximus, hamstrings and quadriceps

Suggested Repetitions: 15 to 20 (or 90 to 120 seconds)

Start/Finish Position: Grasp a dumbbell with each hand. Step forward with your right foot and position your right lower leg so that it's perpendicular to the floor. Elevate your left heel off the floor. Point your feet straight ahead. Keep your torso erect and your right leg almost completely straight. Place most of your bodyweight on your right heel. Straighten your arms and point your palms toward each other.

Performance Description: Lower your body under control to the mid-range position (your right upper leg parallel to the floor). Without bouncing, return to the start/finish position (your right leg almost completely straight). Repeat the exercise for the other side of your body (with your left foot forward).

Training Tips:

- Exert force through your heel, not the ball of your foot.

- Avoid "locking" or "snapping" your knee in the start/finish position.

- If you can't do 15 repetitions, perform this exercise without the dumbbells.

- Use wrist straps if you have difficulty in maintaining your grip on the dumbbells.

STEP-UP

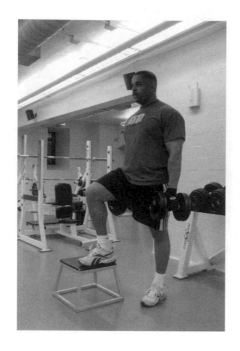

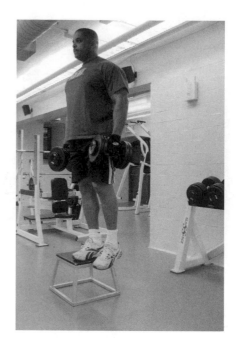

Start/Finish Position   *Mid-Range Position*

Muscles Strengthened: gluteus maximus, hamstrings and quadriceps

Suggested Repetitions: 15 to 20 (or 90 to 120 seconds)

Start/Finish Position: Grasp a dumbbell with each hand. Place your right foot on a step that's about 18 to 24 inches high (or something similar that's stable). Position your right lower leg so that it's perpendicular to the floor. Straighten your left leg. Point your feet straight ahead. Place most of your bodyweight on your right heel. Straighten your arms and point your palms toward each other.

Performance Description: Step up with your right leg until it's almost completely straight. Pause briefly in this mid-range position (your right leg almost completely straight) and then lower your body under control to the start/finish position (your right leg bent). Repeat the exercise for the other side of your body.

Training Tips:

• Avoid using your non-exercising leg to assist your exercising leg.

• Exert force through your heel, not the ball of your foot.

• Avoid "locking" or "snapping" your knee in the mid-range position.

• If you can't do 15 repetitions, perform this exercise without the dumbbells.

• Use wrist straps if you have difficulty in maintaining your grip on the dumbbells.

SEATED CALF RAISE

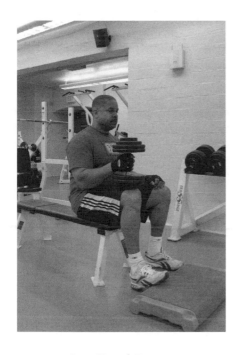

Start/Finish Position

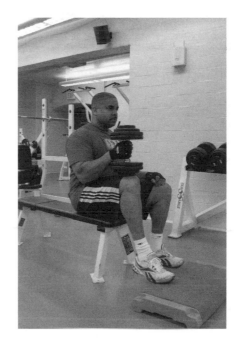

Mid-Range Position

Muscle Strengthened: soleus

Suggested Repetitions: 10 to 15 (or 60 to 90 seconds)

Start/Finish Position: Grasp a dumbbell with your right hand. Sit down near the end of a utility bench (or stool). Place the ball of your right foot on the edge of a step (or something similar that's stable) and lower your heel. Position the dumbbell on the top of your right upper leg near your knee and hold it in place.

Performance Description: Rise up onto your toes as high as possible. Pause briefly in this mid-range position (your ankle straight) and then lower your leg under control to the start/finish position (your heel near the floor). Repeat the exercise for the other side of your body.

Training Tips:

- Use a step or something similar that's at least several inches high to obtain an adequate stretch.

- Avoid this exercise if you have shin splints.

71

STANDING CALF RAISE

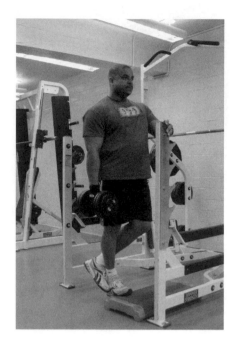

Start/Finish Position

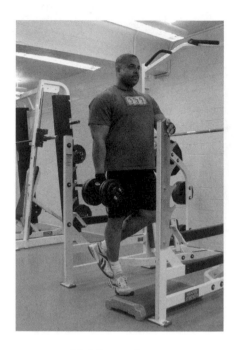

Mid-Range Position

Muscle Strengthened: gastrocnemius

Suggested Repetitions: 10 to 15 (or 60 to 90 seconds)

Start/Finish Position: Grasp a dumbbell with your right hand. Place the ball of your right foot on the edge of a step (or something similar that's stable and offers a place to hold with your left hand to maintain your balance) and lower your heel. Keep your torso erect and straighten your right leg but don't "lock" your knee. Cross your left ankle behind your right ankle.

Performance Description: Rise up onto your toes as high as possible. Pause briefly in this mid-range position (your ankle straight) and then lower your body under control to the start/finish position (your heel near the floor). Repeat the exercise for the other side of your body (with the dumbbell in your left hand).

Training Tips:

• Use a step or something similar that's at least several inches high to obtain an adequate stretch.

• Avoid using your hips and legs. Movement should only occur at your ankle joint.

• Refrain from doing this exercise with a weight placed on your shoulders. This compresses the spinal column.

• If you can't do 10 repetitions, perform this exercise without the dumbbells.

• Use wrist straps if you have difficulty in maintaining your grip on the dumbbell.

• Avoid this exercise if you have shin splints.

DORSI FLEXION

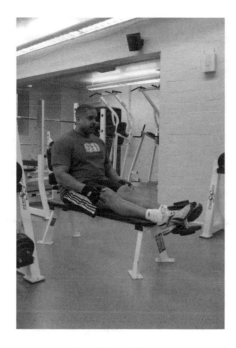

Start/Finish Position

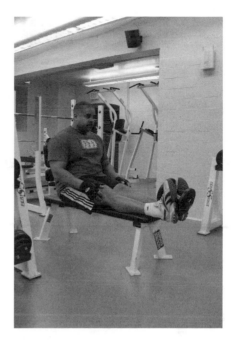

Mid-Range Position

Muscles Strengthened: dorsi flexors

Suggested Repetitions: 10 to 15 (or 60 to 90 seconds)

Start/Finish Position: Grasp a dumbbell with your preferred hand. Sit down near the end of a utility bench and place the dumbbell between your feet. Slide your hips back so that your legs lie across the length of the back pad. Position your heels slightly over the end of the bench and point your toes away from your body.

Performance Description: Keeping your legs flat on the back pad, raise the dumbbell as high as possible. Pause briefly in this mid-range position (your ankles bent) and then lower the dumbbell under control to the start/finish position (your ankles straight).

Training Tips:

- Avoid moving your torso forward and backward. Movement should only occur at your ankle joint.

- This exercise may be contraindicated if you have shin splints.

BENCH PRESS

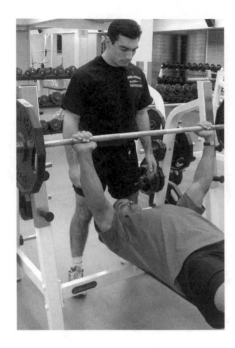

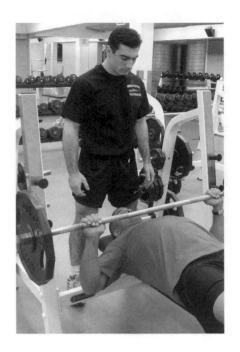

Start/Finish Position   *Mid-Range Position*

Muscles Strengthened: chest, anterior deltoid and triceps

Suggested Repetitions: 5 to 10 (or 30 to 60 seconds)

Start/Finish Position: Lie down on an Olympic supine (flat) bench and place your feet flat on the floor. Grasp a barbell and spread your hands slightly wider than shoulder-width apart. Lift the bar out of the "gun rack" or have a spotter give you assistance. Keep your arms almost completely straight (without "locking" your elbows).

Performance Description: Lower the bar under control to the mid-range position (the bar touching the middle part of your chest). Without bouncing the bar off your chest, push it up to the start/finish position (your arms almost completely straight).

Training Tips:

• Perform this exercise with a spotter.

• Avoid using an excessively wide grip. This reduces your range of motion.

• Keep your hips on the bench.

• If you have low-back pain, place your feet flat on the end of the bench or a stool. This reduces the stress in your low-back region.

• Avoid "locking" or "snapping" your elbows in the start/finish position.

• You can also perform this exercise with dumbbells.

• This exercise may be contraindicated if you have shoulder-impingement syndrome.

INCLINE PRESS

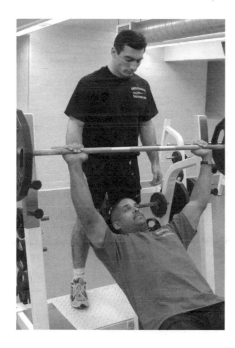

Start/Finish Position

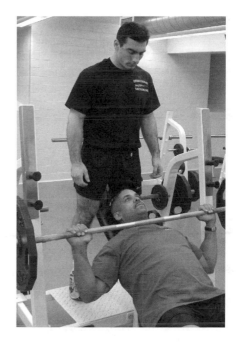

Mid-Range Position

Muscles Strengthened: chest (upper portion), anterior deltoid and triceps

Suggested Repetitions: 5 to 10 (or 30 to 60 seconds)

Start/Finish Position: Sit down on an Olympic incline bench and place your feet flat on the floor (or on the footplate if one is provided). Grasp a barbell and spread your hands slightly wider than shoulder-width apart. Lift the bar out of the "gun rack" or have a spotter give you assistance. Keep your arms almost completely straight (without "locking" your elbows).

Performance Description: Lower the bar under control to the mid-range position (the bar touching the upper part of your chest near your collarbones). Without bouncing the bar off your chest, push it up to the start/finish position (your arms almost completely straight).

Training Tips:

- · Perform this exercise with a spotter.
- Avoid using an excessively wide grip. This reduces your range of motion.
- Keep your hips on the seat pad.
- Avoid "locking" or "snapping" your elbows in the start/finish position.
- You can also perform this exercise with dumbbells.
- This exercise may be contraindicated if you have shoulder-impingement syndrome.

DECLINE PRESS

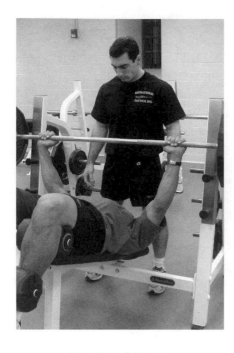

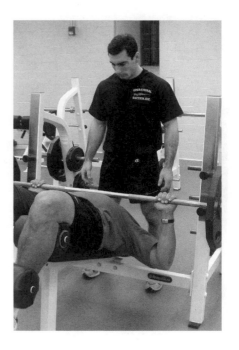

Start/Finish Position   *Mid-Range Position*

Muscles Strengthened: chest (lower portion), anterior deltoid and triceps

Suggested Repetitions: 5 to 10 (or 30 to 60 seconds)

Start/Finish Position: Lie down on an Olympic decline bench and place your legs over the roller pads and against the shin pads. Grasp a barbell and spread your hands slightly wider than shoulder-width apart. Lift the bar out of the "gun rack" or have a spotter give you assistance. Keep your arms almost completely straight (without "locking" your elbows).

Performance Description: Lower the bar under control to the mid-range position (the bar touching the lower part of your chest near the tip of your breastbone). Without bouncing the bar off your chest, push it up to the start/finish position (your arms almost completely straight).

Training Tips:

• Perform this exercise with a spotter.

• Avoid using an excessively wide grip. This reduces your range of motion.

• Keep your hips on the bench.

• Avoid "locking" or "snapping" your elbows in the start/finish position.

• You can also perform this exercise with dumbbells.

• This exercise may be contraindicated if you have shoulder-impingement syndrome.

DIP

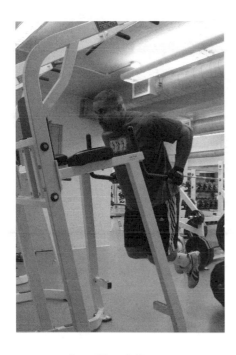

Start/Finish Position

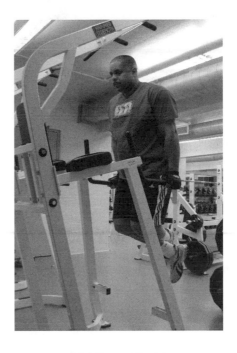

Mid-Range Position

Muscles Strengthened: chest (lower portion), anterior deltoid and triceps

Suggested Repetitions: 5 to 10 (or 30 to 60 seconds)

Start/Finish Position: Grasp the dip bars (or handles) with a parallel grip (your palms facing each other). Bend your arms so that your upper arms are roughly parallel to the floor. Lift your feet off the floor, bend your knees and cross your ankles.

Performance Description: Push your body up until your arms are almost completely straight (without "locking" your elbows). Pause briefly in this mid-range position (your arms almost completely straight) and then lower your body under control to the start/finish position (your arms bent).

Training Tips:

• Avoid swinging your body back and forth. Movement should only occur at your shoulder and elbow joints.

• Avoid "locking" or "snapping" your elbows in the mid-range position.

• If you can do 10 repetitions or more using your bodyweight, increase the workload by attaching additional weight to your waist, performing the exercise with a slower speed of movement or having a spotter apply manual resistance to your waist.

• After reaching muscular fatigue, you can overload your muscles further by stepping up to the mid-range position and lowering your body under control to the start/finish position for 3 to 5 negative-only repetitions.

• This exercise may be contraindicated if you have shoulder-impingement syndrome.

BENT-ARM FLY

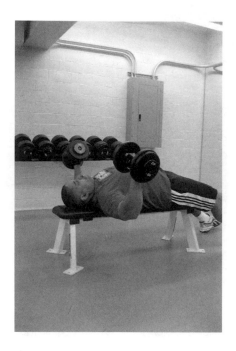

Start/Finish Position

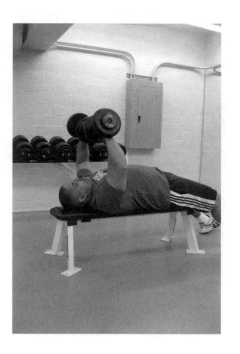

Mid-Range Position

Muscles Strengthened: chest and anterior deltoid

Suggested Repetitions: 5 to 10 (or 30 to 60 seconds)

Start/Finish Position: Grasp a dumbbell with each hand. Lie down on a utility bench and place your feet flat on the floor. Position the dumbbells near your shoulders so that they're even with your chest. Bend your arms so that the angle between your upper and lower arms is about 90 degrees. Point your palms toward your legs.

Performance Description: Keeping the same angle between your upper and lower arms, bring the dumbbells together directly over your chest. Pause briefly in this mid-range position (the dumbbells directly over your chest) and then lower the dumbbells under control to the start/finish position (the dumbbells near your shoulders).

Training Tips:

• This exercise is also referred to as a chest fly and a pec fly.

• Avoid straightening your arms as you raise the dumbbells. This changes the exercise from a bent-arm fly into a bench press. (When raising the dumbbells, imagine that you're hugging a tree.)

• Keep your hips on the bench.

• If you have low-back pain, place your feet on the end of the bench or a stool. This reduces the stress in your low-back region.

• This exercise may be contraindicated if you have shoulder-impingement syndrome.

BENCH ROW

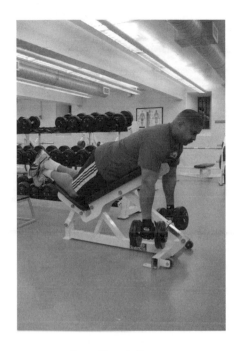

Start/Finish Position

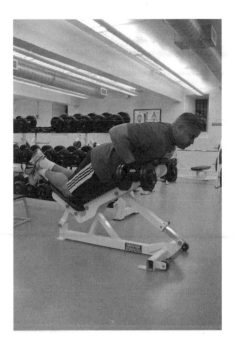

Mid-Range Position

Muscles Strengthened: upper back, biceps and forearms

Suggested Repetitions: 5 to 10 (or 30 to 60 seconds)

Start/Finish Position: Grasp a dumbbell with each hand. Kneel on the seat pad of an adjustable incline bench. Lie forward against the bench and position the dumbbells directly below your torso. Straighten your arms with your palms facing each other.

Performance Description: Pull the dumbbells up to your shoulders. Pause briefly in this mid-range position (your arms bent) and then lower the dumbbells under control to the start/finish position (your arms completely straight).

Training Tips:

- Do this exercise with one limb at a time if you have a shoulder or an arm injury, a gross difference in the strength between your limbs or desire a training variation.

- You can also perform this exercise with your upper arms positioned away from your torso. Doing this involves less of your upper back and more of your posterior deltoid, trapezius and rhomboids. In this case, your upper arms would be perpendicular to your torso in the mid-range position and your palms would be facing backward.

- Use wrist straps if you have difficulty in maintaining your grip on the dumbbells.

- This exercise may be contraindicated if you have hyperextended elbows.

BENT-OVER ROW

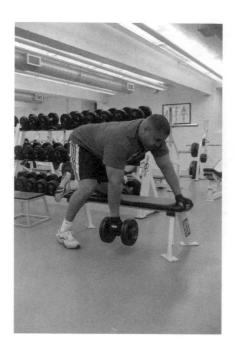

Start/Finish Position

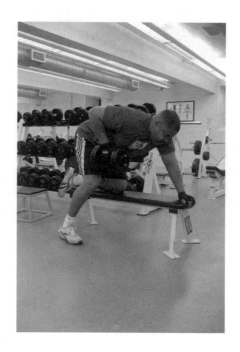

Mid-Range Position

Muscles Strengthened: upper back, biceps and forearms

Suggested Repetitions: 5 to 10 (or 30 to 60 seconds)

Start/Finish Position: Grasp a dumbbell with your right hand. Place your left hand and left knee on a utility bench and position your right foot on the floor at a comfortable distance from the bench. Straighten your right arm with your palm facing the bench.

Performance Description: Pull the dumbbell up to your right shoulder. Pause briefly in this mid-range position (your arm bent) and then lower the dumbbell under control to the start/finish position (your arm completely straight). Repeat the exercise for the other side of your body (with your right hand and right knee on the bench).

Training Tips:

- Avoid using your legs and rotating your torso. Movement should only occur at your shoulder and elbow joints.

- You can also perform this exercise with your upper arm positioned away from your torso. Doing this involves less of your upper back and more of your posterior deltoid, trapezius and rhomboids. In this case, your upper arm would be perpendicular to your torso and your palm would be facing backward in the mid-range position.

- Use wrist straps if you have difficulty in maintaining your grip on the dumbbell.

- This exercise may be contraindicated if you have a hyperextended elbow.

CHIN-UP

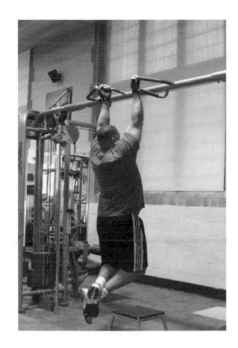

Start/Finish Position

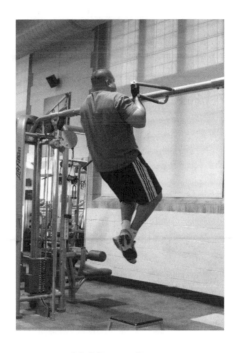

Mid-Range Position

Muscles Strengthened: upper back, biceps and forearms

Suggested Repetitions: 5 to 10 (or 30 to 60 seconds)

Start/Finish Position: Reach up, grasp a chin-up/pull-up bar (or handles) with your palms facing toward you and spread your hands approximately shoulder-width apart. Bring your body to a "dead hang" and cross your ankles.

Performance Description: Pull your body up so that your upper chest touches the bar and draw your elbows backward. Pause briefly in this mid-range position (your arms bent) and then lower your body under control to the start/finish position (your arms completely straight).

Training Tips:

- Avoid swinging your body forward and backward. Movement should only occur at your shoulder and elbow joints.

- If you can't do 5 repetitions using your bodyweight, you can exercise the same muscles in a similar fashion by performing the underhand lat pulldown (as described in Chapter 9).

- If you can do 10 repetitions or more using your bodyweight, increase the workload by attaching additional weight to your waist, performing the exercise with a slower speed of movement or having a spotter apply manual resistance to your waist.

- After reaching muscular fatigue, you can overload your muscles further by stepping up to the mid-range position and lowering your body under control to the start/finish position for 3 to 5 negative-only repetitions.

- Use wrist straps if you have difficulty in maintaining your grip on the bar.

- This exercise may be contraindicated if you have hyperextended elbows.

81

PULL-UP

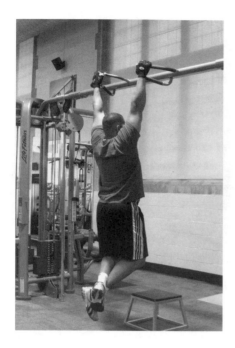

Start/Finish Position

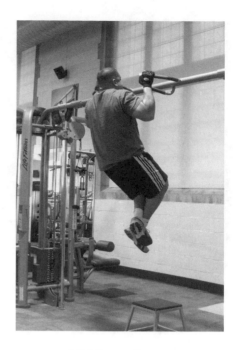

Mid-Range Position

Muscles Strengthened: upper back, biceps and forearms

Suggested Repetitions: 5 to 10 (or 30 to 60 seconds)

Start/Finish Position: Reach up, grasp a chin-up/pull-up bar (or handles) with your palms facing away from you and spread your hands several inches wider than shoulder-width apart. Bring your body to a "dead hang" and cross your ankles.

Performance Description: Pull your body up so that your upper chest touches the bar and draw your elbows backward. Pause briefly in this mid-range position (your arms bent) and then lower your body under control to the start/finish position (your arms straight).

Training Tips:

- Avoid swinging your body forward and backward. Movement should only occur at your shoulder and elbow joints.

- Avoid using an excessively wide grip. This reduces your range of motion.

- If you can't do 5 repetitions using your body-weight, you can exercise the same muscles in a similar fashion by performing the overhand lat pulldown (as described in Chapter 9).

- If you can do 10 repetitions or more using your bodyweight, increase the workload by attaching additional weight to your waist, performing the exercise with a slower speed of movement or having a spotter apply manual resistance to your waist.

- After reaching muscular fatigue, you can overload your muscles further by stepping up to the mid-range position and lowering your body under control to the start/finish position for 3 to 5 negative-only repetitions.

- Performing pull-ups with an overhand grip (your palms facing away from you) isn't as biomechanically efficient as performing chin-ups with an underhand grip (your palms facing toward you). But this exercise is still quite productive with an overhand grip.

- Use wrist straps if you have difficulty in maintaining your grip on the bar.

- You can also perform this exercise with the bar positioned behind your head. However, this may be contraindicated if you have shoulder-impingement syndrome. This exercise may also be contraindicated if you have hyperextended elbows.

PULLOVER

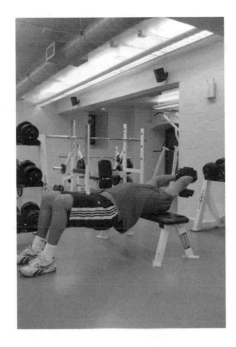

Start/Finish Position

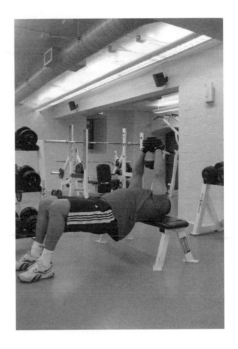

Mid-Range Position

Muscle Strengthened: upper back

Suggested Repetitions: 5 to 10 (or 30 to 60 seconds)

Start/Finish Position: Grasp a dumbbell with both hands. Lie on a utility bench so that your torso is perpendicular to the length of the bench and place your feet flat on the floor. Hold the dumbbell by placing your palms against the innermost plate (not the handle). Position your elbows near or slightly past your head and keep your arms almost completely straight. (A spotter can assist you in positioning a heavy dumbbell.)

Performance Description: Keeping your arms almost completely straight, pull the dumbbell directly over your head. Pause briefly in this mid-range position (the dumbbell directly over your head) and then lower the dumbbell under control to the start/finish position (your elbows near or slightly past your head).

Training Tips:

• You can also perform this exercise with a barbell and an EZ curl bar (spreading your hands about 4 to 6 inches apart).

• This exercise may be contraindicated if you have shoulder-impingement syndrome or low-back pain.

SHOULDER PRESS

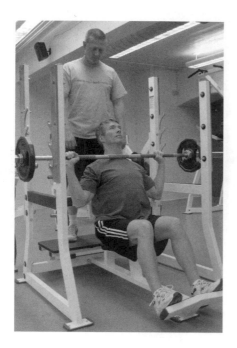

Start/Finish Position

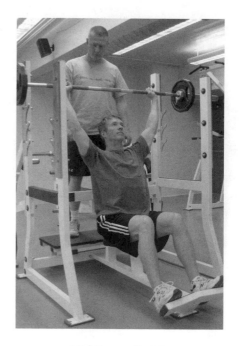

Mid-Range Position

Muscles Strengthened: anterior deltoid and triceps

Suggested Repetitions: 5 to 10 (or 30 to 60 seconds)

Start/Finish Position: Sit down on an Olympic military bench and place your feet flat on the floor (or on the footplate if one is provided). Grasp a barbell and spread your hands slightly wider than shoulder-width apart. Lift the bar out of the "gun rack" or have a spotter give you assistance. Place the bar on the upper part of your chest near your collarbones. (If the bench doesn't have a rack, two spotters can place the bar in the same position.)

Performance Description: Push the bar up until your arms are almost completely straight (without "locking" your elbows). Pause briefly in this mid-range position (your arms almost completely straight) and then lower the bar under control to the start/finish position (your arms bent).

Training Tips:

• This exercise is also referred to as an overhead press, a seated press and a military press.

• Perform this exercise with a spotter.

• Avoid using an excessively wide grip. This reduces your range of motion.

• Keep your hips on the seat pad and your feet flat on the floor.

• Avoid "locking" or "snapping" your elbows in the mid-range position.

• You can also perform this exercise with dumbbells.

• You can also perform this exercise with the bar positioned behind your head. However, this may be contraindicated if you have shoulder-impingement syndrome. This exercise may also be contraindicated if you have low-back pain.

LATERAL RAISE

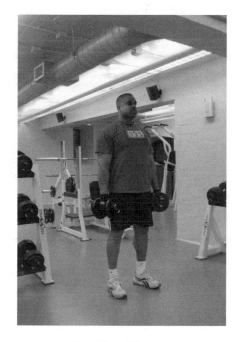

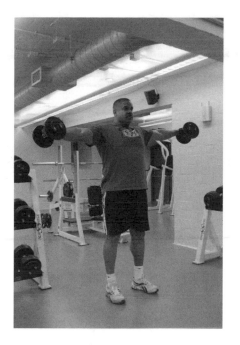

Start/Finish Position

Mid-Range Position

Muscles Strengthened: middle deltoid and trapezius (upper portion)

Suggested Repetitions: 5 to 10 (or 30 to 60 seconds)

Start/Finish Position: Grasp a dumbbell with each hand. Position the dumbbells against the sides of your upper legs with your palms facing each other. Straighten your arms and spread your feet about shoulder-width apart.

Performance Description: Keeping your arms fairly straight, raise the dumbbells sideways until your arms are parallel to the floor. Pause briefly in this mid-range position (your arms parallel to the floor) and then lower the dumbbells under control to the start/finish position (your arms at your sides).

Training Tips:

- Avoid using your legs and moving your torso forward and backward. Movement should only occur at your shoulder joints.

- Raise your arms only to the point at which they're parallel to the floor.

- Your palms should be facing the floor in the mid-range position.

- Do this exercise with one limb at a time if you have a shoulder or an arm injury, a gross difference in the strength between your limbs or desire a training variation.

FRONT RAISE

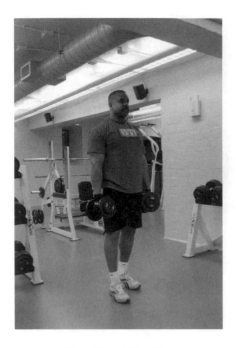

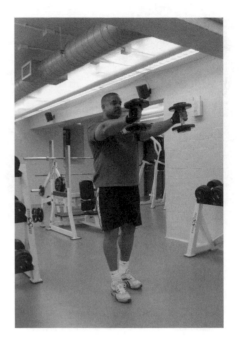

Start/Finish Position   *Mid-Range Position*

Muscle Strengthened: anterior deltoid

Suggested Repetitions: 5 to 10 (or 30 to 60 seconds)

Start/Finish Position: Grasp a dumbbell with each hand. Position the dumbbells against the sides of your upper legs with your palms facing each other. Straighten your arms and spread your feet a comfortable distance apart with one foot slightly in front of the other.

Performance Description: Keeping your arms fairly straight, raise the dumbbells forward until your arms are parallel to the floor. Pause briefly in this mid-range position (your arms parallel to the floor) and then lower the dumbbells under control to the start/finish position (your arms at your sides).

Training Tips:

• Avoid using your legs and moving your torso forward and backward. Movement should only occur at your shoulder joints.

• Raise your arms only to the point at which they're parallel to the floor.

• Your palms should be facing each other in the mid-range position.

• Do this exercise with one limb at a time if you have a shoulder or an arm injury, a gross difference in the strength between your limbs or desire a training variation.

BENT-OVER RAISE

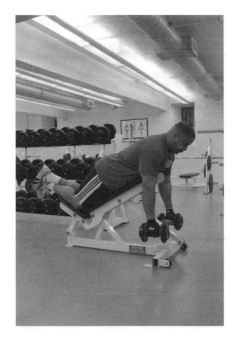

Start/Finish Position

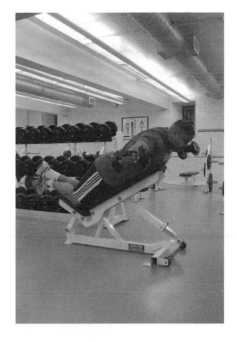

Mid-Range Position

Muscles Strengthened: posterior deltoid, trapezius (middle portion) and rhomboids

Suggested Repetitions: 5 to 10 (or 30 to 60 seconds)

Start/Finish Position: Grasp a dumbbell with each hand. Kneel on the seat pad of an adjustable incline bench. Lie forward against the bench and position the dumbbells directly below your torso. Straighten your arms and point your palms toward each other.

Performance Description: Keeping your arms fairly straight, raise the dumbbells sideways until your arms are parallel to the floor. Pause briefly in this mid-range position (your arms parallel to the floor) and then lower the dumbbells under control to the start/finish position (your hands near the floor).

Training Tips:

- This exercise is also referred to as a posterior raise.

- Raise your arms only to the point at which they're parallel to the floor.

- Your palms should be facing the floor and your upper arms should be perpendicular to your torso in the mid-range position.

INTERNAL ROTATION

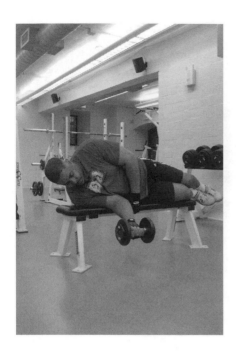

Start/Finish Position

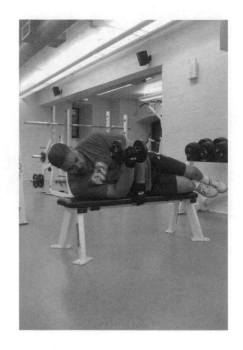

Mid-Range Position

Muscles Strengthened: internal rotators

Suggested Repetitions: 8 to 10 (or 50 to 60 seconds)

Start/Finish Position: Grasp a dumbbell with your right hand. Lie down on a utility bench on your right side and draw your knees toward your torso. Position your right elbow just in front of your torso and bend your right arm so that the angle between your upper and lower arms is about 90 degrees. Point your right palm upward.

Performance Description: Keeping the same angle between your upper and lower arms, pull the dumbbell to your left shoulder. Pause briefly in this mid-range position (your hand near your mid-section) and then lower the dumbbell under control to the start/finish position (your hand away from your mid-section). Repeat the exercise for the other side of your body (with your left side on the bench).

Training Tips:

• Avoid rotating your torso. Movement should only occur at your shoulder joint.

• Refrain from lying directly on your upper arm.

• This exercise can also be done with a resistance band. The band should be secured to an object that won't move such as a machine. While standing, grasp the free handle of the band and pull it horizontally toward your body in the fashion described above.

• Do this exercise on a bench (instead of the floor) to obtain a greater range of motion and permit a better stretch.

EXTERNAL ROTATION

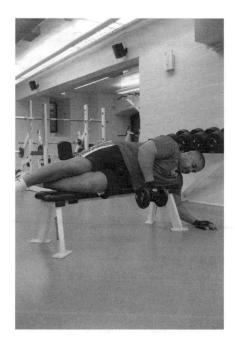

Start/Finish Position

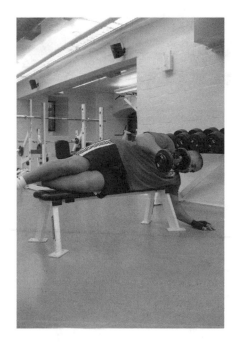

Mid-Range Position

Muscles Strengthened: external rotators

Suggested Repetitions: 8 to 10 (or 50 to 60 seconds)

Start/Finish Position: Grasp a dumbbell with your right hand. Lie down on a utility bench on your left side and draw your knees toward your torso. Position your left arm just in front of your torso and lean back slightly. Keep your right elbow against your side and bend your right arm so that the angle between your upper and lower arms is about 90 degrees. Point your right palm downward.

Performance Description: Keeping the same angle between your upper and lower arms, raise the dumbbell as high as possible. Pause briefly in this mid-range position (your hand away from your mid-section) and then lower the dumbbell under control to the start/finish position (your hand near your mid-section). Repeat the exercise for the other side of your body (with your right side on the bench).

Training Tips:

- Avoid rotating your torso. Movement should only occur at your shoulder joint.

- This exercise can also be done with a resistance band. The band should be secured to an object that won't move such as a machine. While standing, grasp the free handle of the band and pull it horizontally away from your body in the fashion described above.

- Do this exercise on a bench (instead of the floor) to obtain a greater range of motion and permit a better stretch.

UPRIGHT ROW

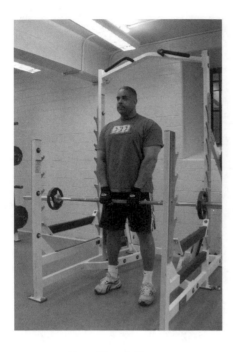

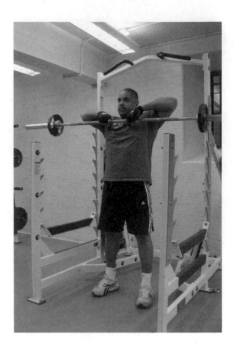

Start/Finish Position

Mid-Range Position

Muscles Strengthened: trapezius (upper portion), biceps and forearms

Suggested Repetitions: 5 to 10 (or 30 to 60 seconds)

Start/Finish Position: Grasp a barbell with your hands spread about 8 to 10 inches apart with your palms facing toward you. Straighten your arms and spread your feet approximately shoulder-width apart.

Performance Description: Pull the bar up until it's just below your chin. (Your elbows should be slightly higher than your hands in this position.) Pause briefly in this mid-range position (your arms bent) and then lower the bar under control to the start/finish position (your arms completely straight).

Training Tips:

- Avoid using your legs and moving your torso forward and backward. Movement should only occur at your shoulder and elbow joints.

- You can also perform this exercise with dumbbells. In this case, grasp the dumbbells with your palms facing toward you and hold them in front of your body about 8 to 10 inches apart.

- Keep the bar close to your body.

- Use wrist straps if you have difficulty in maintaining your grip on the bar.

- This exercise may be contraindicated if you have shoulder-impingement syndrome. However, raising and lowering the bar to the lower part of your chest (near the tip of your breastbone) rather than to the upper part reduces the stress on an impinged shoulder. This exercise may also be contraindicated if you have hyperextended elbows or low-back pain.

SHOULDER SHRUG

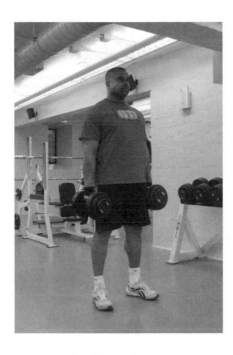

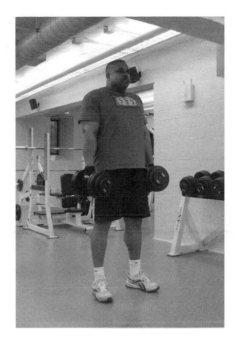

Start/Finish Position   *Mid-Range Position*

Muscle Strengthened: trapezius (upper portion)

Suggested Repetitions: 8 to 10 (or 50 to 60 seconds)

Start/Finish Position: Grasp a dumbbell with each hand. Position the dumbbells against the sides of your upper legs with your palms facing each other. Straighten your arms and spread your feet about shoulder-width apart.

Performance Description: Keeping your arms and legs fairly straight, pull the dumbbells up as high as possible (with the intent of trying to touch your shoulders to your ears as if to say, "I don't know"). Pause briefly in this mid-range position (your shoulders near your ears) and then lower the dumbbells under control to the start/finish position (your shoulders away from your ears).

Training Tips:

- Avoid "rolling" your shoulders in the mid-range position.

- Avoid using your legs and moving your torso forward and backward. Movement should only occur at your shoulder joints.

- You can also perform this exercise with a barbell and trap bar. When doing this exercise with a barbell, grasp the bar with both hands approximately shoulder-width apart with your palms facing toward you; when doing this exercise with a trap bar, use a parallel grip.

- Do this exercise with one limb at a time if you have a shoulder or an arm injury, a gross difference in the strength between your limbs or desire a training variation.

- Use wrist straps if you have difficulty in maintaining your grip on the dumbbells.

- This exercise may be contraindicated if you have hyperextended elbows or low-back pain.

SCAPULAE ADDUCTION

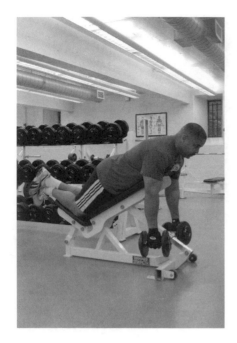

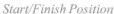

Start/Finish Position

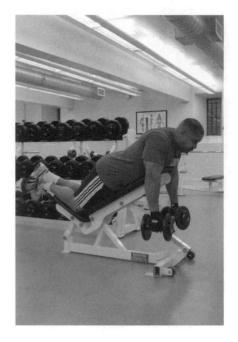

Mid-Range Position

Muscles Strengthened: trapezius (middle portion) and rhomboids

Suggested Repetitions: 8 to 10 (or 50 to 60 seconds)

Start/Finish Position: Grasp a dumbbell with each hand. Kneel on the seat pad of an adjustable incline bench. Lie forward against the bench and position the dumbbells directly below your torso. Straighten your arms with your palms facing each other.

Performance Description: Keeping your arms fairly straight, pull the dumbbells up as high as possible (with the intent of trying to "pinch" your shoulder blades together). Pause briefly in this mid-range position (your shoulder blades together) and then lower the dumbbells under control to the start/finish position (your shoulder blades apart).

Training Tips:

• Do this exercise with one limb at a time if you have a shoulder or an arm injury, a gross difference in the strength between your limbs or desire a training variation.

• Use wrist straps if you have difficulty in maintaining your grip on the dumbbells.

• This exercise may be contraindicated if you have hyperextended elbows.

BICEP CURL

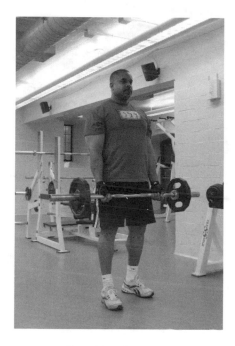

Start/Finish Position

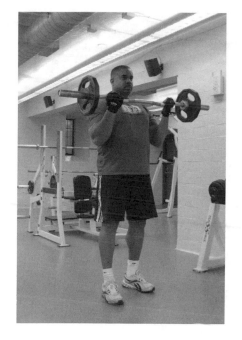

Mid-Range Position

Muscles Strengthened: biceps and forearms

Suggested Repetitions: 5 to 10 (or 30 to 60 seconds)

Start/Finish Position: Grasp an EZ curl barbell with your hands spaced slightly wider than shoulder-width apart and your palms facing away from you. Straighten your arms and spread your feet a comfortable distance apart with one foot slightly in front of the other.

Performance Description: Pull the bar below your chin. Pause briefly in this mid-range position (your arms bent) and then lower the bar under control to the start/finish position (your arms completely straight)

Training Tips:

- Keep your elbows against the sides of your torso.

- Avoid using your legs and moving your torso forward and backward. Movement should only occur at your elbow joints.

- You can also perform this exercise with a barbell and dumbbells. When doing this exercise with dumbbells, use a parallel grip (your palms facing each other) in the start/finish position. As you raise the dumbbells, gradually supinate (turn) your hands so that they're facing toward your shoulders in the mid-range position. Reverse this action when you return the dumbbells to the start/finish position.

- Do this exercise with one limb at a time if you have a shoulder or an arm injury, a gross difference in the strength between your limbs or desire a training variation.

- This exercise may be contraindicated if you have hyperextended elbows.

TRICEP EXTENSION

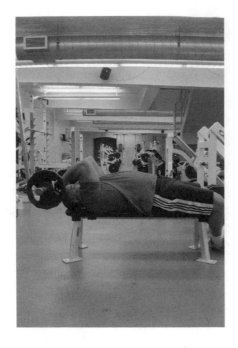

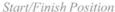

Start/Finish Position

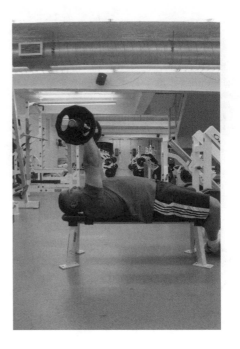

Mid-Range Position

Muscle Strengthened: triceps

Suggested Repetitions: 5 to 10 (or 30 to 60 seconds)

Start/Finish Position: Grasp an EZ curl bar with your hands spread about 4 to 6 inches apart with your palms facing toward you. Lie down on a utility bench and place your feet flat on the floor. Position your upper arms so that they're perpendicular to the floor and point your elbows toward your knees. Lower the bar until it's near your forehead.

Performance Description: Push the bar up until your arms are almost completely straight. Pause briefly in this mid-range position (your arms almost completely straight) and then lower the bar under control to the start/finish position (your arms bent).

Training Tips:

• Keep your upper arms perpendicular to the floor and your elbows pointed toward your knees.

• Keep your hips on the bench.

• If you have low-back pain, place your feet on the end of the bench or a stool. This reduces the stress in your low-back region.

• You can also perform this exercise while sitting or standing. In both cases, keep your upper arms perpendicular to the floor and raise and lower the bar behind your head.

• You can also perform this exercise with a barbell and dumbbells.

• Do this exercise with one limb at a time if you have a shoulder or an arm injury, a gross difference in the strength between your limbs or desire a training variation.

• This exercise may be contraindicated if you have shoulder-impingement syndrome.

WRIST FLEXION

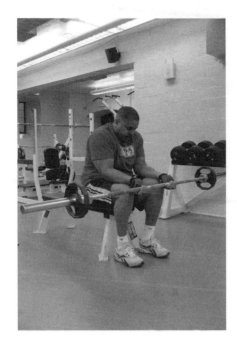

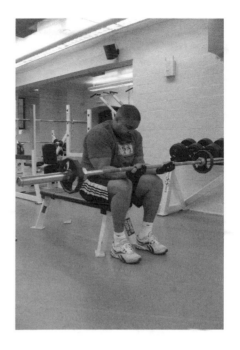

Start/Finish Position   *Mid-Range Position*

Muscles Strengthened: wrist flexors

Suggested Repetitions: 8 to 10 (or 50 to 60 seconds)

Start/Finish Position: Grasp a barbell with your hands spread about 4 to 6 inches apart and your palms facing away from you. Position your thumbs underneath the bar alongside your fingers. Sit down near the end of a utility bench and place the back of your forearms on your upper legs so that your wrists are over your kneecaps. Lean forward slightly so that the angle between your upper and lower arms is about 90 degrees or less.

Performance Description: Pull the bar up as high as possible. Pause briefly in this mid-range position (your wrists bent) and then lower the bar under control to the start/finish position (your wrists extended).

Training Tips:

• Keep your forearms on your upper legs.

• Do this exercise with your thumbs underneath the bar. This increases your range of motion.

• Avoid using your legs and moving your torso forward and backward. Movement should only occur at your wrist joints.

• Do this exercise with one limb at a time if you have an arm injury, a gross difference in the strength between your limbs or desire a training variation.

• You can also perform this exercise with dumbbells.

WRIST EXTENSION

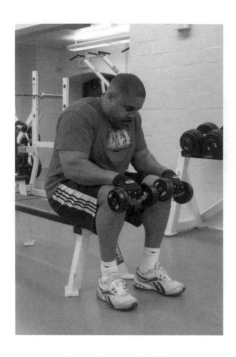

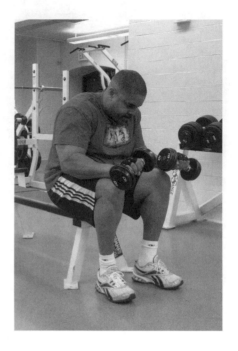

Start/Finish Position   *Mid-Range Position*

Muscles Strengthened: wrist extensors

Suggested Repetitions: 8 to 10 (or 50 to 60 seconds)

Start/Finish Position: Grasp a dumbbell with each hand. Sit down near the end of a utility bench and place the front of your forearms on your upper legs so that your wrists are over your kneecaps and your palms are facing down. Lean forward slightly so that the angle between your upper and lower arms is about 90 degrees or less.

Performance Description: Pull the dumbbells up as high as possible. Pause briefly in this mid-range position (your wrists extended) and then lower the dumbbells under control to the start/finish position (your wrists bent).

Training Tips:

• Keep your forearms on your upper legs.

• Avoid using your legs and moving your torso forward and backward. Movement should only occur at your wrist joints.

• Do this exercise with dumbbells rather than a barbell. This makes it more comfortable on your wrist joints.

• Do this exercise with one limb at a time if you have an arm injury, a gross difference in the strength between your limbs or desire a training variation.

FINGER FLEXION

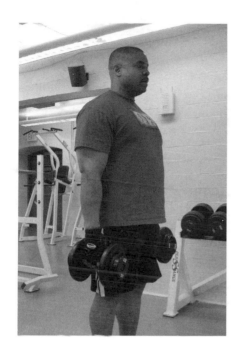

Start/Finish Position

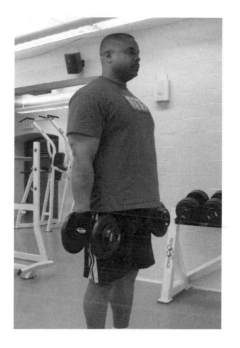

Mid-Range Position

Muscles Strengthened: finger flexors

Suggested Repetitions: 8 to 10 (or 50 to 60 seconds)

Start/Finish Position: Grasp a dumbbell with each hand. Position the dumbbells against the sides of your upper legs with your palms facing each other. Straighten your arms and spread your feet about shoulder-width apart. Allow the dumbbells to roll down your hands to your fingertips.

Performance Description: Keeping your arms fairly straight, pull the dumbbells up to your thumbs. Pause briefly in this mid-range position (your fingers flexed) and then lower the dumbbells under control to the start/finish position (your fingers extended).

Training Tips:

- Avoid using your legs and arms. Movement should only occur at your finger joints.

- Squeeze the dumbbells as hard as possible in the mid-range position.

- Lower the dumbbells all the way down to your fingertips.

- You can also perform this exercise with a barbell (keeping the bar in front of your legs and grasping it with either your palms facing toward you or away from you).

- Do this exercise with one limb at a time if you have an arm injury, a gross difference in the strength between your limbs or desire a training variation.

ABDOMINAL CRUNCH

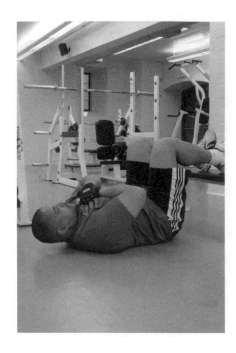

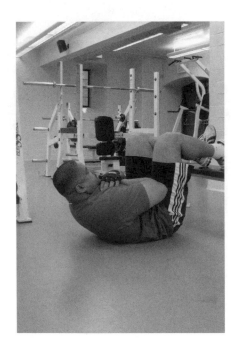

Start/Finish Position   *Mid-Range Position*

Muscle Strengthened: rectus abdominis

Suggested Repetitions: 8 to 10 (or 50 to 60 seconds)

Start/Finish Position: Lie down on the floor and place the back of your lower legs on a utility bench (or stool). Position your upper legs so that they're perpendicular to the floor and the angle between your upper and lower legs is about 90 degrees. Fold your arms across your chest and bring your head toward your chest so that the upper portion of your shoulder blades doesn't touch the floor.

Performance Description: Pull your torso as close to your upper legs as possible. Pause briefly in this mid-range position (your torso bent) and then lower your torso under control to the start/finish position (your torso straight).

Training Tips:

• Avoid touching the floor with your shoulder blades. This removes the load from your abdominals.

• Avoid snapping your head forward. Movement should only occur at your hip joint and mid-section.

• If you can do 10 repetitions or more using your bodyweight, increase the workload by holding additional weight against your chest, performing the exercise with a slower speed of movement or having a spotter apply manual resistance to your shoulders.

• After reaching muscular fatigue, you can overload your muscles further by grasping the backs of your upper legs, pulling your torso to the mid-range position and lowering your torso under control to the start/finish position for 3 to 5 negative-only repetitions.

• This exercise may be contraindicated if you have low-back pain.

KNEE-UP

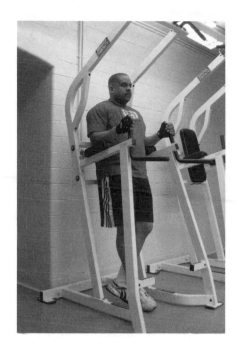

Start/Finish Position

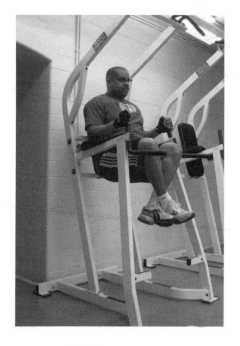

Mid-Range Position

Muscles Strengthened: iliopsoas and rectus abdominis (lower portion)

Suggested Repetitions: 8 to 10 (or 50 to 60 seconds)

Start/Finish Position: Place your lower arms on the forearm pads. Grasp the handles. Straighten your legs and cross your ankles

Performance Description: Pull your knees up as close to your chest as possible. Pause briefly in this mid-range position (your knees near your chest) and then lower your legs under control to the start/finish position (your legs hanging down).

Training Tips:

* Avoid swinging your body forward and backward. Movement should only occur at your hip and knee joints.

* If you can do 10 repetitions or more using your bodyweight, increase the workload by performing the exercise with a slower speed of movement or having a spotter apply manual resistance to your upper legs.

SIDE BEND

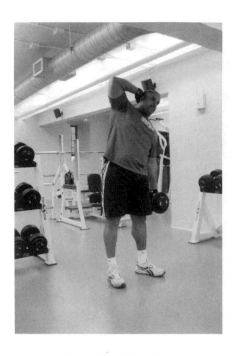

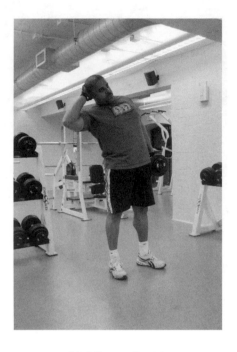

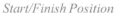

Start/Finish Position   *Mid-Range Position*

Muscles Strengthened: obliques and erector spinae

Suggested Repetitions: 8 to 10 (or 50 to 60 seconds)

Start/Finish Position: Grasp a dumbbell with your left hand. Position the dumbbell against the side of your upper leg with your palm facing your leg. Spread your feet about shoulder-width apart. Place your right palm against the right side of your head. Keep your hips in the same position and bend your torso to the left as far as possible.

Performance Description: Without moving your hips, bring your torso to the right as far as possible. Pause briefly in this mid-range position (your torso bent to the right) and then lower the dumbbell under control to the start/finish position (your torso bent to the left). Repeat the exercise for the other side of your body.

Training Tips:

• Avoid moving your hips. Movement should only occur at your mid-section.

• Refrain from bending forward at the waist.

• Keep your feet flat on the floor.

• Use wrist straps if you have difficulty in maintaining your grip on the dumbbell.

• This exercise may be contraindicated if you have low-back pain.

BACK EXTENSION

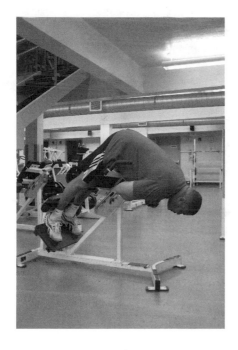

Start/Finish Position

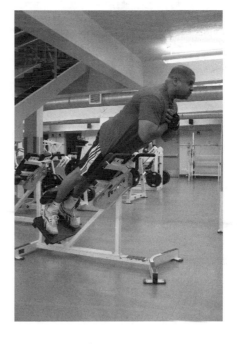

Mid-Range Position

Muscles Strengthened: erector spinae, gluteus maximus and hamstrings

Suggested Repetitions: 10 to 15 (or 60 to 90 seconds)

Start/Finish Position: Place your feet flat on the footboard and the back of your lower legs against the leg pads. Position your pelvis against the hip pads so that your navel is above the edges. Allow your torso to hang down and fold your arms across your chest.

Performance Description: Raise your torso until it's aligned with your upper legs. Pause briefly in this mid-range position (your torso straight) and then lower your torso under control to the start/finish position (your torso bent)

Training Tips:

• Avoid hyperextending your torso (leaning backward excessively) in the mid-range position.

• Avoid snapping your head backward. Movement should only occur at your hip joint and mid-section.

• If you can do 15 repetitions or more using your bodyweight, increase the workload by holding additional weight against your chest, performing the exercise with a slower speed of movement or having a spotter apply manual resistance to your upper back.

• This exercise may be contraindicated if you have low-back pain.

STIFF-LEG DEADLIFT

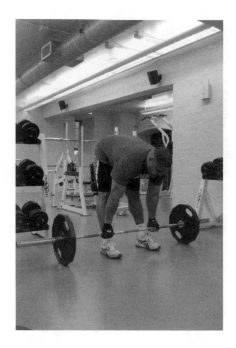

Start/Finish Position

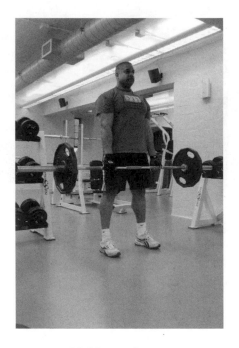

Mid-Range Position

Muscles Strengthened: erector spinae, gluteus maximus and hamstrings

Suggested Repetitions: 10 to 15 (or 60 to 90 seconds)

Start/Finish Position: Spread your feet slightly narrower than shoulder-width apart. Reach down and grasp a bar on the inside of your legs with an alternating grip (your dominant palm facing forward and non-dominant palm facing backward). Straighten your legs but don't "lock" your knees. Place most of your bodyweight on your heels. Straighten your arms.

Performance Description: Stand upright by straightening your torso. Pause briefly in this mid-range position (your torso straight) and then lower the bar under control to the start/finish position (your torso bent).

Training Tips:

• Keep your arms and legs straight as you perform this exercise. Unlike the deadlift, your lower back should do most of the work.

• Exert force through your heels, not the balls of your feet.

• Avoid "locking" or "snapping" your knees in the mid-range position. Also, avoid hyperextending your torso (leaning backward excessively) in the mid-range position.

• Refrain from bouncing the weight off the floor between repetitions.

• You can also perform this exercise with dumbbells.

• Use wrist straps if you have difficulty in maintaining your grip on the bar.

• This exercise may be contraindicated if you have low-back pain, hyperextended elbows or an exceptionally long torso and/or legs.

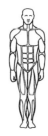

9 Machine Exercises

The two most popular types of machines are selectorized and plate-loaded. With a selectorized machine, adjustments in resistance are made by inserting a selector pin or key into a stack of flat weight plates that travel up and down metal guide rods; with a plate-loaded machine, adjustments in resistance are made by adding or removing Olympic plates from "horns" that are attached to the movement arms.

There's some debate as to who introduced machines to the fitness community on a wide scale. Legend has it that the first Nautilus® machine – a prototype plate-loaded pullover – was built by Arthur Jones in 1948 on a front porch in Tulsa, Oklahoma. But it wasn't until late 1970 – after 27 different versions of the pullover machine were built and tested – that Nautilus® actually sold and delivered a machine to a customer. (It was – you guessed it – a plate-loaded pullover.)

In 1957, the Universal Gym Company developed the first multi-station selectorized machine. Invented by Harold Zinkin, this revolutionary machine featured a number of different exercises (or stations) with separate stacks of weight plates that could accommodate multiple users at one time. The machine proved to be immensely popular for several decades, especially in high schools and YMCAs.

In the early 1980s, Nautilus® began to manufacture and sell a complete "line" of plate-loaded machines which at the time had chrome-plated frames and were referred to as leverage machines. These Nautilus® machines were actually the forerunners of the Hammer Strength® machines that were introduced in 1988 and produced in the same manufacturing plant in Mexia, Texas. (Also of historical note is that Nautilus® acquired Universal Gym in 2006 but soon thereafter discontinued the brand.)

So compared to the venerable barbell, selectorized and plate-loaded machines have a relatively short history. But since machines of high quality were first unveiled, their use and popularity have grown considerably. Besides Nautilus® and Hammer Strength®, there are currently several other major manufacturers of selectorized and plate-loaded machines including Cybex®, Life Fitness® and MedX®.

ADVANTAGES OF MACHINES

In comparison to free weights, machines offer the following advantages:

1. Machines allow you to perform some exercises that can't be done with free weights.

This includes hip abduction, hip adduction, leg curl, leg extension and lat pulldown as well as those for the neck. These machine exercises and others have a valuable role in a comprehensive strength program.

2. Most machines provide variable resistance.

The idea of variable resistance was actually proposed by Max Herz of Hungary in 1898. As an exercise is performed, the biomechanical leverage of your skeletal system changes which makes the movement feel easier in some positions and harder in others. (Plotting these changes on a graph reveals what's known as a strength curve.)

A properly designed machine automatically varies the resistance to match the changes in your biomechanical leverage. In positions of inferior leverage (and inferior strength), the machine creates a mechanical advantage and a lower level of resistance; as your skeletal system moves into a position of superior leverage (and superior strength), the machine creates a mechanical disadvantage and a higher level of resistance. The end result is greater muscular effort throughout the range of motion (ROM).

During a typical free-weight exercise, there's adequate resistance for your muscles in their weakest positions but not enough in their strongest positions. Because of this, the amount of resistance that you can use is limited to that which you can handle in your position of least leverage. There, however, a few free-weight exercises that provide somewhat adequate resistance throughout most of the ROM including wrist flexion/extension, shoulder shrug and calf raise.

3. Most machines don't require you to balance the weight.

Not having to balance the weight means that it will be easier for you to concentrate on the proper performance of the exercise. Some individuals – particularly those who have very little experience in strength training – might worry more about balancing the weight effectively than about performing the exercise properly. Furthermore, you're likely to spend excessive energy in balancing the weight. Because synergistic muscles aren't involved when the weight is balanced, machines can also work the targeted muscles to a greater degree.

4. Workouts are usually more time-efficient when machines are employed.

Some individuals don't have an abundance of free time to spend in the fitness center. The resistance on selectorized machines can be set by moving a pin to select a weight rather than by fiddling around changing plates. Of course, plates must be changed when using plate-loaded machines.

5. In general, machines can provide direct resistance over a greater ROM compared to a similar free-weight exercise.

For example, a machine pullover can offer direct resistance over as much as 270 degrees ROM around your shoulder joint. In contrast, a barbell or dumbbell pullover can offer direct

resistance over about 100 degrees ROM around your shoulder joint. Therefore, a pullover done with a machine is much more efficient than a pullover done with free weights because the targeted muscles are loaded over a greater ROM. This holds true for just about all machine exercises compared to their free-weight counterparts.

6. Machines are more practical than free weights during rehabilitative training.

Suppose that you injured your left knee. Many exercises with free weights would be quite difficult or uncomfortable – if not impossible – to perform. However, you could still train your entire torso, your right leg and possibly even both hips if you have access to machines. Actually, you could exercise on most machines with very little discomfort even if your arm or leg was immobilized in a cast. For instance, if your wrist was casted such that you were unable to grasp a barbell or dumbbell, you could still perform many upper-body exercises with machines including the pec fly, pullover and lateral raise.

7. Machines allow you to train alone in a relatively safe manner.

Any barbell exercise that involves lifting a weight overhead – such as a bench press, incline press or shoulder press – should only be done under the watchful eye of a competent spotter. Doing so reduces the potential for an unexpected mishap such as getting trapped under a weighted bar. With machines, you can't get pinned by a weight in a precarious position. It should be noted that with dumbbells, you can't "get stuck" either since you can simply lower the weights to the floor.

THE EXERCISES

This chapter describes and illustrates the safest and most productive exercises that can be performed with machines. (Generic descriptions are given in this chapter that can be applied to equipment from different manufacturers.) Included in the discussions of each exercise are the muscle(s) involved (if two or more muscles are involved, the first one listed is the prime mover), suggested repetitions (the time that the targeted muscles should be loaded is shown in parentheses), start/finish position, performance description and training tips for making the exercise safer and more productive.

These 36 exercises are described in this chapter: leg press, hip extension, hip flexion, hip abduction, hip adduction, prone leg curl, seated leg curl, leg extension, seated calf raise, calf extension, dorsi flexion, chest press, seated dip, pec fly, seated row, underhand lat pulldown, overhand lat pulldown, pullover, shoulder press, lateral raise, rear deltoid, internal rotation, external rotation, upright row, scapulae adduction, bicep curl, tricep extension, wrist flexion, wrist extension, abdominal crunch, side bend, torso rotation, back extension, neck flexion, neck extension and neck lateral flexion.

LEG PRESS

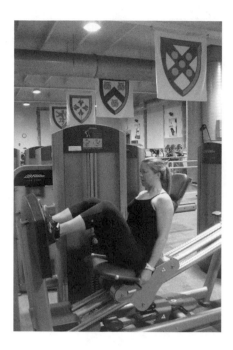

Start/Finish Position

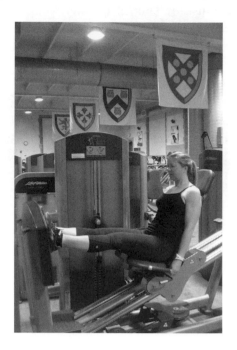

Mid-Range Position

Muscles Strengthened: gluteus maximus, hamstrings and quadriceps

Suggested Repetitions: 15 to 20 (or 90 to 120 seconds)

Start/Finish Position: Adjust the seat carriage so that the angle between your upper and lower legs will be about 90 degrees. Sit down and place your feet on the footplate so that they're slightly wider than shoulder-width apart. Position your lower legs so that they're parallel to the floor. Grasp the handles that are located on the sides of the seat pad.

Performance Description: Push the footplate forward until your legs are almost completely straight (without "locking" your knees). Pause briefly in this mid-range position (your legs almost completely straight) and then lower the weight under control to the start/finish position (your legs bent).

Training Tips:

- The angle of the back pad can be adjusted on some machines. As the back pad is positioned less upright, there's more emphasis on the gluteus maximus (your buttocks). Also note that when the back pad is less upright, the seat must be moved closer to the footplate to maintain the same range of motion as when the back pad is more upright.

- Exert force through your heels, not the balls of your feet.

- Avoid "locking" or "snapping" your knees in the mid-range position.

- You can also perform this exercise with a plate-loaded machine.

- Do this exercise with one limb at a time if you have a hip, leg, knee or ankle injury, a gross difference in the strength between your limbs or desire a training variation.

HIP EXTENSION

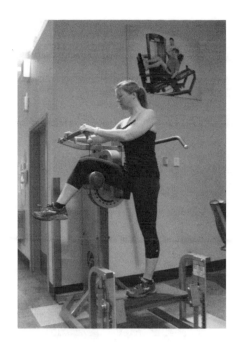

Start/Finish Position

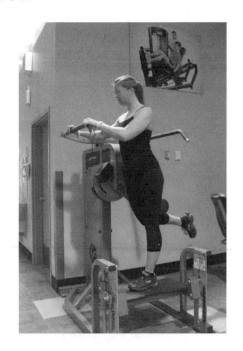

Mid-Range Position

Muscles Strengthened: gluteus maximus and hamstrings

Suggested Repetitions: 15 to 20 (or 90 to 120 seconds)

Start/Finish Position: Adjust the platform so that your hip will be aligned with the axis of rotation. Adjust the movement arm to accommodate your level of flexibility. Place your right upper leg on top of the roller pad. Keep your torso erect and straighten your left leg. Grasp the bar with both hands.

Performance Description: Drive your leg backward while gradually straightening it. Pause briefly in this mid-range position (your leg completely straight) and then lower the weight under control to the start/finish position (your leg bent). Repeat the exercise for the other side of your body.

Training Tips:

• Avoid moving your torso forward and backward. Movement should only occur at your hip and knee joints.

• Attempt to raise the weight as high as possible in the mid-range position to ensure that you're obtaining a maximum contraction of the target muscles.

107

HIP FLEXION

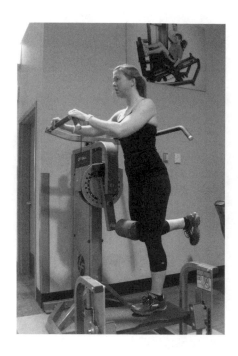

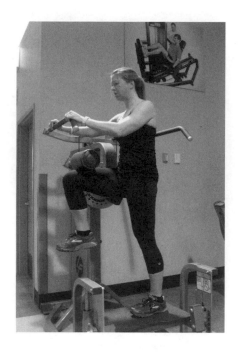

Start/Finish Position   *Mid-Range Position*

Muscle Strengthened: iliopsoas

Suggested Repetitions: 15 to 20 (or 90 to 120 seconds)

Start/Finish Position: Adjust the platform so that your hip will be aligned with the axis of rotation. Adjust the movement arm to accommodate your level of flexibility. Place your right upper leg behind the roller pad. Keep your torso erect and straighten your left leg. Grasp the bar with both hands.

Performance Description: Bring your knee toward your chest while gradually bending your leg. Pause briefly in this mid-range position (your knee near your chest) and then lower the weight under control to the start/finish position (your leg hanging down). Repeat the exercise for the other side of your body.

Training Tips:

• Avoid moving your torso forward and backward. Movement should only occur at your hip and knee joints.

• Attempt to raise the weight as high as possible in the mid-range position to ensure that you're obtaining a maximum contraction of the target muscles.

HIP ABDUCTION

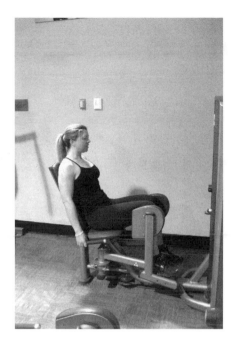

Start/Finish Position

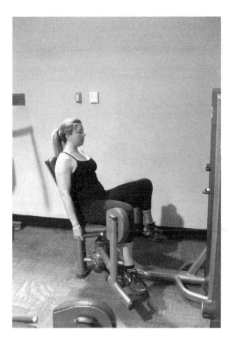

Mid-Range Position

Muscles Strengthened: gluteus medius and gluteus minimus

Suggested Repetitions: 10 to 15 (or 60 to 90 seconds)

Start/Finish Position: Sit down, place your legs on the thigh pads and position your feet on the foot pegs. Grasp the handles that are located on the sides of the seat pad.

Performance Description: Spread your legs apart as far as possible. Pause briefly in this mid-range position (your legs apart) and then lower the weight under control to the start/finish position (your legs together).

Training Tips:

* The angle of the back pad can be adjusted on some machines. In this case, adjust the back pad so that it's as upright as possible.

* Attempt to raise the weight as high as possible in the mid-range position to ensure that you're obtaining a maximum contraction of the target muscles.

* You can also perform this exercise with a plate-loaded machine.

HIP ADDUCTION

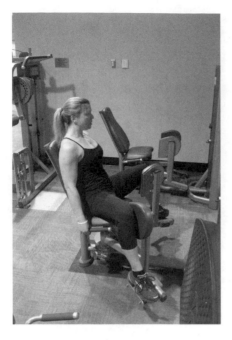

Start/Finish Position

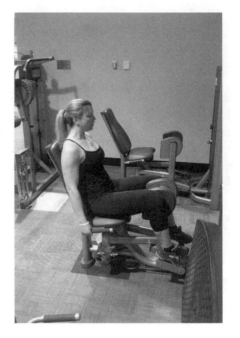

Mid-Range Position

Muscles Strengthened: hip adductors

Suggested Repetitions: 10 to 15 (or 60 to 90 seconds)

Start/Finish Position: Adjust the movement arms to accommodate your level of flexibility. Sit down, place your legs on the thigh pads and position your feet on the foot pegs. Grasp the handles that are located on the sides of the seat pad.

Performance Description: Bring your legs as close together as possible. Pause briefly in this mid-range position (your legs together) and then lower the weight under control to the start/finish position (your legs apart).

Training Tips:

• The angle of the back pad can be adjusted on some machines. In this case, adjust the back pad so that it's as upright as possible.

• Attempt to raise the weight as high as possible in the mid-range position to ensure that you're obtaining a maximum contraction of the target muscles.

• You can also perform this exercise with a plate-loaded machine.

PRONE LEG CURL

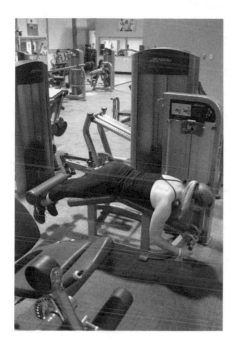 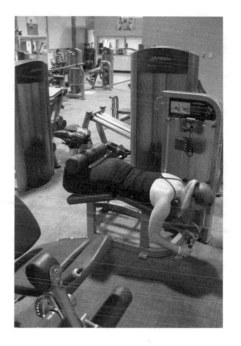

Start/Finish Position   *Mid-Range Position*

Muscles Strengthened: hamstrings

Suggested Repetitions: 10 to 15 (or 60 to 90 seconds)

Start/Finish Position: Adjust the roller pad so that it will be just above your heels. Adjust the movement arm to accommodate your level of flexibility. Lie face down and place your lower legs underneath the roller pad. Position the tops of your kneecaps just over the edge of the thigh pad. (By doing this, your knees will be aligned with the axis of rotation.) Grasp the handles that are located in front of the chest pad.

Performance Description: Pull your heels as close to your hips as possible. Pause briefly in this mid-range position (your heels near your hips) and then lower the weight under control to the start/finish position (your legs completely straight).

Training Tips:

- Avoid raising your torso. Movement should only occur at your knee joints.

- The angle between your upper and lower legs should be about 90 degrees or less in the mid-range position.

- Attempt to raise the weight as high as possible in the mid-range position to ensure that you're obtaining a maximum contraction of the target muscles.

- You can also perform this exercise with a plate-loaded machine.

- Do this exercise with one limb at a time if you have a leg, knee or ankle injury, a gross difference in the strength between your limbs or desire a training variation.

- This exercise may be contraindicated if you have hyperextended knees or low-back pain.

111

SEATED LEG CURL

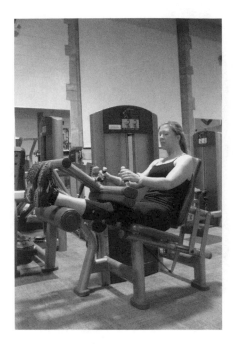

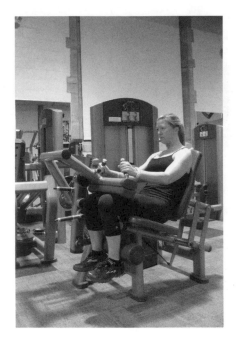

Start/Finish Position   *Mid-Range Position*

Muscles Strengthened: hamstrings

Suggested Repetitions: 10 to 15 (or 60 to 90 seconds)

Start/Finish Position: Adjust the back pad so that your knees will be aligned with the axis of rotation. Adjust the roller pad so that that it will be just above your heels. Adjust the movement arm to accommodate your level of flexibility. Sit down and place your lower legs on top of the roller pad. Lower the thigh pad so that it presses against your upper legs. Grasp the handles that are located above the thigh pad (or on the sides of the seat pad).

Performance Description: Pull your heels as close to your hips as possible. Pause briefly in this mid-range position (your heels near your hips) and then lower the weight under control to the start/finish position (your legs completely straight). Raise the thigh pad when you finish performing the exercise.

Training Tips:

• Performing this exercise in the seated position produces less stress in the low-back region than performing it in the prone position.

• Avoid moving your torso forward and backward. Movement should only occur at your knee joints.

• The angle between your upper and lower legs should be about 90 degrees or less in the mid-range position.

• Attempt to raise the weight as high as possible in the mid-range position to ensure that you're obtaining a maximum contraction of the target muscles.

• You can also perform this exercise with a plate-loaded machine.

• Do this exercise with one limb at a time if you have a leg, knee or ankle injury, a gross difference in the strength between your limbs or desire a training variation.

• This exercise may be contraindicated if you have hyperextended knees.

LEG EXTENSION

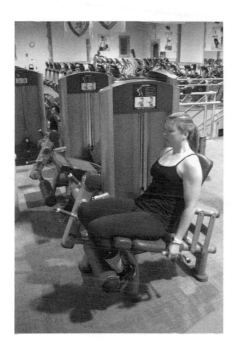

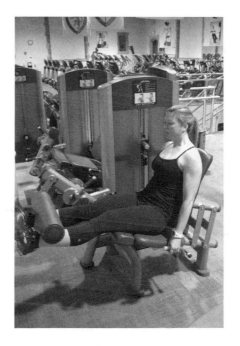

Start/Finish Position

Mid-Range Position

Muscles Strengthened: quadriceps

Suggested Repetitions: 10 to 15 (or 60 to 90 seconds)

Start/Finish Position: Adjust the back pad so that your knees will be aligned with the axis of rotation. Adjust the roller pad so that it will be just above your instep. Adjust the movement arm to accommodate your level of flexibility. Sit down and place your lower legs behind the roller pad. Fasten the waist belt (if one is provided). Grasp the handles that are located on the sides of the seat pad.

Performance Description: Straighten your legs as completely as possible. Pause briefly in this mid-range position (your legs completely straight) and then lower the weight under control to the start/finish position (your legs bent).

Training Tips:

- Avoid moving your torso forward and backward. Movement should only occur at your knee joints.

- Attempt to raise the weight as high as possible in the mid-range position to ensure that you're obtaining a maximum contraction of the target muscles.

- You can also perform this exercise with a plate-loaded machine.

- Do this exercise with one limb at a time if you have a leg, knee or ankle injury, a gross difference in the strength between your limbs or desire a training variation.

113

SEATED CALF RAISE

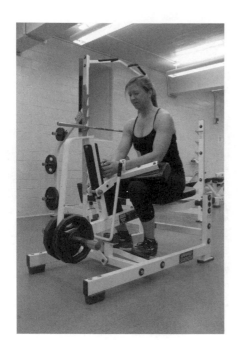

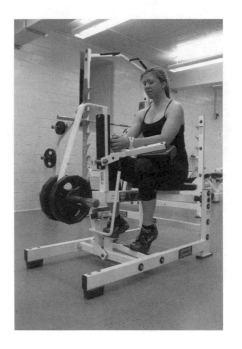

Start/Finish Position   *Mid-Range Position*

Muscle Strengthened: soleus

Suggested Repetitions: 10 to 15 (or 60 to 90 seconds)

Start/Finish Position: Sit down, place the balls of your feet on the edge of the footplate and lower your heels. Lower the thigh pads so that they press against your upper legs. Rise up onto your toes slightly and push the lever arm to the left. (This frees the movement arm so that you have a full range of motion.) Grasp the handle (or hold onto the sides of the seat pad) and lower your heels.

Performance Description: Rise up onto your toes as high as possible. Pause briefly in this mid-range position (your ankles straight) and then lower the weight under control to the start/finish position (your heels near the floor). Rise up onto your toes slightly and push the lever arm to the right when you finish performing the exercise. (This holds the movement arm in place so that you can exit the machine.)

Training Tips:

- Avoid using your arms and moving your torso forward and backward. Movement should only occur at your ankle joints.

- Attempt to raise the weight as high as possible in the mid-range position to ensure that you're obtaining a maximum contraction of the target muscles.

- Do this exercise with one limb at a time if you have a leg, knee or ankle injury, a gross difference in the strength between your limbs or desire a training variation.

- Avoid this exercise if you have shin splints.

CALF EXTENSION

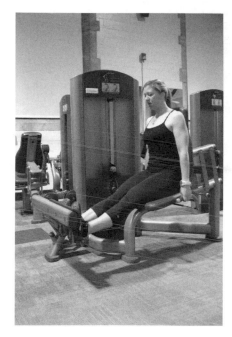

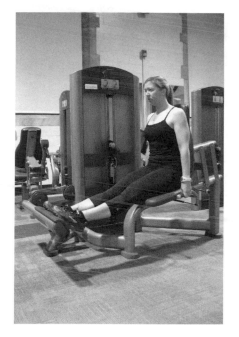

Start/Finish Position   *Mid-Range Position*

Muscle Strengthened: gastrocnemius

Suggested Repetitions: 10 to 15 (or 60 to 90 seconds)

Start/Finish Position: Adjust the back pad to accommodate the length of your legs. Sit down, place the balls of your feet on the edge of the footplate and lower your heels. Straighten your legs but don't "lock" your knees. Grasp the handles that are located on the sides of the seat pad.

Performance Description: Extend your ankles as far as possible. Pause briefly in this mid-range position (your ankles straight) and then lower the weight under control to the start/finish position (your ankles bent).

Training Tips:

• Avoid using your hips and legs. Movement should only occur at your ankle joints.

• Attempt to raise the weight as high as possible in the mid-range position to ensure that you're obtaining a maximum contraction of the target muscles.

• Do this exercise with one limb at a time if you have a leg, knee or ankle injury, a gross difference in the strength between your limbs or desire a training variation.

• Avoid this exercise if you have shin splints.

115

DORSI FLEXION

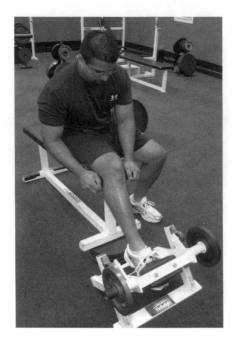

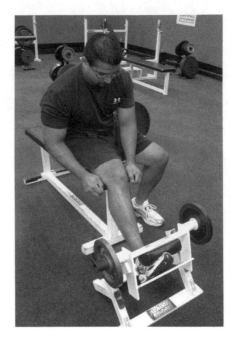

Start/Finish Position   *Mid-Range Position*

Muscles Strengthened: dorsi flexors

Suggested Repetitions: 10 to 15 (or 60 to 90 seconds)

Start/Finish Position: Sit down near the end of a utility bench (or a stool). Place the back of your right knee against the end of the pad. Position your right foot on the footplate so that the ankle pad is against your instep. Grasp the sides of the bench.

Performance Description: Keeping your leg flat on the bench, pull your right foot up as high as possible. Pause briefly in this mid-range position (your ankle bent) and then lower the weight under control to the start/finish position (your ankle straight). Repeat the exercise for the other side of your body.

Training Tips:

• Avoid moving your torso forward and backward. Movement should only occur at your ankle joint.

• Attempt to raise the weight as high as possible in the mid-range position to ensure that you're obtaining a maximum contraction of the target muscles.

• This exercise may be contraindicated if you have shin splints.

CHEST PRESS

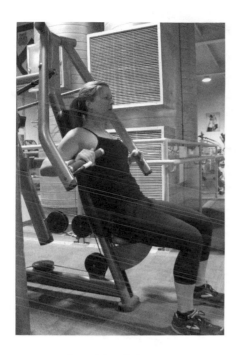

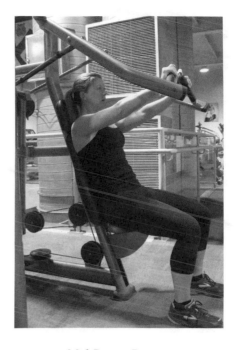

Start/Finish Position

Mid-Range Position

Muscles Strengthened: chest, anterior deltoid and triceps

Suggested Repetitions: 5 to 10 (or 30 to 60 seconds)

Start/Finish Position: Adjust the seat pad so that your hands will be just below your shoulders in the start/finish position. Adjust the movement arms to accommodate your level of flexibility. Sit down and place your feet flat on the floor. Grasp the handles with a narrow grip.

Performance Description: Push the handles forward until your arms are almost completely straight (without "locking" your elbows). Pause briefly in this mid-range position (your arms almost completely straight) and then lower the weight under control to the start/finish position (your hands near your shoulders).

Training Tips:

• The back pad can be adjusted on some machines. Moving it forward increases the range of motion and allows a greater stretch.

• Multiple grips are available on some machines. A parallel grip reduces the stress in your shoulder joints.

• Keep your hips on the seat pad and your torso against the back pad. Movement should only occur at your shoulder and elbow joints.

• Avoid "locking" or "snapping" your elbows in the mid-range position.

• You can also perform this exercise with a plate-loaded machine.

• Do this exercise with one limb at a time if you have a shoulder or an arm injury, a gross difference in the strength between your limbs or desire a training variation.

• This exercise may be contraindicated if you have shoulder-impingement syndrome.

SEATED DIP

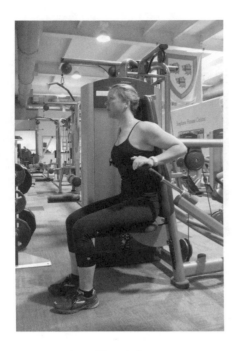

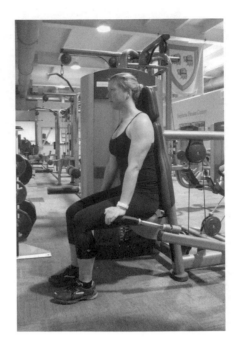

Start/Finish Position

Mid-Range Position

Muscles Strengthened: chest, anterior deltoid and triceps

Suggested Repetitions: 5 to 10 (or 30 to 60 seconds)

Start/Finish Position: Adjust the seat pad so that your hands will be just below your shoulders in the start/finish position. Adjust the movement arms to accommodate the width of your shoulders. Sit down and place your feet flat on the floor. Grasp the handles.

Performance Description: Push the handles down until your arms are almost completely straight (without "locking" your elbows). Pause briefly in this mid-range position (your arms almost completely straight) and then lower the weight under control to the start/finish position (your arms bent).

Training Tips:

- Keep your hips on the seat pad and your torso against the back pad. Movement should only occur at your shoulder and elbow joints.

- Avoid "locking" or "snapping" your elbows in the mid-range position.

- You can also perform this exercise with a plate-loaded machine.

- Do this exercise with one limb at a time if you have a shoulder or an arm injury, a gross difference in the strength between your limbs or desire a training variation.

- This exercise may be contraindicated if you have shoulder-impingement syndrome.

PEC FLY

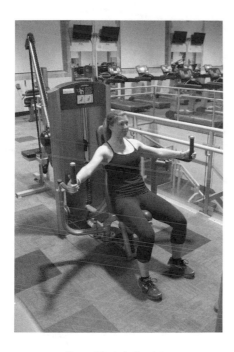

Start/Finish Position

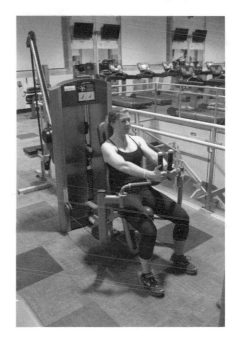

Mid-Range Position

Muscles Strengthened: chest and anterior deltoid

Suggested Repetitions: 5 to 10 (or 30 to 60 seconds)

Start/Finish Position: Adjust the seat pad so that your elbows will be slightly lower than your shoulders in the start/finish position. Adjust the movement arms to accommodate your level of flexibility. Sit down and place your feet flat on the floor. Grasp the handles with a parallel grip (your palms facing each other).

Performance Description: Keeping your arms fairly straight, bring the handles as close together as possible. Pause briefly in this mid-range position (your hands together) and then lower the weight under control to the start/finish position (your hands apart).

Training Tips:

- This exercise is also referred to as a chest fly.

- Keep your hips on the seat pad and your torso against the back pad. Movement should only occur at your shoulder joints.

- You can also perform this exercise with a plate-loaded machine.

- Do this exercise with one limb at a time if you have a shoulder or an arm injury, a gross difference in the strength between your limbs or desire a training variation.

- This exercise may be contraindicated if you have shoulder-impingement syndrome.

SEATED ROW

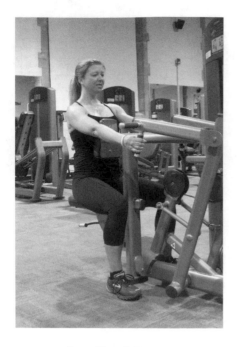

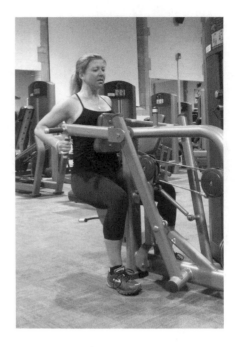

Start/Finish Position   *Mid-Range Position*

Muscles Strengthened: upper back, biceps and forearms

Suggested Repetitions: 5 to 10 (or 30 to 60 seconds)

Start/Finish Position: Adjust the chest pad so that your arms will be completely straight in the start/finish position. Adjust the seat pad so that your hands will be just below your shoulders in the mid-range position. Sit down, lean forward against the chest pad and place your feet flat on the floor (or on the footplate if one is provided). Grasp the handles with a parallel grip (your palms facing each other).

Performance Description: Pull the handles just below your shoulders. Pause briefly in this mid-range position (your arms bent) and then lower the weight under control to the start/finish position (your arms completely straight).

Training Tips:

- You can also perform this exercise with your upper arms positioned away from your torso using an overhand grip. Doing this involves less of your upper back and more of your posterior deltoid, trapezius and rhomboids. In this case, your upper arm would be perpendicular to your torso and your palms would be facing down in the mid-range position.

- Avoid moving your torso forward and backward. Movement should only occur at your shoulder and elbow joints.

- Attempt to raise the weight as high as possible in the mid-range position to ensure that you're obtaining a maximum contraction of the target muscles.

- You can also perform this exercise with a plate-loaded machine.

- Do this exercise with one limb at a time if you have a shoulder or an arm injury, a gross difference in the strength between your limbs or desire a training variation.

- Use wrist straps if you have difficulty in maintaining your grip on the handles.

- This exercise may be contraindicated if you have hyperextended elbows.

UNDERHAND LAT PULLDOWN

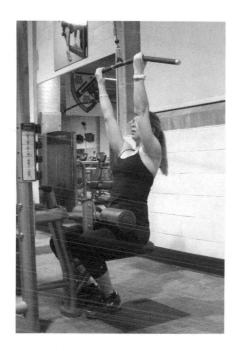

Start/Finish Position

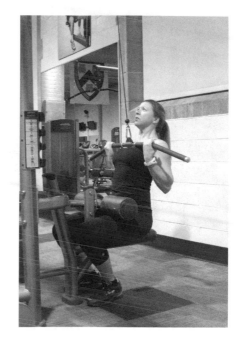

Mid-Range Position

Muscles Strengthened: upper back, biceps and forearms

Suggested Repetitions: 5 to 10 (or 30 to 60 seconds)

Start/Finish Position: Reach up, grasp a bar with your palms facing toward you and spread your hands approximately shoulder-width apart. Sit down, position your upper legs under the roller pads and place your feet flat on the floor. Lean back slightly.

Performance Description: Pull the bar down to your upper chest and draw your elbows backward. Pause briefly in this mid-range position (your arms bent) and then lower the weight under control to the start/finish position (your arms completely straight).

Training Tips:

• Avoid moving your torso forward and backward. Movement should only occur at your shoulder and elbow joints.

• Attempt to raise the weight as high as possible in the mid-range position to ensure that you're obtaining a maximum contraction of the target muscles.

• You can also perform this exercise with a plate-loaded machine.

• Do this exercise with one limb at a time (with a handle instead of a bar) if you have a shoulder or an arm injury, a gross difference in the strength between your limbs or desire a training variation.

• Use wrist straps if you have difficulty in maintaining your grip on the bar.

• This exercise may be contraindicated if you have hyperextended elbows.

OVERHAND LAT PULLDOWN

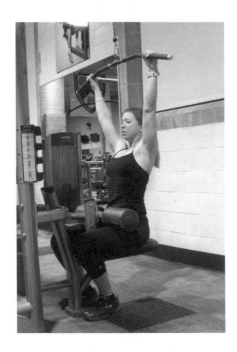

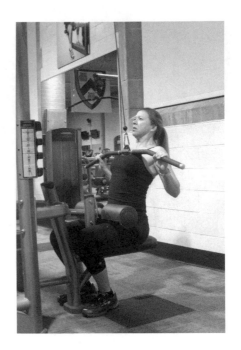

Start/Finish Position   *Mid-Range Position*

Muscles Strengthened: upper back, biceps and forearms

Suggested Repetitions: 5 to 10 (or 30 to 60 seconds)

Start/Finish Position: Reach up, grasp a bar with your palms facing away from you and space your hands several inches wider than shoulder-width apart. Sit down, position your upper legs under the roller pads and place your feet flat on the floor. Lean back slightly.

Performance Description: Pull the bar down to your upper chest and draw your elbows backward. Pause briefly in this mid-range position (your arms bent) and then lower the weight under control to the start/finish position (your arms completely straight).

Training Tips:

- Avoid moving your torso forward and backward. Movement should only occur at your shoulder and elbow joints.

- Avoid using an excessively wide grip. This reduces your range of motion.

- Attempt to raise the weight as high as possible in the mid-range position to ensure that you're obtaining a maximum contraction of the target muscles.

- You can also perform this exercise with a plate-loaded machine.

- Do this exercise with one limb at a time (with a handle instead of a bar) if you have a shoulder or an arm injury, a gross difference in the strength between your limbs or desire a training variation.

- Performing a lat pulldown with an overhand grip (your palms facing away from you) isn't as biomechanically efficient as performing a lat pulldown with an underhand grip (your palms facing toward you). But this exercise is still quite productive when done with an overhand grip.

- Use wrist straps if you have difficulty in maintaining your grip on the bar.

- You can also perform this exercise with the bar positioned behind your head. However, this may be contraindicated if you have shoulder-impingement syndrome. This exercise may also be contraindicated if you have hyperextended elbows.

PULLOVER

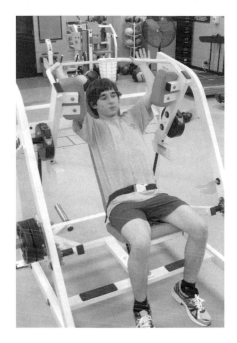

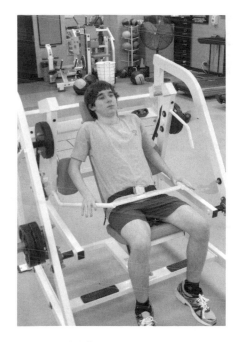

Start/Finish Position   *Mid-Range Position*

Muscle Strengthened: upper back

Suggested Repetitions: 5 to 10 (or 30 to 60 seconds)

Start/Finish Position: Adjust the seat pad so that the side part of your shoulders will be aligned with the axis of rotation in the start/finish position. Sit down and place your feet flat on the floor. Fasten the waist belt (if one is provided). Position the back of your upper arms on the elbow pads. Place your palms on the bar and open your hands (extend your fingers).

Performance Description: Pull the bar down to your mid-section. Pause briefly in this mid-range position (the bar against your mid-section) and then lower the weight under control to the start/finish position (your elbows near or slightly past your head).

Training Tips:

- Avoid moving your torso forward and backward. Movement should only occur at your shoulder joints.

- Exert force against the elbow pads with your upper arms, not your hands. This isolates your upper back.

- If you're unable to keep your upper arms against the elbow pads, you can grasp the bar with an underhand grip and pull with your hands instead of your upper arms. This doesn't allow you to isolate your upper back but it will make the exercise more comfortable for you to perform.

- Attempt to raise the weight as high as possible in the mid-range position to ensure that you're obtaining a maximum contraction of the target muscles.

- You can also perform this exercise with a selectorized machine.

- Do this exercise with one limb at a time if you have a shoulder or an arm injury, a gross difference in the strength between your limbs or desire a training variation.

- This exercise may be contraindicated if you have shoulder-impingement syndrome.

SHOULDER PRESS

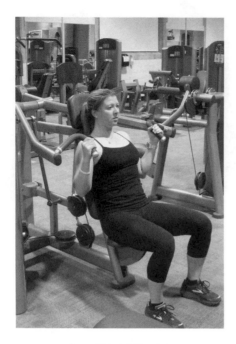

Start/Finish Position

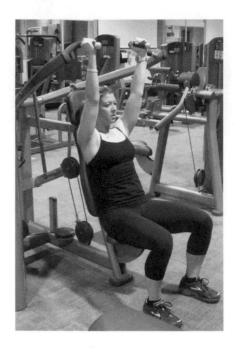

Mid-Range Position

Muscles Strengthened: anterior deltoid and triceps

Suggested Repetitions: 5 to 10 (or 30 to 60 seconds)

Start/Finish Position: Adjust the seat pad so that your hands will be near your shoulders in the start/finish position. Sit down and place your feet flat on the floor. Reach up and grasp the handles with a parallel grip (your palms facing each other).

Performance Description: Push the handles up until your arms are almost completely straight (without "locking" your elbows). Pause briefly in this mid-range position (your arms almost completely straight) and then lower the weight under control to the start/finish position (your arms bent).

Training Tips:

• This exercise is also referred to as an overhead press, a seated press and a military press.

• Multiple grips are available on some machines. A parallel grip reduces the stress in your shoulder joints.

• Keep your hips on the seat pad and your feet flat on the floor.

• Avoid "locking" or "snapping" your elbows in the mid-range position.

• You can also perform this exercise with a plate-loaded machine.

• Do this exercise with one limb at a time if you have a shoulder or an arm injury, a gross difference in the strength between your limbs or desire a training variation.

• This exercise may be contraindicated if you have shoulder-impingement syndrome or low-back pain.

LATERAL RAISE

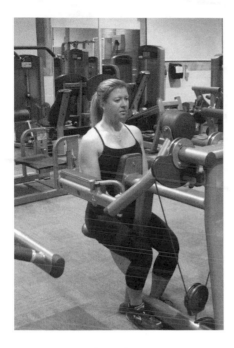

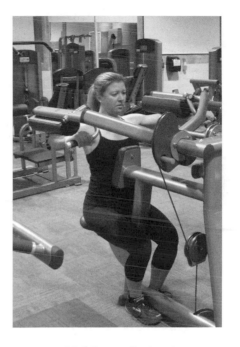

Start/Finish Position   *Mid-Range Position*

Muscles Strengthened: middle deltoid and trapezius (upper portion)

Suggested Repetitions: 5 to 10 (or 30 to 60 seconds)

Start/Finish Position: Adjust the seat pad so that the front part of your shoulders will be aligned with the axis of rotation in the start/finish position. Sit down and place your feet flat on the floor. Position your upper arms against the forearm pads. Grasp the handles with a parallel grip (your palms facing each other).

Performance Description: Raise your arms sideways until they're parallel to the floor. Pause briefly in this mid-range position (your arms parallel to the floor) and then lower the weight under control to the start/finish position (your arms at your sides).

Training Tips:

• Keep your hips on the seat pad and your feet flat on the floor. Movement should only occur at your shoulder joints.

• Raise your arms only to the point where they're parallel to the floor.

• Your palms should be facing the floor in the mid-range position.

• You can also perform this exercise with a plate-loaded machine.

• Do this exercise with one limb at a time if you have a shoulder or an arm injury, a gross difference in the strength between your limbs or desire a training variation.

REAR DELTOID

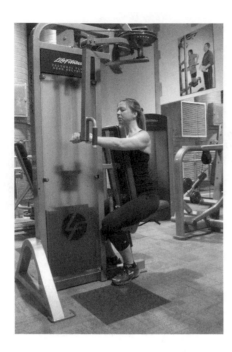

Start/Finish Position

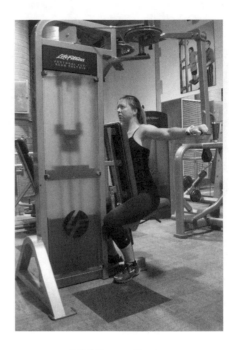

Mid-Range Position

Muscles Strengthened: posterior deltoid, trapezius (middle portion) and rhomboids

Suggested Repetitions: 5 to 10 (or 30 to 60 seconds)

Start/Finish Position: Adjust the seat pad so that your elbows will be slightly lower than your shoulders in the start/finish position. Adjust the movement arms to accommodate your level of flexibility. Sit down and place your feet flat on the floor. Grasp the handles.

Performance Description: Keeping your arms fairly straight, pull the handles back as far as possible. Pause briefly in this mid-range position (your hands apart) and then lower the weight under control to the start/finish position (your hands together).

Training Tips:

• Avoid moving your torso forward and backward. Movement should only occur at your shoulder joints.

• Attempt to raise the weight as high as possible in the mid-range position to ensure that you're obtaining a maximum contraction of the target muscles.

• You can also perform this exercise with a plate-loaded machine.

• Do this exercise with one limb at a time if you have a shoulder or an arm injury, a gross difference in the strength between your limbs or desire a training variation.

INTERNAL ROTATION

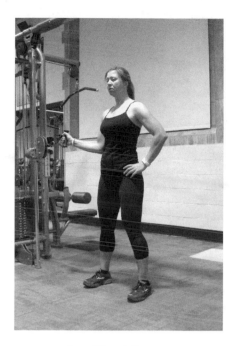

Start/Finish Position

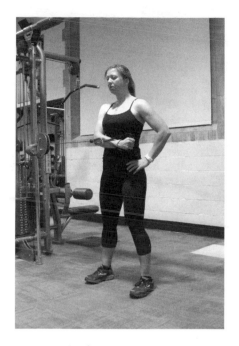

Mid-Range Position

Muscles Strengthened: internal rotators

Suggested Repetitions: 8 to 10 (or 50 to 60 seconds)

Start/Finish Position: Adjust the pulley so that it's even with your right elbow. Grasp a handle with your right hand. Position your body so that your right side faces the pulley. Place your left hand on your left hip and spread your feet about shoulder-width apart. Place your right elbow against the right side of your torso and bend your right arm so that the angle between your upper and lower arms is about 90 degrees. (By doing this, your right lower arm will be parallel to the floor.) Position the handle away from your mid-section.

Performance Description: Keeping the same angle between your upper and lower arms, pull the handle to your mid-section. Pause briefly in this mid-range position (your hand near your mid-section) and then lower the weight under control to the start/finish position (your hand away from your mid-section). Repeat the exercise for the other side of your body.

Training Tips:

• Keep your elbow against the side of your torso and your lower arm parallel to the floor.

• Avoid rotating your torso. Movement should only occur at your shoulder joint.

• You can also perform this exercise with a plate-loaded machine.

EXTERNAL ROTATION

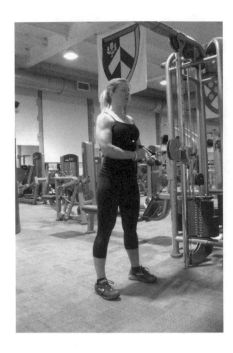

Start/Finish Position

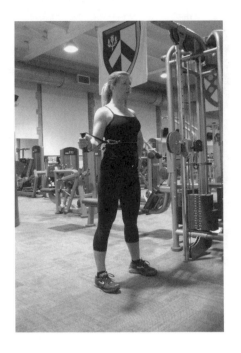

Mid-Range Position

Muscles Strengthened: external rotators

Suggested Repetitions: 8 to 10 (or 50 to 60 seconds)

Start/Finish Position: Adjust the pulley so that it's even with your right elbow. Grasp a handle with your right hand. Position your body so that your left side faces the pulley. Place your left hand on your left hip and spread your feet about shoulder-width apart. Place your right elbow against the right side of your torso and bend your right arm so that the angle between your upper and lower arms is about 90 degrees. (By doing this, your right lower arm will be parallel to the floor.) Position the handle near your mid-section.

Performance Description: Keeping the same angle between your upper and lower arms, pull the handle away from your mid-section. Pause briefly in this mid-range position (your hand away from your mid-section) and then lower the weight under control to the start/finish position (your hand near your mid-section). Repeat the exercise for the other side of your body.

Training Tips:

• Keep your elbow against the side of your torso and your lower arm parallel to the floor.

• Avoid rotating your torso. Movement should only occur at your shoulder joint.

• You can also perform this exercise with a plate-loaded machine.

UPRIGHT ROW

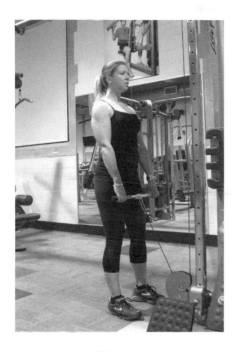

Start/Finish Position

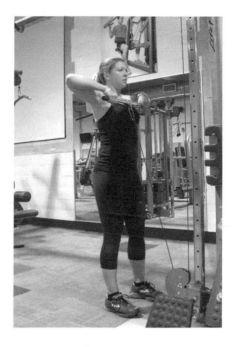

Mid-Range Position

Muscles Strengthened: trapezius (upper portion), biceps and forearms

Suggested Repetitions: 5 to 10 (or 30 to 60 seconds)

Start/Finish Position: Adjust the pulley so that it's near the floor. Grasp a bar with your hands spaced about 8 to 10 inches apart and your palms facing you. Straighten your arms and spread your feet approximately shoulder-width apart.

Performance Description: Pull the bar up until it's just below your chin. (Your elbows should be slightly higher than your hands in this position.) Pause briefly in this mid-range position (your arms bent) and then lower the weight under control to the start/finish position (your arms completely straight).

Training Tips:

• Avoid using your legs and moving your torso forward and backward. Movement should only occur at your shoulder and elbow joints.

• Keep the bar close to your body.

• You can also perform this exercise with a plate-loaded machine.

• Do this exercise with one limb at a time (with a handle instead of a bar) if you have a shoulder or an arm injury, a gross difference in the strength between your limbs or desire a training variation.

• Use wrist straps if you have difficulty in maintaining your grip on the bar.

• This exercise may be contraindicated if you have shoulder-impingement syndrome. However, raising and lowering the bar to the lower part of your chest (near the tip of your breastbone) rather than to the upper part reduces the stress on an impinged shoulder. This exercise may also be contraindicated if you have low-back pain or hyperextended elbows.

SCAPULAE ADDUCTION

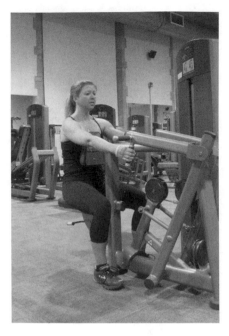

Start/Finish Position

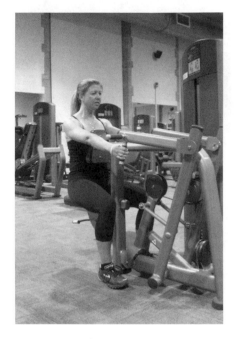

Mid-Range Position

Muscles Strengthened: trapezius (middle portion) and rhomboids

Suggested Repetitions: 8 to 10 (or 50 to 60 seconds)

Start/Finish Position: Adjust the chest pad so that your arms will be completely straight in the start/finish position. Adjust the seat pad so that your arms will be parallel to the floor in the start/finish position. Sit down, lean forward against the chest pad and place your feet flat on the floor (or on the footplate if one is provided). Grasp the handles with a parallel grip (your palms facing each other).

Performance Description: Keeping your arms fairly straight, pull the handles back as far as possible (with the intent of trying to "pinch" your shoulder blades together). Pause briefly in this mid-range position (your shoulder blades together) and then lower the weight under control to the start/finish position (your shoulder blades apart).

Training Tips:

- Avoid moving your torso forward and backward. Movement should only occur at your shoulder and elbow joints.

- Attempt to raise the weight as high as possible in the mid-range position to ensure that you're obtaining a maximum contraction of the target muscles.

- You can also perform this exercise with a plate-loaded machine.

- Do this exercise with one limb at a time if you have a shoulder or an arm injury, a gross difference in the strength between your limbs or desire a training variation.

- Use wrist straps if you have difficulty in maintaining your grip on the handles.

- This exercise may be contraindicated if you have hyperextended elbows.

BICEP CURL

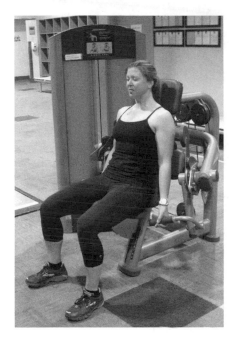

Start/Finish Position

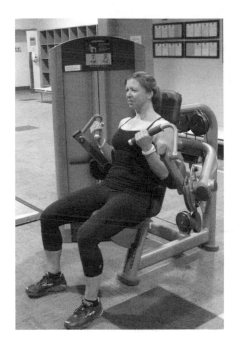

Mid-Range Position

Muscles Strengthened: biceps and forearms

Suggested Repetitions: 5 to 10 (or 30 to 60 seconds)

Start/Finish Position: Adjust the seat pad so that your elbows will be aligned with the axis of rotation in the start/finish position. Sit down and place your feet flat on the floor. Position your upper arms against the arm pads. Grasp the handles with your palms facing forward.

Performance Description: Pull the handles up to your shoulders. Pause briefly in this mid-range position (your arms bent) and then lower the weight under control to the start/finish position (your arms completely straight).

Training Tips:

- Avoid using your legs and moving your torso forward and backward. Movement should only occur at your elbow joints.

- Keep your upper arms against the arm pads.

- Attempt to raise the weight as high as possible in the mid-range position to ensure that you're obtaining a maximum contraction of the target muscles.

- You can also perform this exercise with a cable column and plate-loaded machine.

- Do this exercise with one limb at a time if you have a shoulder or an arm injury, a gross difference in the strength between your limbs or desire a training variation.

- This exercise may be contraindicated if you have hyperextended elbows.

TRICEP EXTENSION

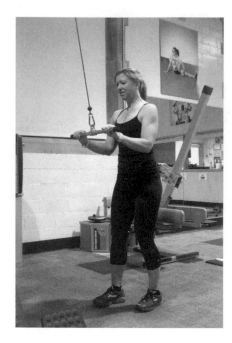
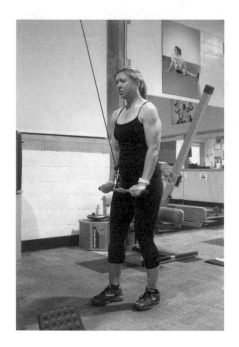

Start/Finish Position   *Mid-Range Position*

Muscle Strengthened: triceps

Suggested Repetitions: 5 to 10 (or 30 to 60 seconds)

Start/Finish Position: Reach up and grasp a bar with your hands spaced about 4 to 6 inches apart and your palms facing downward. Pull the bar down and position your elbows against the sides of your torso. Spread your feet a comfortable distance apart with one foot slightly in front of the other.

Performance Description: Push the bar down until your arms are completely straight. Pause briefly in this mid-range position (your arms completely straight) and then lower the weight under control to the start/finish position (your arms bent).

Training Tips:

• Keep your elbows against the sides of your torso.

• You can also perform this exercise with a selectorized machine.

• Do this exercise with one limb at a time (with a handle instead of a bar) if you have a shoulder or an arm injury, a gross difference in the strength between your limbs or desire a training variation.

WRIST FLEXION

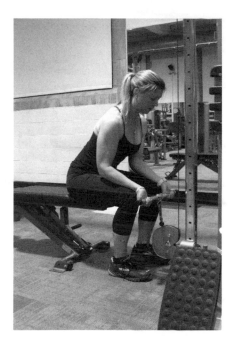

Start/Finish Position

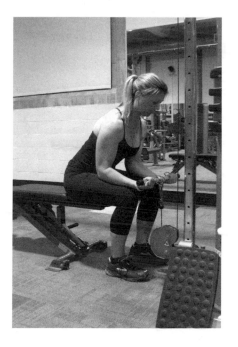

Mid-Range Position

Muscles Strengthened: wrist flexors

Suggested Repetitions: 8 to 10 (or 50 to 60 seconds)

Start/Finish Position: Adjust the pulley so that it's near the floor. Reach down and grasp a bar with your hands spread about 4 to 6 inches apart and your palms facing away from you. Position your thumbs underneath the bar alongside your fingers. Sit down near the end of a utility bench and place the back of your forearms on your upper legs so that your wrists are over your kneecaps. Lean forward slightly so that the angle between your upper and lower arms is about 90 degrees or less.

Performance Description: Pull the bar up as high as possible. Pause briefly in this mid-range position (your wrists bent) and then lower the weight under control to the start/finish position (your wrists extended).

Training Tips:

- Keep your forearms on your upper legs.

- Do this exercise with your thumbs underneath the bar. This increases your range of motion.

- Avoid using your legs and moving your torso forward and backward. Movement should only occur at your wrist joints.

- Attempt to raise the weight as high as possible in the mid-range position to ensure that you're obtaining a maximum contraction of the target muscles.

- Do this exercise with one limb at a time (with a handle instead of a bar) if you have a shoulder or an arm injury, a gross difference in the strength between your limbs or desire a training variation.

WRIST EXTENSION

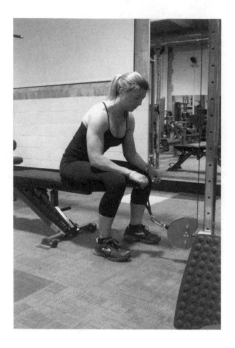

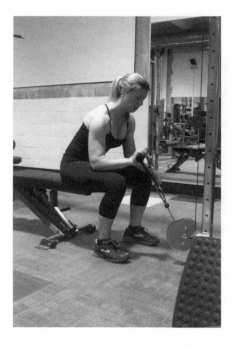

Start/Finish Position   *Mid-Range Position*

Muscle Strengthened: wrist extensors

Suggested Repetitions: 8 to 10 (or 50 to 60 seconds)

Start/Finish Position: Adjust the pulley so that it's near the floor. Reach down and grasp a handle with your right hand. Sit down near the end of a utility bench and place the front of your right forearm on your right upper leg so that your wrist is over your kneecap and your palm is facing down. Lean forward slightly so that the angle between your upper and lower arms is about 90 degrees or less.

Performance Description: Pull the handle up as high as possible. Pause briefly in this mid-range position (your wrist extended) and then lower the weight under control to the start/finish position (your wrist bent). Repeat the exercise for the other side of your body.

Training Tips:

• Keep your forearm on your upper leg.

• Avoid using your leg and moving your torso forward and backward. Movement should only occur at your wrist joint.

• Attempt to raise the weight as high as possible in the mid-range position to ensure that you're obtaining a maximum contraction of the target muscles.

• Do this exercise with a handle rather than a bar. This makes it more comfortable on your wrist joint.

134

ABDOMINAL CRUNCH

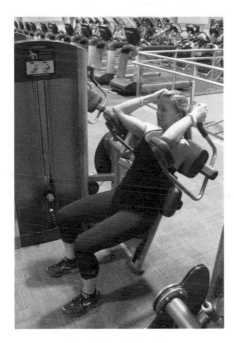

Start/Finish Position

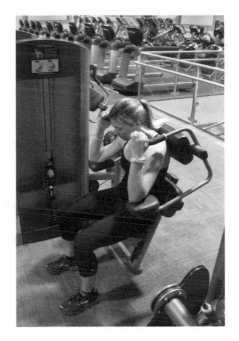

Mid-Range Position

Muscle Strengthened: rectus abdominis

Suggested Repetitions: 8 to 10 (or 50 to 60 seconds)

Start/Finish Position: Adjust the seat pad so that your navel ("belly button") will be aligned with the axis of rotation in the start/finish position. Sit down and place your feet flat on the floor. Position the back of your upper arms on the elbow pads. Place your palms on the handles and open your hands (extend your fingers).

Performance Description: Pull your torso as close to your upper legs as possible. Pause briefly in this mid-range position (your torso bent) and then lower the weight under control to the start/finish position (your torso straight).

Training Tips:

- Avoid snapping your head forward. Movement should only occur at your hip joint and mid-section.

- Exert force against the elbow pads with your upper arms, not your hands. This isolates your abdominals.

- If you're unable to keep your upper arms against the elbow pads, you can grasp the handles with a parallel grip (your palms facing each other) and pull with your hands instead of your upper arms. This doesn't allow you to isolate your abdominals but it will make the exercise more comfortable for you to perform.

- Attempt to raise the weight as high as possible in the mid-range position to ensure that you're obtaining a maximum contraction of the target muscles.

- You can also perform this exercise with a plate-loaded machine.

- This exercise may be contraindicated if you have low-back pain or shoulder-impingement syndrome.

135

SIDE BEND

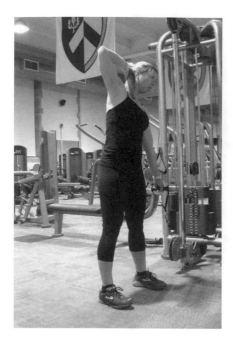

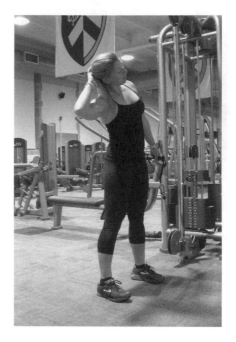

Start/Finish Position   *Mid-Range Position*

Muscles Strengthened: obliques and erector spinae

Suggested Repetitions: 8 to 10 (or 50 to 60 seconds)

Start/Finish Position: Adjust the pulley so that it's near the floor. Reach down and grasp a handle with your left hand. Position your body so that your left side faces the pulley. Position the handle near the side of your upper leg with your palm facing your leg. Spread your feet about shoulder-width apart. Place your right palm against the right side of your head. Keep your hips in the same position and bend your torso to the left as far as possible.

Performance Description: Without moving your hips, bring your torso to the right as far as possible. Pause briefly in this mid-range position (your torso bent to the right) and then lower the weight under control to the start/finish position (your torso bent to the left). Repeat the exercise for the other side of your body.

Training Tips:

• Avoid moving your hips. Movement should only occur at your mid-section.

• Refrain from bending forward at the waist.

• Keep your feet flat on the floor.

• Attempt to raise the weight as high as possible in the mid-range position to ensure that you're obtaining a maximum contraction of the target muscles.

• Use wrist straps if you have difficulty in maintaining your grip on the handle.

• This exercise may be contraindicated if you have low-back pain.

TORSO ROTATION

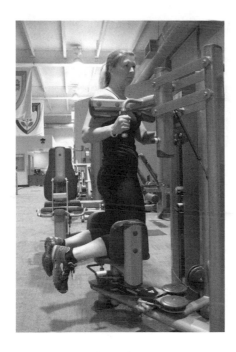

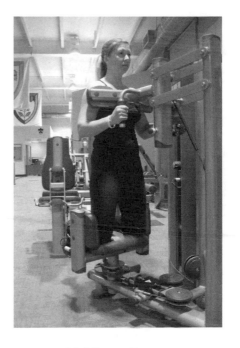

Start/Finish Position   *Mid-Range Position*

Muscles Strengthened: obliques and erector spinae

Suggested Repetitions: 8 to 10 (or 50 to 60 seconds)

Start/Finish Position: Adjust the chest pads so that they will be centered on your chest in the start/finish position. Adjust the movement arm clockwise to accommodate your level of flexibility. Kneel down on the knee pad and position the side part of your thighs against the thigh pads. Grasp the handles with a parallel grip (your palms facing each other).

Performance Description: Rotate your torso to the right as far as possible. Pause briefly in this mid-range position (your torso rotated to the right) and then lower the weight under control to the start/finish position (your torso rotated to the left). Repeat the exercise for the other side of your body (adjusting the movement arm counterclockwise to accommodate your level of flexibility).

Training Tips:

- Attempt to raise the weight as high as possible in the mid-range position to ensure that you're obtaining a maximum contraction of the target muscles.

- This exercise may be contraindicated if you have low-back pain.

137

BACK EXTENSION

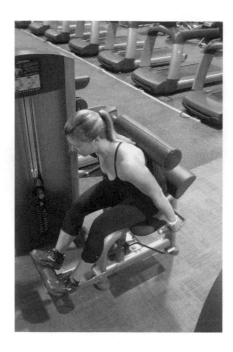

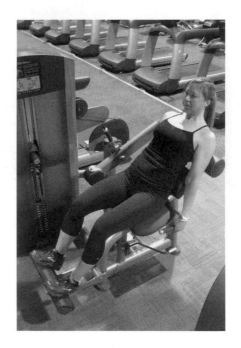

Start/Finish Position

Mid-Range Position

Muscles Strengthened: erector spinae, gluteus maximus and hamstrings

Suggested Repetitions: 10 to 15 (or 60 to 90 seconds)

Start/Finish Position: Adjust the movement arm to accommodate your level of flexibility. Adjust the footplate so that your legs will be almost completely straight in the start/finish position. Sit down and place your feet flat on the footplate. Position your upper back against the roller pad. Grasp the handles that are located on the sides of the seat pad.

Performance Description: Extend your torso backward until it's aligned with your upper legs. Pause briefly in this mid-range position (your torso straight) and then lower the weight under control to the start/finish position (your torso bent).

Training Tips:

• Avoid snapping your head backward. Movement should only occur at your hip joint and mid-section.

• Keep your hips on the seat pad and your feet flat on the footplate.

• This exercise may be contraindicated if you have low-back pain.

NECK FLEXION

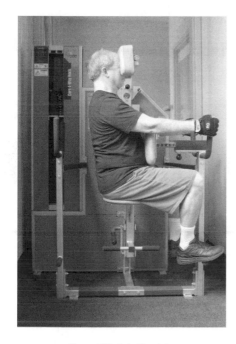

Start/Finish Position

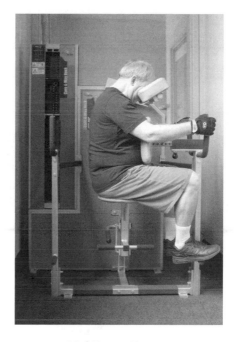

Mid-Range Position

Muscle Strengthened: sternocleidomastoideus

Suggested Repetitions: 8 to 10 (or 50 to 60 seconds)

Start/Finish Position: Adjust the seat pad so that your laryngeal prominence ("Adam's apple") will be aligned with the axis of rotation in the start/finish position. Adjust the torso pad so that your torso will be even with the axis of rotation in the start/finish position. Adjust the movement arm so that your head will be perpendicular to the floor in the start/finish position. Sit down, position the front part of your head against the head pad and place your feet flat on the floor (or on the foot pedal if one is provided). Grasp the handles with a parallel grip (your palms facing each other).

Performance Description: Pull your head as close to your chest as possible. Pause briefly in this mid-range position (your chin near your chest) and then lower the weight under control to the start/finish position (your head perpendicular to the floor).

Training Tips:

- Avoid moving your head backward beyond the point at which it's perpendicular to the floor.

- Avoid moving your torso forward and backward. Movement should only occur at your neck.

- Keep your hips on the seat pad and your feet flat on the floor.

- Attempt to raise the weight as high as possible in the mid-range position to ensure that you're obtaining a maximum contraction of the target muscles.

- You can also perform this exercise with a plate-loaded machine.

NECK EXTENSION

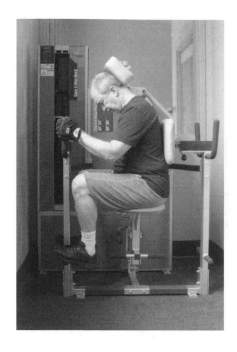

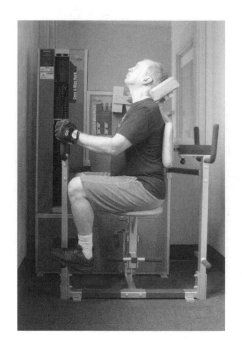

Start/Finish Position   *Mid-Range Position*

Muscles Strengthened: neck extensors and trapezius (upper portion)

Suggested Repetitions: 8 to 10 (or 50 to 60 seconds)

Start/Finish Position: Adjust the seat pad so that your laryngeal prominence ("Adam's apple") will be aligned with the axis of rotation in the start/finish position. Adjust the torso pad so that your torso will be even with the axis of rotation in the start/finish position. Adjust the movement arm to accommodate your level of flexibility. Sit down, position the back part of your head against the head pad and place your feet flat on the floor (or on the foot pedal if one is provided). Grasp the handles with a parallel grip (your palms facing each other). Position your chin near your chest.

Performance Description: Extend your head backward as far as possible. Pause briefly in this mid-range position (your neck extended) and then lower the weight under control to the start/finish position (your chin near your chest).

Training Tips:

- Avoid moving your torso forward and backward. Movement should only occur at your neck.

- Keep your hips on the seat pad and your feet flat on the floor.

- Attempt to raise the weight as high as possible in the mid-range position to ensure that you're obtaining a maximum contraction of the target muscles.

- You can also perform this exercise with a plate-loaded machine.

NECK LATERAL FLEXION

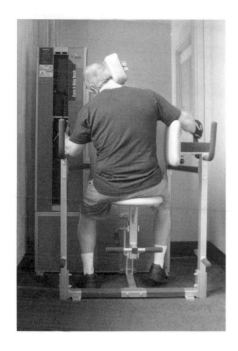

Start/Finish Position

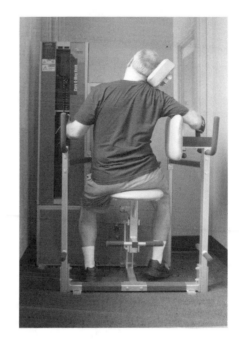

Mid-Range Position

Muscle Strengthened: sternocleidomastoideus

Suggested Repetitions: 8 to 10 (or 50 to 60 seconds)

Start/Finish Position: Adjust the seat pad so that your laryngeal prominence ("Adam's apple") will be aligned with the axis of rotation in the start/finish position. Adjust the torso pad so that it doesn't restrict your range of motion. Adjust the movement arm to accommodate your level of flexibility. Sit down, position the right side of your head against the head pad and place your feet flat on the floor (or on the foot pedal if one is provided). Grasp the handles with a parallel grip (your palms facing each other). Position your head so that it's near your left shoulder.

Performance Description: Pull your head to your right shoulder. Pause briefly in this mid-range position (your head near your right shoulder) and then lower the weight under control to the start/finish position (your head near your left shoulder). Repeat the exercise for the other side of your body.

Training Tips:

• Avoid moving your torso. Movement should only occur at your neck.

• Keep your hips on the seat pad and your feet flat on the floor.

• Attempt to raise the weight as high as possible in the mid-range position to ensure that you're obtaining a maximum contraction of the target muscles.

• You can also perform this exercise with a plate-loaded machine.

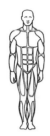

10 Manual-Resistance Exercises

Manual resistance has been referred to as a productive alternative for developing strength with little or no equipment. It's an extremely effective way of strength training in which one individual supplies the resistance for another individual.

Surprisingly, manual resistance – aka partner resistance – has actually been around for quite a long time. The origins of these exercises can be traced back to the Swedish system of gymnastics which was developed by Per Henrik Ling in the early 1800s. In one of the first accounts of manual resistance that dates back about 200 years, Ling stated that "Resistance may consist of gravity, the opposing force of antagonizing muscles, or that which is exerted by another person." In an 1862 magazine article that was written by Dr. Dio Lewis, a physician, several exercises were described in which an individual pulled one or two wooden gymnastic rings that were held by another person who offered resistance. In that article, Dr. Lewis wrote, "In most exercises there must be some resistance. How much better that this should be another human being, rather than a pole, ladder or bar!"

Self resistance – a novel version of manual resistance – gained notoriety nearly a century ago. In 1922, Charles Atlas – born as Angelo Siciliano – was awarded the title of "The World's Most Perfectly Developed Man" after beating 774 other men in a physique contest that was held in Madison Square Garden. Atlas claimed to have used self-resistance exercises to develop his award-winning physique (although it seems as if he "supplemented" the exercises with barbells and dumbbells). His system was called Dynamic-Tension and, with the help of Charles Roman, he began an extremely lucrative mail-order business in 1929 to sell the exercises. (Atlas passed away in 1972 but his legacy lives on. His mail-order company continues to thrive more than 80 years after it was established.)

During the late 1970s, manual resistance was refined and galvanized by Dan Riley who was at the time the strength coach at Penn State. Largely because of his early efforts, manual resistance has been used at the scholastic, collegiate and professional levels for many years.

ADVANTAGES AND DISADVANTAGES

Manual resistance has many advantages. First of all, little or no equipment is required. Because of this, the exercises can be done just about anywhere without having to go to a fitness center or weight room. In addition, there's little or no expense. This is an important consideration for those with a limited or tight budget. Manual resistance is also a way of training large numbers of individuals in an extremely time-efficient fashion. (Regardless of the size of the group, one half are the lifters while the other half are the spotters.)

Manual resistance has several disadvantages. The major drawback is that the resistance can't be quantified thereby making it impossible to monitor progress. Another disadvantage of manual resistance is that it requires a competent spotter.

GENERAL TECHNIQUE

In order for manual resistance to be productive, the exercises must be performed with proper technique. The following are general guidelines for the lifter and spotter:

The Lifter

As in lifting any weight, the lifter should perform the repetitions in a smooth, controlled manner without any explosive or jerking movements and throughout the greatest possible range of motion (ROM) that safety allows. The resistance (as applied by the spotter) should be raised in at least one to two seconds and lowered in at least three to four seconds.

The lifter should reach muscular fatigue within about 10 to 15 repetitions for the lower body and 5 to 10 repetitions for the torso. (Muscular fatigue should occur within about 8 to 10 repetitions for torso exercises that have an abbreviated ROM.) It should be noted that these ranges are based on six-second repetitions.

As an alternative to counting repetitions, the exercises can be performed for a prescribed amount of time. In this case, the lifter should reach muscular fatigue within about 60 to 90 seconds for the lower body and about 30 to 60 seconds for the torso. (Muscular fatigue should occur within about 50 to 60 seconds for torso exercises that have an abbreviated ROM.)

Also, the lifter must keep the muscles loaded throughout the entire exercise. Finally, the lifter must communicate to the spotter whether the resistance is too little or too much.

The Spotter

Because an individual is naturally stronger in some positions than others due to the changing biomechanical leverage of the skeletal system, the spotter is responsible for varying the resistance throughout the lifter's entire ROM. In a lateral raise, for instance, you lose leverage as you raise your arms away from the sides of your body. As the lifter's leverage decreases, the spotter must provide less resistance. And since eccentric strength is greater than concentric strength (in the same exercise), the spotter must apply more resistance when the lifter performs the negative phase of each repetition.

The spotter must also regulate the resistance in accordance with the lifter's momentary level of strength. This means that the spotter must furnish less resistance as the lifter fatigues during each repetition. In addition, the spotter must control the speed with which the lifter performs the repetitions. Lastly, the spotter should provide the lifter with feedback on technique and motivate the lifter with words of encouragement.

THE EXERCISES

This chapter describes and illustrates the safest and most productive exercises that can be performed with manual resistance. Included in the discussions of each exercise are the muscle(s) strengthened (if two or more muscles are involved, the first muscle listed is the prime mover), suggested repetitions (the time that the targeted muscles should be loaded is shown in parentheses), start/finish position, performance description and training tips for making the exercise safer and more productive. (Note: In the accompanying photographs, the lifter is wearing the darker shirt.)

These 24 exercises are described in this chapter: hip abduction, hip adduction, prone leg curl, seated leg curl, leg extension, dorsi flexion, push-up, bent-arm fly, bent-over row, seated row, lat pulldown, shoulder press, lateral raise, front raise, bent-over raise, internal rotation, external rotation, bicep curl, tricep extension, wrist pronation, wrist supination, abdominal crunch, neck flexion and neck extension.

HIP ABDUCTION

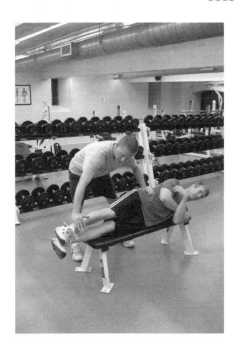

Start/Finish Position

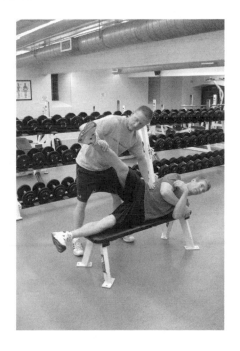

Mid-Range Position

Muscles Strengthened: gluteus medius and gluteus minimus

Suggested Repetitions: 10 to 15 (or 60 to 90 seconds)

Start/Finish Position: Lie down on a utility bench (or the floor) on the left side of your body and straighten your legs. Point your right toes toward your right knee. The spotter should stand or kneel behind you and apply resistance against your right ankle.

Performance Description: Raise your right leg as high as possible as the spotter provides resistance evenly throughout the full range of motion. Pause briefly in this mid-range position (your legs apart) and then resist as the spotter pushes your leg back to the start/finish position (your legs together). Repeat the exercise for the other side of your body (with your right side on the bench).

Training Tips:

- The spotter should apply resistance above your knee if you suffer from a hyperextended knee or other joint pain.

- Refrain from bending forward at the waist.

- Attempt to raise your leg as high as possible in the mid-range position to ensure that you're obtaining a maximum contraction of the target muscles.

- After reaching muscular fatigue, you can overload your muscles further by having the spotter lift your leg to the mid-range position and then push it back to the start/finish position as you resist for 3 to 5 negative-only repetitions.

HIP ADDUCTION

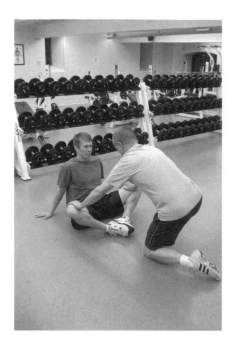

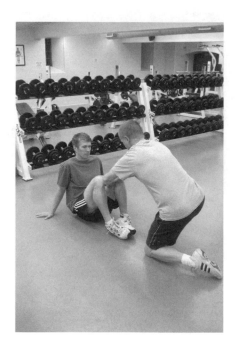

Start/Finish Position

Mid-Range Position

Muscles Strengthened: hip adductors

Suggested Repetitions: 10 to 15 (or 60 to 90 seconds)

Start/Finish Position: Sit down on the floor, bend your legs and place the soles of your feet together. Position your feet close to your hips and spread your knees apart. Place your hands alongside your hips and lean back slightly. The spotter should kneel in front of you and apply resistance against the inside of your knees.

Performance Description: Bring your knees as close together as possible as the spotter provides resistance evenly throughout the full range of motion. Pause briefly in this mid-range position (your knees together) and then resist as the spotter pushes your legs back to the start/finish position (your knees apart).

Training Tips:

- Attempt to bring your knees as close together as possible in the mid-range position to ensure that you're obtaining a maximum contraction of the target muscles.

- After reaching muscular fatigue, you can overload your muscles further by having the spotter lift your legs to the mid-range position and then push them back to the start/finish position as you resist for 3 to 5 negative-only repetitions.

PRONE LEG CURL

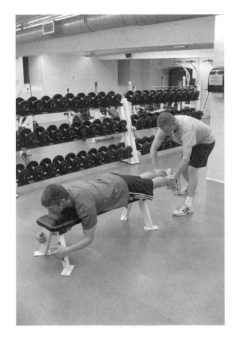

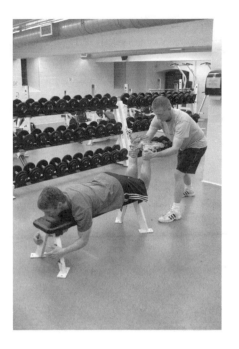

Start/Finish Position   *Mid-Range Position*

Muscles Strengthened: hamstrings

Suggested Repetitions: 10 to 15 (or 60 to 90 seconds)

Start/Finish Position: Lie face down on a utility bench (or the floor) and straighten your legs. Position the tops of your kneecaps just over the edge the back pad. Grasp the front edge of the bench. The spotter should stand or kneel behind you and apply resistance against your heels.

Performance Description: Pull your heels as close to your hips as possible as the spotter provides resistance evenly throughout the full range of motion. Pause briefly in this mid-range position (your heels near your hips) and then resist as the spotter pulls your heels back to the start/finish position (your legs completely straight).

Training Tips:

- Avoid raising your torso. Movement should only occur at your knee joints

- The angle between your upper and lower legs should be about 90 degrees or less in the mid-range position.

- Attempt to bring your heels as close to your hips as possible in the mid-range position to ensure that you're obtaining a maximum contraction of the target muscles.

- Do this exercise with one limb at a time if you have a leg, knee or ankle injury, a gross difference in the strength between your limbs or desire a training variation.

- After reaching muscular fatigue, you can overload your muscles further by having the spotter lift your lower legs to the mid-range position and then pull them back to the start/finish position as you resist for 3 to 5 negative-only repetitions.

- This exercise may be contraindicated if you have hyperextended knees or low-back pain.

SEATED LEG CURL

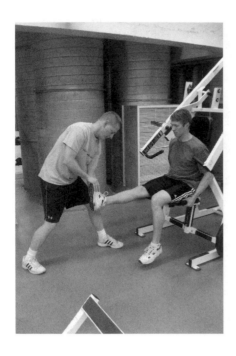

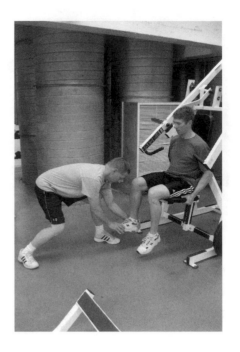

Start/Finish Position   *Mid-Range Position*

Muscles Strengthened: hamstrings

Suggested Repetitions: 10 to 15 (or 60 to 90 seconds)

Start/Finish Position: Sit down on a machine (or table or chair) that's high enough so that your feet don't touch the floor and straighten your right leg. Grasp the sides of the seat pad. The spotter should stand or kneel in front of you and apply resistance against your right heel.

Performance Description: Pull your heel as close to your hip as possible as the spotter provides resistance evenly throughout the full range of motion. Pause briefly in this mid-range position (your heel near your hip) and then resist as the spotter pulls your heel back to the start/finish position (your leg completely straight). Repeat the exercise for the other side of your body.

Training Tips:

• Performing this exercise in the seated position produces less stress in the low-back region than performing it in the prone position.

• Avoid moving your torso forward and backward. Movement should only occur at your knee joint.

• The angle between your upper and lower leg should be about 90 degrees or less in the mid-range position.

• Attempt to bring your heel as close to your hip as possible in the mid-range position to ensure that you're obtaining a maximum contraction of the target muscles.

• After reaching muscular fatigue, you can overload your muscles further by having the spotter bring your lower leg to the mid-range position and then pull it back to the start/finish position as you resist for 3 to 5 negative-only repetitions.

• This exercise may be contraindicated if you have hyperextended knees.

LEG EXTENSION

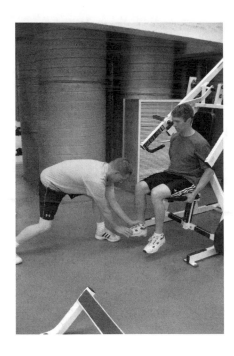

Start/Finish Position

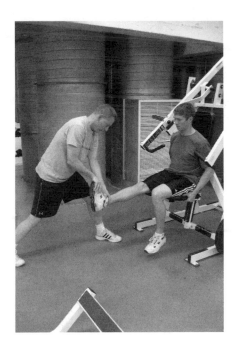

Mid-Range Position

Muscles Strengthened: quadriceps

Suggested Repetitions: 10 to 15 (or 60 to 90 seconds)

Start/Finish Position: Sit down on a machine (or table or chair) that's high enough so that your feet don't touch the floor and bend your right leg. Grasp the sides of the seat pad. The spotter should stand or kneel in front of you and apply resistance against your right instep.

Performance Description: Straighten your right leg as completely as possible as the spotter provides resistance evenly throughout the full range of motion. Pause briefly in this mid-range position (your leg completely straight) and then resist as the spotter pushes your ankle back to the start/finish position (your leg bent). Repeat the exercise for the other side of your body.

Training Tips:

• Avoid moving your torso forward and backward. Movement should only occur at your knee joint.

• Attempt to straighten your leg as high as possible in the mid-range position to ensure that you're obtaining a maximum contraction of the target muscles.

• After reaching muscular fatigue, you can overload your muscles further by having the spotter lift your lower leg to the mid-range position and then push it back to the start/finish position as you resist for 3 to 5 negative-only repetitions.

DORSI FLEXION

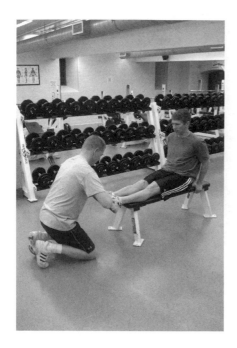

Start/Finish Position

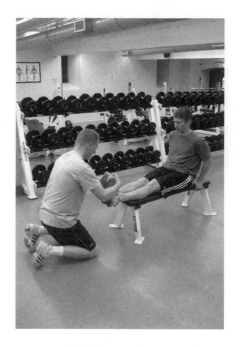

Mid-Range Position

Muscles Strengthened: dorsi flexors

Suggested Repetitions: 10 to 15 (or 60 to 90 seconds)

Start/Finish Position: Sit down on a utility bench. Place your legs across the length of it. Position your heels over the end of the back pad and point your toes away from your body. Grasp the sides of the bench. The spotter should stand or kneel in front of you and apply resistance against your insteps.

Performance Description: Keeping your legs flat on the bench, pull your feet up as high as possible as the spotter provides resistance evenly throughout the full range of motion. Pause briefly in this mid-range position (your ankles bent) and then resist as the spotter pulls your feet back to the start/finish position (your ankles straight).

Training Tips:

• Avoid moving your torso forward and backward. Movement should only occur at your ankle joints.

• Attempt to raise your feet as high as possible in the mid-range position to ensure that you're obtaining a maximum contraction of the target muscles.

• Do this exercise with one limb at a time if you have a leg, knee or ankle injury, a gross difference in the strength between your limbs or desire a training variation.

• After reaching muscular fatigue, you can overload your muscles further by having the spotter bring your feet to the mid-range position and then pull them back to the start/finish position as you resist for 3 to 5 negative-only repetitions.

• This exercise may be contraindicated if you have shin splints.

PUSH-UP

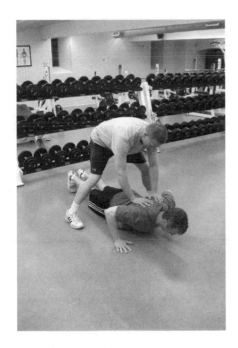

Start/Finish Position

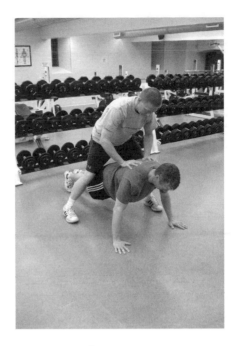

Mid-Range Position

Muscles Strengthened: chest, anterior deltoid and triceps

Suggested Repetitions: 5 to 10 (or 30 to 60 seconds)

Start/Finish Position: Lie face down on the floor, straighten your legs and curl your toes under your feet. Place your palms on the floor and spread your hands slightly wider than shoulder-width apart. The spotter should straddle your torso and apply resistance against your upper back.

Performance Description: Push your body up until your arms are almost completely straight (without "locking" your elbows) as the spotter provides resistance evenly throughout the full range of motion. Pause briefly in this mid-range position (your arms almost completely straight) and then resist as the spotter pushes you back to the start/finish position (your arms bent).

Training Tips:

- Avoid using an excessively wide hand position. This reduces your range of motion.

- Avoid arching your lower back. Your torso should remain aligned with your lower body.

- Avoid "locking" or "snapping" your elbows in the mid-range position.

- If you can't do 5 repetitions using your bodyweight, you can increase your biomechanical leverage by performing this exercise in the kneeling position.

- After reaching muscular fatigue, you can overload your muscles further by having the spotter lift your body to the mid-range position and then push it back to the start/finish position as you resist for 3 to 5 negative-only repetitions.

- This exercise may be contraindicated if you have shoulder-impingement syndrome.

BENT-ARM FLY

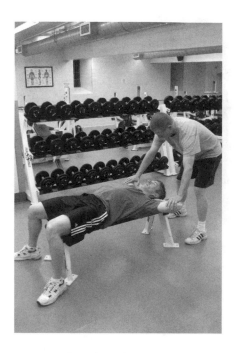

Start/Finish Position

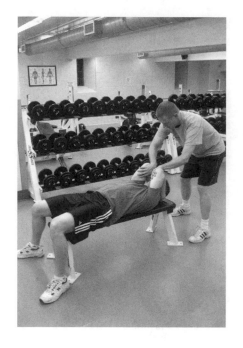

Mid-Range Position

Muscles Strengthened: chest and anterior deltoid

Suggested Repetitions: 5 to 10 (or 30 to 60 seconds)

Start/Finish Position: Lie down on a utility bench (or the floor) and interlock your fingers behind your head. Place your feet flat on the floor. The spotter should stand or kneel behind your head and apply resistance against the inside of your elbows.

Performance Description: Keeping your head against the back pad, bring your elbows as close together as possible as the spotter provides resistance evenly throughout the full range of motion. Pause briefly in this mid-range position (your elbows together) and then resist as the spotter pushes your arms back to the start/finish position (your elbows apart).

Training Tips:

- Keep your head, hips and torso against the back pad and your feet flat on the floor. Movement should only occur at your shoulder joints.

- If you have low-back pain, place your feet flat on the end of the bench or a stool. This reduces the stress in your low-back region.

- Do this exercise with one limb at a time if you have a shoulder or an arm injury, a gross difference in the strength between your limbs or desire a training variation.

- After reaching muscular fatigue, you can overload your muscles further by having the spotter lift your arms to the mid-range position and then push them back to the start/finish position as you resist for 3 to 5 negative-only repetitions.

- This exercise may be contraindicated if you have shoulder-impingement syndrome.

BENT-OVER ROW

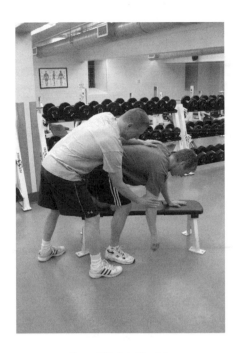
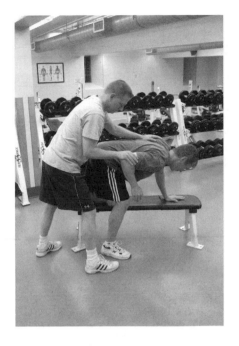

Start/Finish Position   *Mid-Range Position*

Muscle Strengthened: upper back

Suggested Repetitions: 5 to 10 (or 30 to 60 seconds)

Start/Finish Position: Place your left hand and left knee on a utility bench and position your right foot on the floor a comfortable distance from the bench. Position your right arm so that it's perpendicular to the floor and open your right hand (extend your fingers). Straighten your right arm and point your palm toward the bench. The spotter should stand along the right side of your torso and apply resistance against the back of your right upper arm near your elbow.

Performance Description: Pull your elbow up as high as possible as the spotter provides resistance evenly throughout the full range of motion. Pause briefly in this mid-range position (your arm bent) and then resist as the spotter pushes your arm back to the start/finish position (your arm completely straight). Repeat the exercise for the other side of your body (with your right hand and right knee on the bench)

Training Tips:

- Keep your hand open (your fingers extended).

- Avoid using your legs and rotating your torso. Movement should only occur at your shoulder and elbow joints.

- You can also perform this exercise with your upper arm positioned away from your torso. Doing this involves less of your upper back and more of your posterior deltoid, trapezius and rhomboids. In this case, your upper arm would be perpendicular to your torso and your palm would be facing backward in the mid-range position.

- This exercise is a multiple-joint movement when performed with dumbbells but a single-joint movement when performed with manual resistance because the resistance is applied above your elbow, not to your hand.

- After reaching muscular fatigue, you can overload your muscles further by having the spotter lift your arm to the mid-range position and then push it back to the start/finish position as you resist for 3 to 5 negative-only repetitions.

SEATED ROW

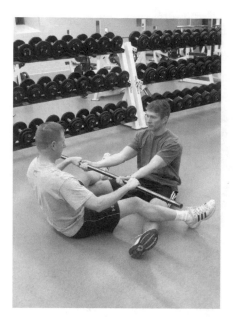

Start/Finish Position

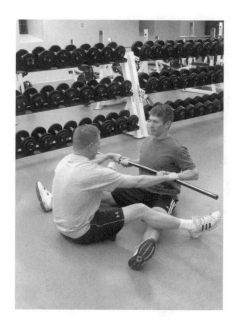

Mid-Range Position

Muscles Strengthened: upper back, biceps and forearms

Suggested Repetitions: 5 to 10 (or 30 to 60 seconds)

Start/Finish Position: Sit down on the floor, straighten your legs and spread them apart. Grasp a long stick (or similar object) with your palms facing up and space your hands approximately shoulder-width apart. Straighten your arms and lean back slightly. The spotter should sit down on the floor between your legs and grasp the stick on the outside of your grip with palms facing down.

Performance Description: Pull the stick to your mid-section as the spotter provides resistance evenly throughout the full range of motion. Pause briefly in this mid-range position (your arms bent) and then resist as the spotter pulls your arms back to the start/finish position (your arms completely straight).

Training Tips:

• The spotter should provide resistance by bending forward and backward at the waist to involve the larger, more powerful muscles of the lower back.

• You can also perform this exercise with your upper arms positioned away from your torso using an overhand grip. Doing this involves less of your upper back and more of your posterior deltoid, trapezius and rhomboids. In this case, your upper arm would be perpendicular to your torso and your palms would be facing down in the mid-range position.

• Avoid using an excessively wide grip. This reduces your range of motion.

• Avoid moving your torso forward and backward. Movement should only occur at your shoulder and elbow joints.

• Do this exercise with one limb at a time if you have a shoulder or an arm injury, a gross difference in the strength between your limbs or desire a training variation.

• Use wrist straps if you have difficulty in maintaining your grip on the stick.

• After reaching muscular fatigue, you can overload your muscles further by having the spotter bring the stick to the mid-range position and then pull it back to the start/finish position as you resist for 3 to 5 negative-only repetitions.

• This exercise may be contraindicated if you have hyperextended elbows.

154

LAT PULLDOWN

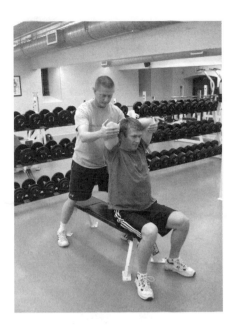

Start/Finish Position

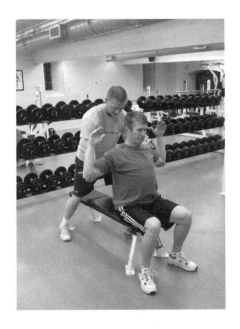

Mid-Range Position

Muscle Strengthened: upper back

Suggested Repetitions: 5 to 10 (or 30 to 60 seconds)

Start/Finish Position: Sit down on a utility bench (or stool or chair) and place your upper arms near the sides of your head. Cross your lower arms above your head and open your hands (extend your fingers). The spotter should stand behind you and apply resistance against the back of your upper arms near your elbows.

Performance Description: Keeping your upper arms aligned with your torso, pull your elbows down to your sides as the spotter provides resistance evenly throughout the full range of motion. Pause briefly in this mid-range position (your upper arms near the sides of your body) and then resist as the spotter pulls your arms back to the start/finish position (your upper arms near the sides of your head).

Training Tips:

- Keep your hands open (your fingers extended).

- Avoid moving your hands in front of your face. Your hands should remain out of your sight.

- This exercise is a multiple-joint movement when performed with a machine but it becomes a single-joint movement when using manual resistance because the load is applied above your elbows, not to your hands.

- Do this exercise with one limb at a time if you have a shoulder or an arm injury, a gross difference in the strength between your limbs or desire a training variation.

- After reaching muscular fatigue, you can overload your muscles further by having the spotter bring your arms to the mid-range position and then pull them back to the start/finish position as you resist for 3 to 5 negative-only repetitions.

- This exercise may be contraindicated if you have shoulder-impingement syndrome.

SHOULDER PRESS

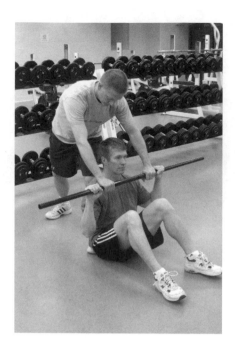

Start/Finish Position

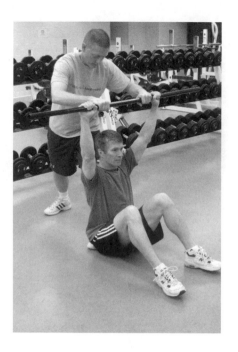

Mid-Range Position

Muscles Strengthened: anterior deltoid and triceps

Suggested Repetitions: 5 to 10 (or 30 to 60 seconds)

Start/Finish Position: Sit down on the floor, bend your legs and place your feet flat on the floor. Grasp a long stick (or similar object) and spread your hands slightly wider than shoulder-width apart. Place the stick on the upper part of your chest near your collarbones. The spotter should stand behind you, place one leg behind your torso for you to lean against and grasp the stick on the inside of your grip with palms facing down.

Performance Description: Push the stick up until your arms are almost completely straight (without "locking" your elbows) as the spotter provides resistance evenly throughout the full range of motion. Pause briefly in this mid-range position (your arms almost completely straight) and then resist as the spotter pushes the stick back to the start/finish position (your arms bent).

Training Tips:

• Avoid using an excessively wide grip. This reduces your range of motion.

• Avoid "locking" or "snapping" your elbows in the mid-range position.

• Do this exercise with one limb at a time if you have a shoulder or an arm injury, a gross difference in the strength between your limbs or desire a training variation.

• After reaching muscular fatigue, you can overload your muscles further by having the spotter lift the stick to the mid-range position and then push it back to the start/finish position as you resist for 3 to 5 negative-only repetitions.

• You can also perform this exercise with the stick positioned behind your head. However, this may be contraindicated if you have shoulder-impingement syndrome. This exercise may also be contraindicated if you have low-back pain.

LATERAL RAISE

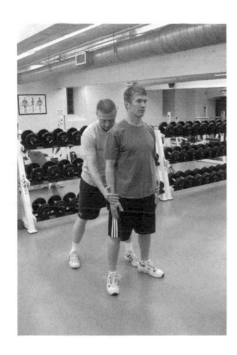

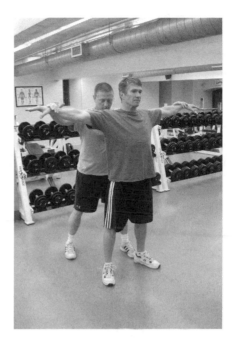

Start/Finish Position   *Mid-Range Position*

Muscles Strengthened: middle deltoid and trapezius (upper portion)

Suggested Repetitions: 5 to 10 (or 30 to 60 seconds)

Start/Finish Position: Position your hands against the sides of your upper legs with your palms facing each other and open your hands (extend your fingers). Straighten your arms and spread your feet about shoulder-width apart. The spotter should stand behind you and apply resistance near your wrists.

Performance Description: Keeping your arms fairly straight, raise them sideways until they're parallel to the floor as the spotter provides resistance evenly throughout the full range of motion. Pause briefly in this mid-range position (your arms parallel to the floor) and then resist as the spotter pushes your arms back to the start/finish position (your arms at your sides).

Training Tips:

- The spotter should apply resistance above your elbows if you suffer from a hyperextended elbow or other joint pain.

- Keep your hands open (your fingers extended).

- Avoid using your legs and moving your torso forward and backward. Movement should only occur at your shoulder joints.

- Raise your arms only to the point at which they're parallel to the floor.

- Your palms should be facing the floor in the mid-range position.

- Do this exercise with one limb at a time if you have a shoulder or an arm injury, a gross difference in the strength between your limbs or desire a training variation.

- After reaching muscular fatigue, you can overload your muscles further by having the spotter lift your arms to the mid-range position and then push them back to the start/finish position as you resist for 3 to 5 negative-only repetitions.

157

FRONT RAISE

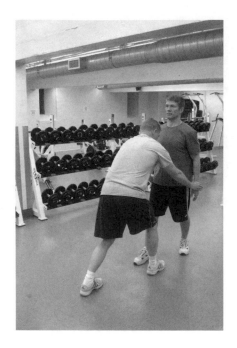

Start/Finish Position

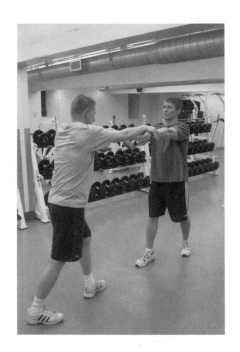

Mid-Range Position

Muscle Strengthened: anterior deltoid

Suggested Repetitions: 5 to 10 (or 30 to 60 seconds)

Start/Finish Position: Position your hands slightly past your hips with your palms facing each other and open your hands (extend your fingers). Straighten your arms and spread your feet a comfortable distance apart with one foot slightly in front of the other. The spotter should stand in front of you, place one foot to the inside of your forward foot and apply resistance against your wrists.

Performance Description: Keeping your arms fairly straight, raise them forward until they're parallel to the floor as the spotter applies resistance evenly throughout the full range of motion. Pause briefly in this mid-range position (your arms parallel to the floor) and then resist as the spotter pushes your arms back to the start/finish position (your arms past your hips).

Training Tips:

- The spotter should apply resistance above your elbows if you suffer from a hyperextended elbow or other joint pain.

- The spotter's front foot should slide backward as you raise your arms up to the mid-range position and forward as you lower your arms to the start/finish position.

- Keep your hands open (your fingers extended).

- Avoid using your legs and moving your torso forward and backward. Movement should only occur at your shoulder joints.

- Raise your arms only to the point at which they're parallel to the floor.

- Your palms should be facing each other in the mid-range position.

- Do this exercise with one limb at a time if you have a shoulder or an arm injury, a gross difference in the strength between your limbs or desire a training variation.

- After reaching muscular fatigue, you can overload your muscles further by having the spotter lift your arms to the mid-range position and then push them back to the start/finish position as you resist for 3 to 5 nega-tive-only repetitions.

BENT-OVER RAISE

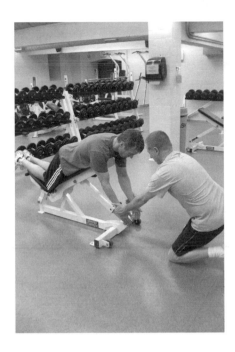

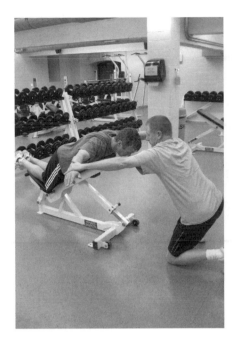

Start/Finish Position   *Mid-Range Position*

Muscles Strengthened: posterior deltoid, trapezius (middle portion) and rhomboids

Suggested Repetitions: 5 to 10 (or 30 to 60 seconds)

Start/Finish Position: Kneel on the seat pad of an adjustable incline bench. Lie forward against the bench, position your arms so that they're perpendicular to your torso and open your hands (extend your fingers). Straighten your arms and point your palms toward each other. The spotter should stand or kneel in front of you and apply resistance against your wrists.

Performance Description: Keeping your arms fairly straight, raise your arms sideways until they're parallel to the floor as the spotter applies resistance evenly throughout the full range of motion. Pause briefly in this mid-range position (your arms parallel to the floor) and then resist as the spotter pushes your arms back to the start/finish position (your arms hanging down).

Training Tips:

- The spotter should apply resistance above your elbows if you suffer from a hyperextended elbow or other joint pain.

- Keep your hands open (your fingers extended).

- Raise your arms only to the point at which they're parallel to the floor.

- Your palms should be facing the floor and your upper arms should be perpendicular to your torso in the mid-range position.

- Do this exercise with one limb at a time if you have a shoulder or an arm injury, a gross difference in the strength between your limbs or desire a training variation.

- After reaching muscular fatigue, you can overload your muscles further by having the spotter lift your arms to the mid-range position and then push them back to the start/finish position as you resist for 3 to 5 negative-only repetitions.

INTERNAL ROTATION

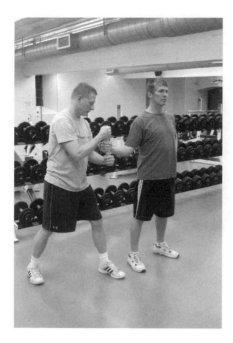

Start/Finish Position

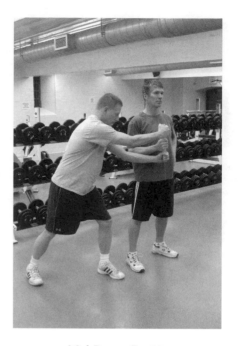

Mid-Range Position

Muscles Strengthened: internal rotators

Suggested Repetitions: 8 to 10 (or 50 to 60 seconds)

Start/Finish Position: Grasp a small stick (or similar object) with your right hand. Place your left hand on your left hip and spread your feet about shoulder-width apart. Place your right elbow against the right side of your torso and bend your right arm so that the angle between your upper and lower arms is about 90 degrees. (By doing this, your right lower arm will be approximately parallel to the floor.) Position the stick away from your mid-section. The spotter should stand alongside you and grasp the stick above and below your right hand.

Performance Description: Keeping the same angle between your upper and lower arms, pull the stick to your mid-section as the spotter applies resistance evenly throughout the full range of motion. Pause briefly in this mid-range position (your hand near your mid-section) and then resist as the spotter pulls the stick back to the start/finish position (your hand away from your mid-section). Repeat the exercise for the other side of your body.

Training Tips:

- Keep your elbow against the side of your torso and your lower arm parallel to the floor.

- Avoid rotating your torso. Movement should only occur at your shoulder joint.

- After reaching muscular fatigue, you can overload your muscles further by having the spotter bring the stick to the mid-range position and then pull it back to the start/finish position as you resist for 3 to 5 negative-only repetitions.

EXTERNAL ROTATION

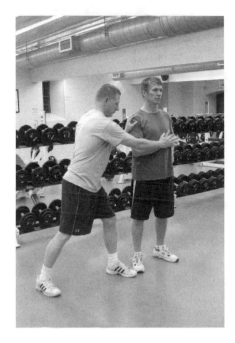

Start/Finish Position

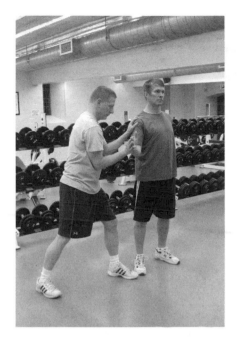

Mid-Range Position

Muscles Strengthened: external rotators

Suggested Repetitions: 8 to 10 (or 50 to 60 seconds)

Start/Finish Position: Place your left hand on your left hip and spread your feet about shoulder-width apart. Place your right elbow against the right side of your torso and bend your right arm so that the angle between your upper and lower arms is about 90 degrees. (By doing this, your right lower arm will be approximately parallel to the floor.) Position your right palm near your mid-section and open your hand (extend your fingers). The spotter should stand alongside you and apply resistance against your right wrist.

Performance Description: Keeping the same angle between your upper and lower arms, push your hand away from your mid-section as the spotter applies resistance evenly throughout the full range of motion. Pause briefly in this mid-range position (your hand away from your mid-section) and then resist as the spotter pushes your hand back to the start/finish position (your hand near your mid-section). Repeat the exercise for the other side of your body.

Training Tips:

- Keep your hand open (your fingers extended).

- Keep your elbow against the side of your torso and your lower arm parallel to the floor.

- Avoid rotating your torso. Movement should only occur at your shoulder joint.

- After reaching muscular fatigue, you can overload your muscles further by having the spotter bring your hand to the mid-range position and then push it back to the start/finish position as you resist for 3 to 5 negative-only repetitions.

BICEP CURL

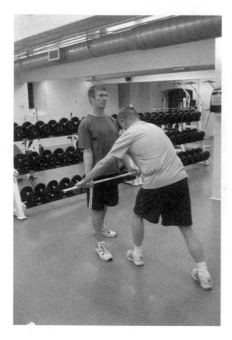

Start/Finish Position

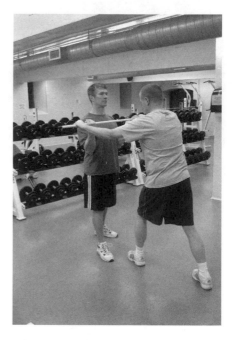

Mid-Range Position

Muscles Strengthened: biceps and forearms

Suggested Repetitions: 5 to 10 (or 30 to 60 seconds)

Start/Finish Position: Grasp a long stick (or similar object) with your hands spaced slightly wider than shoulder-width apart and your palms facing away from you. Spread your feet a comfortable distance apart with one foot slightly in front of the other. Straighten your arms. The spotter should stand in front of you and grasp the stick on the outside of your grip with palms facing down.

Performance Description: Pull the stick below your chin as the spotter applies resistance evenly throughout the full range of motion. Pause briefly in this mid-range position (your arms bent) and then resist as the spotter pulls the stick back to the start/finish position (your arms completely straight).

Training Tips:

- Keep your elbows against the sides of your torso.

- Avoid using your legs and moving your torso forward and backward. Movement should only occur at your elbow joints.

- Do this exercise with one limb at a time if you have a shoulder or an arm injury, a gross difference in the strength between your limbs or desire a training variation.

- After reaching muscular fatigue, you can overload your muscles further by having the spotter lift the stick to the mid-range position and then pull it back to the start/finish position as you resist for 3 to 5 negative-only repetitions.

- This exercise may be contraindicated if you have hyperextended elbows.

TRICEP EXTENSION

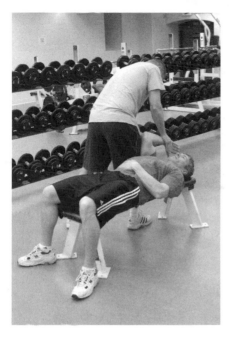

Start/Finish Position

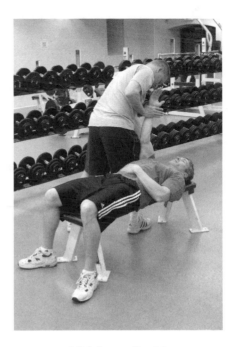

Mid-Range Position

Muscle Strengthened: triceps

Suggested Repetitions: 5 to 10 (or 30 to 60 seconds)

Start/Finish Position: Lie down on a utility bench and place your feet flat on the floor. Position the back of your right upper arm against the spotter's right thigh so that it's perpendicular to the floor and point your right elbow toward your right knee. Place your right hand near the right side of your head with your palm facing your ear and open your hand (extend your fingers). The spotter should apply resistance against your right wrist.

Performance Description: Push your hand up until your arm is almost completely straight as the spotter applies resistance evenly throughout the full range of motion. Pause briefly in this mid-range position (your arm almost completely straight) and then resist as the spotter pushes your lower arm back to the start/finish position (your arm bent). Repeat the exercise for the other side of your body.

Training Tips:

- Keep your hand open (your fingers extended).

- Keep your upper arm perpendicular to the floor and your elbow pointed toward your knee.

- Keep your hips on the bench.

- If you have low-back pain, place your feet on the end of the bench or a stool. This reduces the stress in your low-back region.

- You can also perform this exercise while sitting or standing. In both cases, keep your upper arm perpendicular to the floor and raise and lower your arm behind your head.

- After reaching muscular fatigue, you can overload your muscles further by having the spotter lift your hand to the mid-range position and then push it back to the start/finish position as you resist for 3 to 5 negative-only repetitions.

WRIST PRONATION

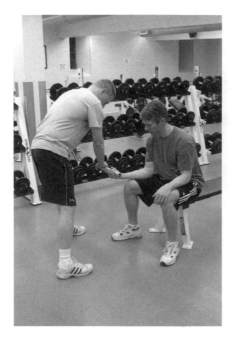

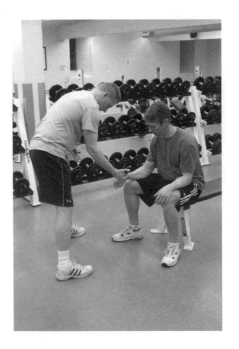

Start/Finish Position   *Mid-Range Position*

Muscles Strengthened: wrist pronators

Suggested Repetitions: 8 to 10 (or 50 to 60 seconds)

Start/Finish Position: Grasp the end of a small stick (or similar object) with your right hand. Sit down near the end of a utility bench and place the back of your right forearm on your right upper leg so that your wrist is over your kneecap and your palm is facing up. Lean forward slightly so that the angle between your upper and lower arms is about 90 degrees or less. The spotter should stand or kneel in front of you and grasp the other end of the stick.

Performance Description: Turn your hand downward as the spotter applies resistance evenly throughout the full range of motion. Pause briefly in this mid-range position (your palm down) and then resist as the spotter pushes the stick back to the start/finish position (your palm up). Repeat the exercise for the other side of your body.

Training Tips:

• Keep your forearm on your upper leg.

• Avoid using your leg and moving your torso forward and backward. Movement should only occur at your wrist joint.

• After reaching muscular fatigue, you can overload your muscles further by having the spotter bring the stick to the mid-range position and then push it back to the start/finish position as you resist for 3 to 5 negative-only repetitions.

WRIST SUPINATION

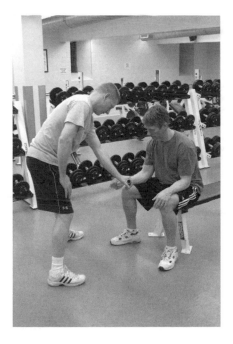

Start/Finish Position

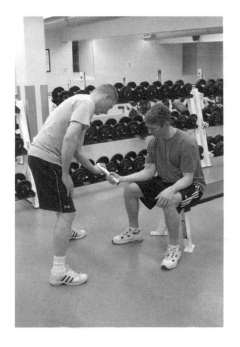

Mid-Range Position

Muscles Strengthened: wrist supinators

Suggested Repetitions: 8 to 10 (or 50 to 60 seconds)

Start/Finish Position: Grasp the end of a small stick (or similar object) with your right hand. Sit down near the end of a utility bench and place the front of your right forearm on your right upper leg so that your wrist is over your kneecap and your palm is facing down. Lean forward slightly so that the angle between your upper and lower arms is about 90 degrees or less. The spotter should stand or kneel in front of you and grasp the other end of the stick.

Performance Description: Turn your hand upward as the spotter applies resistance evenly throughout the full range of motion. Pause briefly in this mid-range position (your palm up) and then resist as the spotter pulls the stick back to the start/finish position (your palm down). Repeat the exercise for the other side of your body.

Training Tips:

• Keep your forearm on your upper leg.

• Avoid using your leg and moving your torso forward and backward. Movement should only occur at your wrist joint.

• After reaching muscular fatigue, you can overload your muscles further by having the spotter bring the stick to the mid-range position and then pull it back to the start/finish position as you resist for 3 to 5 negative-only repetitions.

ABDOMINAL CRUNCH

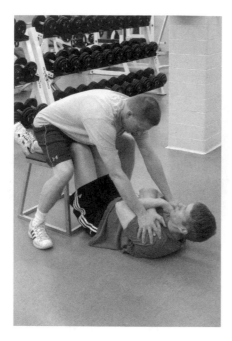

Start/Finish Position

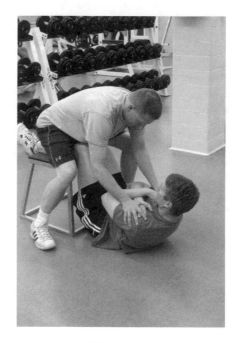

Mid-Range Position

Muscle Strengthened: rectus abdominis

Suggested Repetitions: 8 to 10 (or 50 to 60 seconds)

Start/Finish Position: Lie down on the floor and place the back of your lower legs on a utility bench (or stool). Position your upper legs so that they're perpendicular to the floor and the angle between your upper and lower legs is about 90 degrees. Fold your arms across your chest and bring your head toward your chest so that the upper portion of your shoulder blades doesn't touch the floor. The spotter should sit on your lower legs and apply resistance against the front part of your shoulders.

Performance Description: Pull your torso as close to your upper legs as possible as the spotter applies resistance evenly throughout the full range of motion. Pause briefly in this mid-range position (your torso bent) and then resist as the spotter pushes your torso back to the start/finish position (your torso straight).

Training Tips:

• · Avoid touching the floor with your shoulder blades. This removes the load from your abdominals.

• Avoid snapping your head forward. Movement should only occur at your hip joint and mid-section.

• After reaching muscular fatigue, you can overload your muscles further by having the spotter lift your torso to the mid-range position and then push it back to the start/finish position as you resist for 3 to 5 negative-only repetitions.

• This exercise may be contraindicated if you have low-back pain.

NECK FLEXION

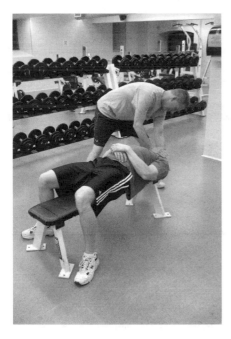
Start/Finish Position

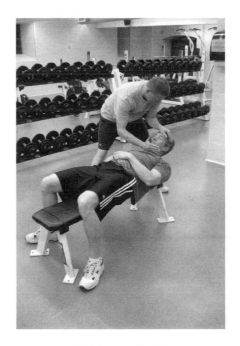
Mid-Range Position

Muscle Strengthened: sternocleidomastoideus

Suggested Repetitions: 8 to 10 (or 50 to 60 seconds)

Start/Finish Position: Lie down on a utility bench and place your feet flat on the floor. Position your head over the end of the back pad. Place your hands on your mid-section. The spotter should stand or kneel alongside your head and apply resistance against your chin with one hand and your forehead with the other.

Performance Description: Pull your head as close to your chest as possible as the spotter applies resistance evenly throughout the full range of motion. Pause briefly in this mid-range position (your chin near your chest) and then resist as the spotter pushes your head back to the start/finish position (your head hanging down).

Training Tips:

• The resistance must be applied carefully since the cervical spine is involved.

• Keep your hips and torso on the bench.

• If you have low-back pain, place your feet flat on the end of the bench or a stool. This reduces the stress in your low-back region.

• You can also perform this exercise while sitting on the floor. In this case, the spotter would sit or kneel behind you and apply resistance against your chin with one hand and your forehead with the other.

• After reaching muscular fatigue, you can overload your muscles further by having the spotter lift your head to the mid-range position and then push it back to the start/finish position as you resist for 3 to 5 negative-only repetitions.

NECK EXTENSION

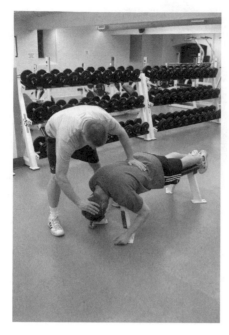

Start/Finish Position

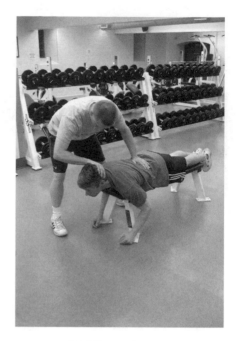

Mid-Range Position

Muscles Strengthened: neck extensors and trapezius (upper portion)

Suggested Repetitions: 8 to 10 (or 50 to 60 seconds)

Start/Finish Position: Lie face down on a utility bench and place your hands on the floor. Position your legs across the length of the back pad and your head over the end of the back pad with your chin near your chest. The spotter should stand or kneel alongside your head and apply resistance against the back of your head with one hand and your back with the other.

Performance Description: Extend your head backward as far as possible as the spotter applies resistance evenly throughout the full range of motion. Pause briefly in this mid-range position (your neck extended) and then resist as the spotter pushes your head back to the start/finish position (your chin near your chest).

Training Tips:

• The resistance must be applied carefully since the cervical spine is involved.

• Keep your torso on the bench.

• You can also perform the exercise while on your hands and knees.

• After reaching muscular fatigue, you can overload your muscles further by having the spotter lift your head to the mid-range position and then push it back to the start/finish position as you resist for 3 to 5 negative-only repetitions.

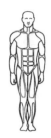

11 Designing and Varying the Strength Program

Your strength program can be designed and varied in countless ways, incorporating a wide assortment of exercises and equipment. But designing and varying the strength program involves much more than merely doing specific exercises and/or using certain equipment.

PROGRAM DESIGN

A number of elements go into program design. What follows are some things that must be considered.

The Training Week

An important aspect of program design is planning the training week. Here are several options for scheduling total-body workouts:

- Do three workouts per week on any non-consecutive days such as Monday/Wednesday/Friday; Monday/Wednesday/Saturday; Tuesday/Thursday/Sunday; or some other combination.

- Do two workouts per week on any non-consecutive days such as Monday/Thursday; Monday/Friday; Tuesday/Friday; Tuesday/Saturday; or some other combination. Note that the two workouts should be scheduled so that the time between them is roughly the same. If the two workouts for the week are on Monday and Thursday, for example, then an individual would have 72 hours between Monday and Thursday and then 96 hours between Thursday and Monday. This is more favorable than if the two workouts for the week are on Monday and Wednesday. Here, an individual would have 48 hours between Monday and Wednesday and then 120 hours between Wednesday and Monday.

- Do one workout every third day such as Monday, Thursday, Sunday, Wednesday, Saturday, Tuesday, Friday and so on. In a three-week period, then, an individual will get seven workouts: One week in which three workouts are done and two weeks in which two workouts are done.

Workouts can be performed three times per week, two times per week, every third day or with whatever scheme is most appropriate for each individual based on age, maturation, personal preferences, social situations and academic and athletic/recreational obligations. Keep in mind that all of these factors will change over time. As a result, it's not always practical to employ a rigid schedule or regular pattern of days to do strength training. The idea, though, is to implement the schedule that best meets your needs and maintains your enthusiasm while giving your body sufficient time to recover from previous workouts so as to avoid overtraining.

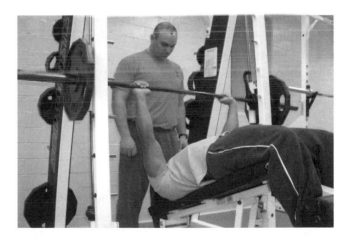

Implement the schedule that best meets your needs and maintains your enthusiasm while giving your body sufficient time to recover from previous workouts.

Volume of Exercises

Recall from Chapter 4 that most people can perform a total-body workout using no more than about 14 exercises. In this case, you should do one exercise for your hips, hamstrings, quadriceps, calves/dorsi flexors, biceps, triceps, abdominals and lower back. Since your shoulder joint permits freedom of movement at a variety of angles, you should perform two exercises for your chest, upper back and shoulders.

If you participate in a combat sport – such as football, rugby, boxing, judo and wrestling – your workout should include an additional two to four exercises for your neck to strengthen and protect your cervical area against catastrophic injury. If you participate in sports or activities that require grip strength – such as baseball, golf and tennis – you should include one exercise for your lower arms (forearms).

There's nothing inherently wrong with doing additional exercises in order to emphasize a particular muscle. But if your level of strength begins to plateau in one or more exercises, it's probably because you're overtraining: You're unable to recover from the volume of your training.

Also keep in mind that placing too much emphasis on one muscle may eventually produce abnormal development and/or create an imbalance between two muscles which can predispose you to injury. For instance, too much emphasis on your chest may lead to a round-shouldered appearance; too much emphasis on your quadriceps may make you susceptible to problems with your hamstrings.

Agonists and Antagonists

At this point, it's necessary to define two terms: agonist and antagonist. An agonist is a muscle that causes movement; an antagonist is a muscle that opposes movement of the agonist. As an example, consider your biceps and triceps. Your biceps on the front of your upper arm bend (or flex) your elbow and your triceps on the back of your upper arm straighten (or extend) your elbow. When one of these muscles acts as an agonist, the other acts as an antagonist. (Note: An agonist is also referred to as a prime mover.)

In general, your muscles are arranged in pairs that have opposing positions and functions. In addition to the biceps-triceps partnership, other agonist/antagonist pairings include your hip abductors and hip adductors; hamstrings and quadriceps; calves and dorsi flexors; chest and upper back; anterior deltoid and posterior deltoid; wrist flexors and wrist extensors; and abdominals and lower back.

It's important to provide agonist/antagonist muscles with an equal – or nearly equal – amount of stimulus. In doing so, you'll ensure that you're not overemphasizing one muscle or underemphasizing another. This, in turn, will reduce your risk of producing abnormal development or creating an imbalance between two muscles. Therefore, you should perform approximately the same volume of training – roughly the same number of exercises, sets and repetitions – for pairs of agonist/antagonist muscles. In short, don't emphasize a particular muscle without also addressing its antagonistic counterpart with a similar volume of training.

Types of Movements

Essentially, there are two types of movements: single joint and multiple joint. A single-joint movement (aka a simple movement or primary movement) involves action of one joint. A good example is a pullover in which the upper arm moves about the shoulder joint. The advantage of a single-joint movement is that it usually provides muscle isolation.

A multiple-joint movement (aka compound movement or secondary movement) involves action of more than one joint. A good example is a lat pulldown in which the upper arm moves about the shoulder joint and the lower arm moves about the elbow joint. The advantage of a multiple-joint movement is that it engages a relatively large amount of muscle mass in one exercise.

Whenever you do two or more exercises for a large muscle of your torso – your chest, upper back or shoulders – at least one of them should be a single-joint movement. Why is this important?

Multiple-joint movements have a distinct disadvantage, namely a "weak link." When you fatigue in a multiple-joint movement, it's because the resistance has been filtered through a smaller, weaker muscle that exhausts well before a larger, stronger muscle has received a sufficient workload. In an exercise such as the lat pulldown, your biceps are the smaller muscle – the proverbial weak link – and, therefore, will fatigue long before your upper back. In fact, your forearms might fatigue even earlier than your biceps. As a result, your biceps and forearms get an adequate workload but your upper back – which is really the target of the exercise – gets an inadequate workload. So if the exercises that you do for your torso consist entirely of multiple-joint movements, your smaller muscles would receive much more of the workload than your larger muscles.

By including single-joint and multiple-joint movements in your workout, you can obtain the benefits of both types of movements: You get the advantage of a single-joint movement in that you can isolate a large muscle without being hindered by the limited strength of a small muscle. And you get the advantage of a multiple-joint movement in that you can address a relatively large amount of muscle mass in one exercise.

Multiple-joint movements have another disadvantage. In a multiple-joint movement, not all muscles are exercised throughout a full range of motion. For instance, the leg press is a multiple-joint movement that involves the hips, quadriceps and hamstrings. When doing this exercise, you'll "feel" it in your hips and quadriceps but not so much in your hamstrings since the range of motion for that muscle is limited. On the other hand, a leg curl is a single-joint movement that stimulates the hamstrings over a much greater range of motion.

This doesn't mean that it would be totally wrong if you only perform multiple-joint movements for a particular muscle. Your workouts will be more efficient and productive, however, if you do a single-joint movement to

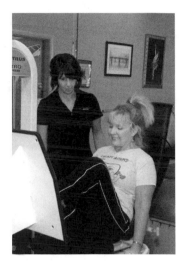

The advantage of a multiple-joint movement is that it engages a relatively large amount of muscle mass in one exercise. (Photo by Pilar Martinez.)

offset the limitations of a multiple-joint movement.

Order of Exercise

As a reminder, you should train your muscles from largest to smallest. Generally speaking, the order of exercise in a total-body workout would be hips, upper legs (hamstrings and quadriceps), lower legs (calves or dorsi flexors), torso (chest, upper back and shoulders), upper arms (biceps and triceps), abdominals and lower back.

If included, exercises for your neck should be done at the beginning of your workout or just after your lower body (prior to exercises for your torso); exercises for your lower arms (forearms) should be done just after your upper arms.

The aforementioned order of exercise would still apply to a split routine (in which your muscles are split into several workouts instead of one total-body workout). In a workout that's designed to target only your chest, shoulders and triceps, for example, you should still address those muscles from largest to smallest.

Exercise Options

Summaries of exercises that can be done with free weights (barbells and dumbbells), machines (selectorized and plate-loaded) and manual resistance appear in Appendices A, B and C, respectively. Naturally, your exercise options are based on the available equipment.

Given the wide assortment of exercise options, the design of a workout can have almost an infinite number of possibilities. The only limits are the equipment and your imagination.

PROGRAM VARIATION

At some point in your strength training, you'll likely reach a plateau in your performance. Quite often, this is a result of overtraining. In this case, your volume of training is so great that your muscular system is overstressed (or overworked). In effect, the demands of your training have exceeded your ability to recover. Here, you simply need to reduce your volume of training (in terms of the number of workouts, exercises and/or sets).

Sometimes, however, your performance will plateau because you're doing the same thing over and over again for lengthy periods of time. In this case, your strength program has become a form of unproductive manual labor that's monotonous, dull and unchallenging.

Simply checking your records will reveal if you've reached a plateau. You should review your records carefully, however. If you think that you've plateaued in a certain exercise, you must consider your performance in earlier exercises of that workout. For instance, suppose that you did 10 repetitions with 120 pounds on the leg extension for five consecutive workouts. At first glance, it may not seem as if your quadriceps have gotten any stronger. But what if the resistance that you used on the leg press increased from 250 pounds to 275 pounds during those same five workouts? This means that the load on your hips, hamstrings and quadriceps increased by 10% or an average of 2% per workout. In other words, your quadriceps were increasingly more pre-fatigued by the leg press in your workouts each time prior to performing the leg extension. If true, there's little doubt that your quadriceps did get stronger. In fact, simply being able to duplicate your past performances on the leg extension would actually be quite a feat, although that wouldn't be readily apparent. Similarly, if the resistance that you used on the bicep curl plateaus, it could be because your biceps are being exposed to increasingly heavier loads earlier in your workout when you do multiple-joint movements for your torso such as the lat pulldown, seated row or upright row. So, you

must examine your entire workout in order to determine whether or not you have indeed reached a plateau.

Keep in mind that unless you're a beginner, you won't be able to improve your performance in every exercise from one workout to the next. Be that as it may, you should observe gradual improvements in your performance over the course of several weeks. If you fail to make a progression in an exercise by this time – in the amount of resistance and/or the number of repetitions – you should vary some aspect of your strength program.

There are several ways that this may be accomplished. In general, you can vary three main components of your strength program: your workouts, exercises and sets/repetitions.

Varying Workouts

There are a number of ways that you can vary your workouts. For instance, you can change your workouts on a daily basis by doing different workouts on different days such as Workout A on Monday, Workout B on Wednesday and Workout C on Friday. You can also change your workouts on a weekly or monthly basis. Or you can simply change them as needed.

Regardless, the idea is to vary your workouts on a fairly regular basis. Some strength coaches have many different workouts for their athletes with varying themes. For example, the athletes might be assigned barbell-only, dumbbell-only, iso-lateral, "no-hands," "no-feet," pre-exhaustion or negative-only workouts.

Varying Exercises

You have three basic options available to vary your exercises: Specifically, you can rearrange the order, change the equipment and alternate the exercises.

Rearrange the Order

One of the easiest ways that you can integrate variety into your training is to rearrange the order in which you do exercises for a particular muscle. Suppose, for example, that you desire a change in the way that you train your chest. If you've been doing the bench press followed by the bent-arm fly, you can add variety by simply switching the two exercises. In other words, you can perform the bent-arm fly first and the bench press second.

Be aware that whenever you change the order in which you do exercises, you must adjust the levels of resistance. So if you do the bent-arm fly first (instead of second), your chest and shoulders will be fresh and, therefore, you should increase the resistance in that exercise. And if you do the bench press second (instead of first), your chest and shoulders will be fatigued and, therefore, you must decrease the resistance in that exercise.

An additional possibility is to rearrange the order in which you train your muscles. Rather than go from chest to upper back to shoulders, you might start with shoulders, proceed to upper back and then finish with chest. So a six-exercise sequence for your torso of bench press, bent-arm fly, seated row, pullover, shoulder press and shoulder shrug could be changed to shoulder shrug, shoulder press, pullover, seated row, bent-arm fly and bench press. In fact, these six exercises alone could be rearranged for 720 different sequences. [Six exercises can be placed in six different ordered positions. The first exercise that's chosen can be put in six possible spots, the second exercise can be put in one of the five remaining spots, the third exercise can be put in one of the four remaining spots and so on. Therefore, the total number of possible arrangements for six exercises is 6 x 5 x 4 x 3 x 2 x 1 = 720.] Once again, remember that you'll need to adjust the levels of resistance any time that you rearrange the order of exercises.

Change the Equipment

Another way that you can vary the exercises is to change the equipment that you use. Say that you've been doing the bicep curl with a barbell for quite some time and, consequently, desire a change of pace. In this situation, you can perform a bicep curl with another type of equipment such as dumbbells, machines (selectorized or plate-loaded) or manual resistance. There's even variety within selectorized machines since some have one dependent movement arm while others

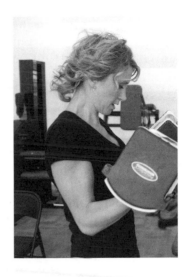

A change of pace from a bicep curl with a barbell is to do the exercise with another type of equipment such as dumbbells, machines or manual resistance. (Photo provided by Luke Carlson.)

have two independent movement arms (meaning that they function separately). Obviously, the extent to which you can change the equipment depends on what's available.

Alternate the Exercises

A third means of varying exercises is to alternate them with other ones that employ the same muscles. Consider this: The seated row is a multiple-joint movement that engages your upper back, biceps and forearms. And so do other multiple-joint movements that involve rowing, chinning and pulling. This includes the bench row, bent-over row, chin-up, pull-up, underhand lat pulldown and overhand lat pulldown. Therefore, any of these exercises are potential substitutes for the seated row. Once again, the availability of equipment will determine how much you can alternate the exercises.

Besides providing for variety, periodically alternating your exercises (and/or equipment) has another advantage: It allows you to train your muscles through different ranges of motion. In this way, you can target your muscles in a more complete and comprehensive manner.

Varying Sets/Repetitions

A final component of your strength program that you can vary is the way that you do a set which essentially is the way that you do a repetition. Ordinarily, repetitions are done in a bilateral manner, meaning with both limbs at the same time. But you can do at least six other variations including negative-only, negative-accentuated, duosymmetric-polycontractile, unilateral, modified-cadence and extended-pause repetitions.

A few words of caution: Although the ensuing ways of varying a repetition may sound simple, a reasonably high level of skill is required to do them in a manner that's safe and productive. Because of this, you shouldn't attempt to employ these advanced applications in your strength program until you can demonstrate proper technique when you do repetitions in a bilateral fashion.

Negative-Only Repetitions

You can perform repetitions in a negative-only manner by having a partner raise the resistance and you lower it. Essentially, the partner does the positive (or concentric) work and the lifter does the negative (or eccentric) work. To illustrate, here's how you'd do negative-only repetitions on the leg curl: With no help from you, your partner brings the movement arm to the mid-range position (your heels near your hips). Then, your partner releases the movement arm and you slowly lower the resistance to the start/finish position (your legs straight). Repeat the procedure for the desired number of repetitions.

As noted in Chapter 4, your eccentric strength is always greater than your concentric strength in the same exercise. In other words, you can always lower a greater amount of resistance than you can raise (again, in the same exercise). This means that you can use more resistance for repetitions that are done in a negative-only manner than you can for repetitions that are done in a traditional manner. How much more? If you're performing negative-only repetitions for the first time, start with about 10% more resistance than you're normally capable of handling. So if you most recently used 150 pounds on an exercise in the traditional manner, increase the resistance by about 15 pounds – to 165 pounds – for your first attempt at a set of negative-only repetitions. When you attain the maximum number of negative-only

repetitions, you should increase the resistance for your next workout.

To achieve the best results, negative-only repetitions should be done slowly. In general, each negative-only repetition should be performed in about six to eight seconds, depending on the range of motion. (An exercise with a large range of motion should take longer to complete than an exercise with a short one.) Chapter 4 discusses appropriate time frames for training your muscles in the anaerobic domain. For most of the population, this is about 90 to 120 seconds for a hip exercise, 60 to 90 seconds for a leg exercise and 30 to 60 seconds for a torso exercise. Based on these windows of time, then, an eight-second negative-only repetition would translate into repetition ranges of about 11 to 15 for the hips, 8 to 11 for the legs and 4 to 8 for the torso.

Performing negative-only repetitions is extremely demanding. For this reason, they shouldn't be done in any given exercise more than once per week.

Negative-Accentuated Repetitions

The major disadvantage of negative-only repetitions is that at least one other person is almost always required to lift the weight. For the most part, you can do negative-only repetitions without needing help from someone else in a handful of exercises that involve your bodyweight as resistance such as push-ups, dips, chin-ups, pull-ups and abdominal crunches. As an example, you can do negative-only chin-ups by stepping or climbing up to the mid-range position (your arms bent) and lowering your body under control to the start/finish position (your arms completely straight). Stated otherwise, your lower body does the positive work and your upper body does the negative work.

The value of negative-accentuated repetitions is that they emphasize the eccentric component of an exercise yet they can be performed without any assistance from another individual. When doing negative-accentuated repetitions, the positive work is shared by both limbs but the negative work is done by only one limb. In other words, the resistance is raised with both arms or legs and then lowered with only one arm or leg. As a result, the resistance is literally twice as much during the negative phase as it is during the positive phase.

Although it's impossible to perform negative-accentuated repetitions with a barbell, most machines permit you to do so. For instance, you'd perform negative-accentuated repetitions on the leg extension as follows: Using both legs, raise the resistance to the mid-range position (your legs completely straight) and pause briefly. Move your left leg away from the roller pad and hold the resistance momentarily with your right leg. Lower the resistance slowly and steadily to the start/finish position (your leg bent) with your right leg. Raise the resistance to the mid-range position with both legs and continue the preceding sequence using your left leg to lower the resistance. Repeat the procedure for the desired number of repetitions.

Similar to negative-only repetitions, the resistance should be lowered in about six to eight seconds. As a starting point, use about 70% of the resistance that you normally handle in the traditional fashion. So if you most recently used 100 pounds on an exercise, start with about 70 pounds for negative-accentuated repetitions. In the case of negative-accentuated exercise, appropriate repetition ranges for most of the population are about 15 to 20 for the hips, 10 to 15 for the legs and 5 to 10 for the torso. (Note that these are the total repetitions for both limbs, not the total repetitions for each limb.)

One final point: It's important that you maintain a stable position when doing negative-accentuated repetitions. In particular, avoid twisting or turning your torso to safeguard your lower back.

Duosymmetric-Polycontractile Repetitions

The term duosymmetric-polycontractile – or duo-poly, for short – was first introduced in the mid-1970s as a style of performing repetitions with machines that had independent movement arms, something that was fairly unique at the time. Nowadays, many machines are available with independent movement arms thereby giving you the option of executing duo-poly repetitions.

If you have access to a bicep-curl machine with independent movement arms, you can perform duo-poly repetitions in this manner: Using both arms, raise the resistance to the mid-range position (your arms bent) and pause briefly. Lower the resistance to the start/finish position (your arm completely straight) with your right arm while keeping your left arm in the mid-range position. Raise the resistance to the mid-range position with your right arm and pause briefly. Lower the resistance to the start/finish position with your left arm while keeping your right arm in the mid-range position. Repeat the procedure for the desired number of repetitions. Incidentally, you can also perform duo-poly repetitions for your biceps with dumbbells in the manner described here.

Unilateral Repetitions

As a variation in the repetition style, many exercises can be done in a unilateral manner, meaning with one limb at a time. Dr. Ken Leistner – who has been a recognized and respected authority on strength training since the mid-1970s – states, "One-limb work is effective because, in almost all cases, it is more intense than the same exercise done with two limbs working simultaneously."

Besides making the exercise more intense, unilateral repetitions are advisable for those who have a strength imbalance between one side of

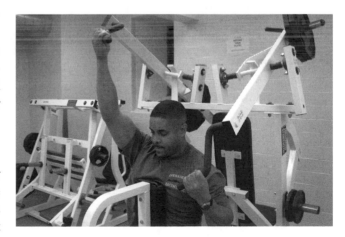

Besides making the exercise more intense, unilateral repetitions are advisable for those who have a strength imbalance between one side of their body and the other. (Photo by Peter Silletti.)

their body and the other. Unilateral repetitions are also recommended for individuals with hypertension since it dampens the blood-pressure response that's associated with strength training.

Machines that are equipped with independent movement arms allow you to do unilateral repetitions. In addition, you can do unilateral repetitions with dumbbells and manual resistance.

Modified-Cadence Repetitions

Another option is to vary the cadence or speed with which you normally perform your repetitions. One cadence that continues to receive a considerable amount of attention is the SuperSlow® Protocol which was introduced by Ken Hutchins in the early 1980s. The basic cadence for SuperSlow® repetitions is to raise the resistance in 10 seconds and lower it in 5 seconds. (In shorthand, this would be written as a 10/5 speed with the first digit indicating the number of seconds to do the positive phase and the second digit indicating the number of seconds to do the negative phase.)

Other popular variations of repetition speed include 4/4, 8/8 and 10/10. A single set consisting of one 30/30 repetition can also be done; in other words, one repetition that takes 60 seconds to complete with 30 seconds allotted for the positive phase and 30 seconds for the negative phase. Keep in mind that you'll need to adjust your repetition ranges any time that you modify the duration of a repetition.

Extended-Pause Repetitions

As pointed out in Chapter 4, it's important to pause briefly in the mid-range position of each repetition. There are at least three reasons for emphasizing the mid-range position. First, it enables you to strengthen an otherwise weak position in your range of motion. Second, it allows you to focus your attention on your muscles when they're fully contracted. Third, it permits a smooth transition between the raising and lowering of the weight thereby helping to reduce the influence of momentum.

As a repetition variation, the brief pause in the mid-range position can be done for a slightly longer duration, perhaps in three or four seconds. Using this technique is also an excellent tool to employ with beginners in the initial stages of training in order for them to understand the concept and value of pausing in the mid-range position. Once again, remember that you'll need to adjust your repetition ranges any time that you modify the duration of a repetition.

Note that an extended pause in the mid-range position essentially involves a mild isometric contraction that tends to elevate blood pressure beyond that which is normally encountered in strength training. As such, individuals who have hypertension shouldn't employ this technique.

PRACTICAL APPLICATIONS

Based on the information contained here and in Chapter 4, three sample total-body workouts are shown in Figure 11.1; a sample two-day split routine is shown in Figure 11.2. These sample workouts will give you some ideas for designing and varying your strength program.

How often should a strength program be varied? For the most part, this depends on the individual. But in general, people who are just initiating a strength program or haven't been doing one for too long probably won't require much variety; early on, the program is still too novel to be monotonous or dull. Those who are more experienced will need to vary their strength program in some way on a regular basis.

Figure 11.1: Sample total-body workouts

WORKOUT A	WORKOUT B	WORKOUT C
Neck Flexion (MR)	Neck Lateral Flexion/R (SM)	Neck Extension (SM)
Neck Extension (MR)	Neck Lateral Flexion/L (SM)	Neck Flexion (MR)
Leg Press (PM)	Hip Adduction (SM)	Hip Abduction (MR)
Prone Leg Curl (SM)	Seated Leg Curl (SM)	Prone Leg Curl (PM)
Leg Extension (MR)	Leg Extension (SM)	Leg Extension (PM)
Standing Calf Raise (DB)	Dorsi Flexion (MR)	Seated Calf Raise (PM)
Dip (BW)	Bent-Arm Fly (DB)	Incline Press (BB)
Bent-Arm Fly (MR)	Bench Press (BB)	Pec Fly (SM)
Chin-Up (BW)	Pullover (EZ)	Bent-Over Row (DB)
Pullover (PM)	Seated Row (PM)	Pullover (DB)
Shoulder Press (BB)	Internal Rotation (MR)	Shoulder Shrug (TB)
Lateral Raise (SM)	External Rotation (MR)	Upright Row (BB)
Bicep Curl (MR)	Bicep Curl (EZ)	Tricep Extension (MR)
Tricep Extension (CC)	Tricep Extension (DB)	Bicep Curl (DB)
Wrist Flexion (BB)	Wrist Extension (DB)	Wrist Flexion (DB)
Side Bend (DB)	Abdominal Crunch (MR)	Torso Rotation (SM)
Back Extension (BW)	Back Extension (SM)	Back Extension (BW)

Equipment Codes: BB = Barbell; BW = Bodyweight; CC = Cable Column; DB = Dumbbells; EZ = EZ Curl Bar; MR = Manual Resistance; PM = Plate-Loaded Machine; SM = Selectorized Machine; TB = Trap Bar

Figure 11.2: Sample two-day split routine

WORKOUT A	WORKOUT B
Deadlift (TB)	Neck Flexion (MR)
Seated Leg Curl (PM)	Neck Extension (PM)
Leg Extension (SM)	Chest Press (SM)
Calf Extension (SM)	Bent-Arm Fly (DB)
Pullover (PM)	Shoulder Press (BB)
Pull-Up (BW)	Bent-Over Raise (MR)
Bicep Curl (CC)	Tricep Extension (EZ)
Wrist Flexion (BB)	Torso Rotation (SM)
	Back Extension (SM)

Equipment Codes: BB = Barbell; BW = Bodyweight; CC = Cable Column; DB = Dumbbells; EZ = EZ Curl Bar; MR = Manual Resistance; PM = Plate-Loaded Machine; SM = Selectorized Machine; TB = Trap Bar

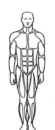

12 Rehabilitative Training

Injuries are an unforeseen, inevitable and unfortunate fact of life. In spite of how much you prepare, many injuries are purely the result of being in the wrong place at the wrong time.

In general, injuries can be either traumatic or non-traumatic. Traumatic injuries are more serious and severe such as fractures of bones and tears of muscle or connective tissue. Quite often, these types of injuries require surgical intervention. On the other hand, non-traumatic injuries are less serious and severe such as tendinitis and bursitis. Sometimes, these types of injuries simply result from overuse. No matter what kind of injury, it's important for you to consult with a qualified sportsmedical specialist such as an orthopedic physician, physical therapist or athletic trainer.

In many instances, an individual who suffers an injury ends up eliminating all forms of physical training, including those that involve uninjured body parts. Yet, it's extremely important to continue some type of physical training whenever possible even in the event of an injury.

According to many authorities, a muscle begins to lose strength (and size) if it doesn't receive an adequate amount of stimulation within about 96 hours of a previous workout. There's some anecdotal evidence suggesting that it may be a bit longer than this time frame, at least for some individuals. But it's clear that a loss of strength (and size) will occur after some period of extended inactivity. Moreover, the rate of strength loss is most rapid during the first few weeks. Because of this, rehabilitative training can prevent a significant loss of not only strength (and size) but also aerobic, anaerobic and metabolic fitness. This, of course, is provided that the training can be done in a pain-free – or nearly pain-free – manner.

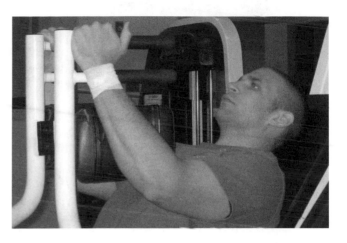

It's extremely important to continue some type of physical training whenever possible even in the event of an injury.

Regardless of whether the injury is traumatic or non-traumatic, it will have some degree of impact on your physical training; some injuries – especially those that are traumatic – might not permit any physical training whatsoever. Nevertheless, you can often train parts of your body that aren't related to the afflicted area. And in many cases, you may even be able to address the injured body part directly.

PRUDENT METHODS

There are several different options and adjustments that you can use to continue training an injured area or body part in a safe, sensible and pain-free manner. It should be noted that these methods aren't intended for those injuries that are viewed as being very serious or extremely painful. As such, you should receive approval from a qualified sportsmedical specialist before initiating any prescription for rehabilitative training.

You can perform rehabilitative training by considering and then applying the following nine guidelines:

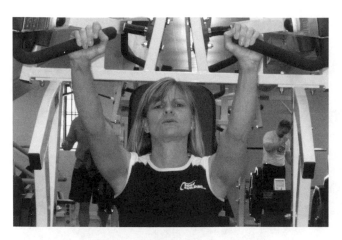

If you want to continue training an injured body part, your first step is to decrease the amount of resistance that you normally use in exercises that involve the afflicted area.

1. Lighten the weight.

If you want to continue training an injured body part, your first step is to decrease the amount of resistance that you normally use in exercises that involve the afflicted area. This is usually the easiest and most straightforward recommendation.

Suppose that you have a knee injury and, as a result, you experience pain in your patellar tendon when doing the leg extension with your usual level of resistance. Decreasing the amount of weight will produce less stress on the tendon and perhaps allow you to perform the exercise in a pain-free – or nearly pain-free – manner. The amount that you reduce the weight depends on the extent and nature of your injury.

2. Slow the speed of movement.

Often done in conjunction with decreasing the amount of weight for an exercise is using a slower speed of movement. Slowing the repetition speed decreases the orthopedic stress that's placed on a given joint.

As the injury heals, you can gradually return to your preferred speed of movement. Then again, you may find that the slower speed of movement is more appealing and continue using it after you complete your rehabilitative training. Or perhaps you might even adopt the slower speed of movement to train other body parts that

aren't injured. Incidentally, slowing down the speed of movement also requires using a reduced amount of weight thereby lowering the orthopedic stress even further.

3. Change the exercise angle.

If pain persists during certain exercises that involve an injured body part, it may be possible for you to change the angle of the exercise. This essentially alters – and restricts – the angle through which your limb is moved.

You can use this option with many exercises for your torso, particularly those that involve your shoulder joint. This is especially important because the mobility and instability of the shoulder make it highly prone to injury. In fact, one of the most frequently injured body parts is the shoulder. A common problem in this joint is known as shoulder-impingement syndrome, a general term used to describe pain that's often characterized as tightness or pinching in the shoulder.

Suppose that you have slight shoulder impingement when doing the bench press. In some cases, changing the angle of the exercise from supine (flat) to decline – in other words, switching from the bench press to the decline press – will produce significantly less orthopedic stress on your shoulder joint.

Likewise, some people experience pain due to shoulder impingement when moving the bar behind their head during the shoulder press and overhand lat pulldown. Generally speaking, the discomfort in both of these exercises can be lessened considerably by changing the angle of the push and pull. This can be done by performing the exercises with the bar traveling in front of the head rather than behind the head.

This option has limited – though useful – applications for aerobic and anaerobic training. If you have low-back pain, for example, you can pedal a cycle in a recumbent position rather than an upright one. The angle of the seat places the torso in a position that decreases the amount of stress in the lower back. (And the seat itself provides support for the lower back which also decreases the stress.)

4. Use a different grip or hand position.

Many times, there's less orthopedic stress when you use a different grip or hand position. Once again, this is extremely relevant when addressing the shoulder joint. If you have a slight pain in your shoulder when doing an exercise such as the bench press, it's quite possible that there will be a significant reduction in pain by simply changing the position of your hands from that used with a barbell to a parallel grip (palms facing each other) with dumbbells. In exercises for your torso, changing the position of your hands in this way causes the head of your humerus (your upper-arm bone) to rotate laterally which may relieve the stress in your shoulder joint.

As noted in Chapter 8, every exercise that can be performed with a barbell can also be performed with dumbbells. These exercises include the bench press, incline press, decline press, shoulder press, upright row, shoulder shrug, bicep curl, tricep extension, wrist flexion and stiff-leg deadlift. As such, you have an option for varying the position of your hands in exercises for just about every major muscle in your torso. Additionally, some machines offer more than one grip/hand position.

5. Perform different exercises.

Yet another option for rehabilitative training is to perform different exercises that require the same muscle groups. For instance, if you simply can't perform any type of lat pulldown without experiencing shoulder pain or discomfort then perhaps you can employ another exercise that addresses the same muscles albeit in a pain-free manner. In this situation, a seated row or bench row can be substituted for the lat pulldown. Both of these exercises involve the same major muscles, namely your upper back, biceps and forearms.

This guideline can also be applied to aerobic and anaerobic training. If you can't run due to a sprained ankle, for example, you may be able to perform aerobic and anaerobic training with a non-weightbearing activity such as an upright or a recumbent cycle.

6. Bypass the injured area.

Some exercises with machines and manual resistance allow you to apply the resistance above a joint so that it doesn't involve an injured area. Presume that you sprained your wrist and, consequently, exercises for your torso are difficult or uncomfortable – if not impossible – to perform with barbells and dumbbells. In this case, however, you could still use machines and manual resistance to perform a variety of exercises that target the major muscles of your torso without involving your wrist joint. Machine exercises that bypass the wrist area include the pec fly (aka the chest fly), pullover and lateral raise; manual-resistance exercises that bypass the wrist area include the bent-arm fly, front raise, lateral raise and bent-over raise. Actually, you could still perform the aforementioned exercises and others with machines and manual resistance even if your wrist was immobilized in a cast.

Also consider this: If you ruptured your patellar tendon or medial collateral ligament and your leg was placed in a knee immobilizer, it wouldn't be possible for you to perform any multiple-joint movements that address your hips such as the deadlift or leg press. It would be possible, however, to avoid your knee joint and train your hips in a safe and effective fashion – despite the immobilizer – by doing a single-joint

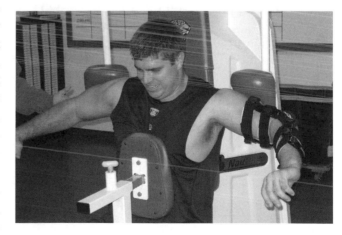

Some exercises with machines and manual resistance allow you to apply the resistance above a joint so that it doesn't involve an injured area. (Photo provided by Mark Asanovich.)

181

movement with machines or manual resistance such as hip abduction or hip adduction.

7. Limit the range of motion.

There's a good possibility that pain only occurs at certain points in your range of motion (ROM) such as the start/finish position or mid-range position of the repetition. In either case, you can restrict your ROM for the exercise. For example, an injury such as a hyperextended elbow is especially painful in the start/finish position of the bicep curl. In this instance, you should stop short of lowering the weight all the way down; by the same token, if pain occurs in the mid-range position, you should stop short of full flexion or extension. As the injured area heals over a period of time, you can gradually and carefully increase your ROM until it's possible for you to perform repetitions that are pain-free throughout a full ROM.

Nowadays, many machines offer range-limiting devices. This enables you to restrict your ROM in a precise, repeatable manner. As a matter of fact, the ROM can sometimes be adjusted in fractional increments without exiting the machine. By the way, it's a good idea to document your ROM (as well as the resistance and repetitions) during rehabilitative training in order to monitor your progress.

Sometimes, your pain-free ROM may be restricted to a specific joint angle plus or minus a few degrees. In this case, you can perform an isometric contraction of varying durations to train your muscles at pain-free positions. One way to accomplish this is to use your good limb to raise the weight to the pain-free position of your injured limb. At this point, you'd transfer or "hand off" the weight to your injured limb. Then, you'd exert force against this resistance without changing the angle of your injured limb. You can also exert force isometrically against another person who's applying manual resistance.

This option can be incorporated during aerobic and anaerobic training. If you have knee pain while cycling, you can lower the height of the seat thereby reducing the ROM of your knee joint.

8. Exercise the good limb.

If all else fails, you can still train your unaffected limb. Here's an example: Suppose that you had shoulder surgery and, as a result, your left arm was placed in a sling. Obviously, the sling wouldn't allow you to perform any exercises that involved any ROM whatsoever for the left side of your torso. Even so, you could do exercises for the right side of your torso.

This is of great consequence to the rehabilitative process because many studies have shown that training a muscle on one side of the body has some effect on the contralateral muscle (the same muscle on the opposite side of the body). This phenomenon – which first came to light way back in 1894 – has been referred to by several different names including bilateral transfer, cross education and cross transfer.

Although the effect is small, the effect is real. A review and meta-analysis of 13 studies and updated findings of another three studies examined the contralateral effect. After pooling the data of these 16 studies, the researchers determined that strength in the untrained limb improved by an average of 7.6%.

Just how well this bodes for rehabilitative training was graphically demonstrated in a rather novel study. In the study, two groups of subjects had their non-dominant wrist, thumb and hand immobilized in a fiberglass cast for a period of 21 days. During that time, one group trained their dominant (non-casted) arm five days per week and the other group did not. The group that didn't train their non-casted arm showed a 14.7% decrease in the strength of their casted arm. Meanwhile, the group that trained their non-casted arm showed a 2.2% increase in the strength of their casted arm (as well as a 23.8% increase in the strength of their non-casted arm). In addition, the group that didn't train their non-casted arm had a 4.3% decrease in the size of their casted arm. Meanwhile, the group that trained their non-casted arm had a 1.1% decrease in the size of their casted arm (as well as a 2.9% increase in the size of their non-casted arm).

In summary, those who trained their non-casted arm experienced an increase in strength

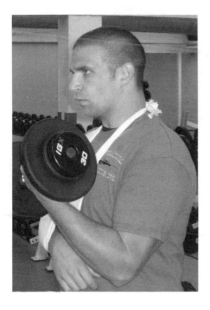

Many studies have shown that training a muscle on one side of the body has some effect on the contralateral muscle (the same muscle on the opposite side of the body).

in their casted (untrained) arm and a smaller decrease in size in their casted arm compared to those who didn't train their non-casted arm.

Researchers have explored a number of possible mechanisms - muscular, neural, spinal cord, cortical and subcortical – but don't know the exact reason why the contralateral effect occurs. For instance, support for a muscular mechanism comes from studies that have found some degree of muscle activity in the untrained limb; and support for a neural mechanism comes from studies that have found a significant increase in strength without a significant increase in size. Actually, the collective efforts of two or more mechanisms may be responsible for this phenomenon.

Machines with independent movement arms enable you to do unilateral training – exercising one limb at a time – in a safe and comfortable fashion. You can also use dumbbells and manual resistance for unilateral training.

9. Exercise unaffected body parts.

In the event that you can't train an injured area due to an unreasonable amount of pain or discomfort, you can still perform exercises for your uninjured body parts. So, if you have a hip or knee injury that doesn't allow you to do any exercises for your lower body, you can train your entire torso (provided that the exercises are done

while you're sitting or lying and not standing). Likewise, if you have a dislocated shoulder or a torn rotator cuff that doesn't allow you to do any exercises for your torso, you can train your entire lower body along with your arms and mid-section (provided that the exercises don't indirectly produce shoulder pain).

Once again, this guideline is also appropriate for aerobic and anaerobic training. Suppose that you have a hip, a leg or an ankle injury that prohibits you from doing any aerobic or anaerobic training for your lower body. A few commercial devices are available that enable you to do aerobic and anaerobic training exclusively with the muscles of your torso such as a rope-climbing machine or an upper-body ergometer. (An ergometer is a device that measures work.)

PRUDENT CHOICES

In many instances, you can exercise an injured area or body part in a safe, prudent and pain-free manner. This will prevent a significant loss in strength (and size) as well as aerobic, anaerobic and metabolic fitness. And even though you may not be able to exercise an injured area due to an excessive amount of pain or discomfort, you can still train your uninjured body parts. Once the injured area heals, you can reintroduce exercises that were previously painful to perform.

Remember, though, that the critical factor in the prudent administration of rehabilitative training is pain-free – or nearly pain-free – exercise/activity. That said, it's important to understand that there's a distinct difference between muscular pain and joint pain. Muscular pain isn't necessarily cause for alarm; it's an indication that you're doing high-intensity work and your muscles are being fatigued. Joint pain, however, is something else altogether. Localized pain in a joint usually means that there's some type of structural malady. If you experience pain in your joints while exercising, you're merely aggravating your condition and perhaps even causing further damage by brutalizing the joint infrastructure. Simply, an exercise that produces joint pain must be avoided or altered.

How important is rehabilitative training? According to Ken Mannie, who has more than 25 years of experience as a strength coach in the collegiate ranks, "Our philosophy . . . has always been that strength training is a vital constituent in the rehab process and that all training options for an injured area will be considered before deciding not to address the area."

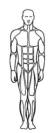

13 Flexibility Training

Flexibility can be defined as the range of motion (ROM) throughout which your joints can move. The best way for you to maintain – or improve – the ROM of your joints is to perform specific stretches to elongate the surrounding muscles.

Flexibility training is undoubtedly the simplest and most effortless type of physical training that you can perform; the exertion level is relatively low and relaxation is an absolute requirement. However, many people often overlook or underemphasize flexibility training.

Increasing flexibility serves at least two purposes. First, being more flexible enables you to exert your strength over a greater ROM. Second, improving your flexibility allows you to move your joints through a greater ROM which makes it easier for you to assume body positions that are otherwise difficult. This, of course, is an advantage in numerous sports including gymnastics, dancing, diving, figure skating and martial arts.

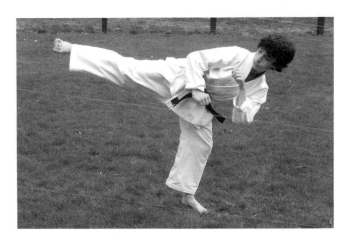

Greater flexibility is an advantage in numerous sports including martial arts. (Photo by John Quigley.)

It should be noted that although stretching after an activity might "feel good," there's no scientific evidence that it reduces muscular soreness. This is also true of stretching before an activity.

FACTORS THAT AFFECT FLEXIBILITY

The most significant contributor to decreased flexibility seems to be inactivity. Obviously, you can avoid at least some loss of flexibility by simply participating in physical training on a regular basis. But besides inactivity, there are many other factors that affect your ROM, some over which you have little or no control.

There's a distinct relationship between your age and your flexibility. The greatest increase in flexibility usually occurs up to and between the ages of 7 and 12. During early adolescence, flexibility tends to level off and thereafter begins to decline with increasing age. Consequently, one of the goals of flexibility training is to slow or perhaps reverse this decline.

Flexibility is also related to gender. Some men are more flexible than some women but, in general, women are more flexible than men (and they retain this advantage throughout life).

In addition, flexibility is influenced by several genetic (or inherited) characteristics such as the insertion points of your tendons as well as your percentage of body fat (especially that which is around your mid-section). Your ROM also has genetic limitations that are structural which include your bones, tendons, ligaments and skin along with the extensibility of your muscles.

As you may already be painfully aware, previous injury to a muscle or connective tissue can affect your ROM. Furthermore, immobilizing a joint during rehabilitation may cause

185

connective tissue to adapt to its shortest functional length thereby reducing the ROM of the joint.

Finally, your body temperature is another factor that influences your flexibility. Muscles and connective tissue that are warmed up will be more flexible and extensible than muscles and connective tissue that are not. Because of this, some authorities recommend that stretching should be performed after you've completed your physical training when your body temperature is higher.

ASSESSING FLEXIBILITY

It's difficult to assess flexibility in a fair manner. For one thing, some measurements of flexibility can be misleading. A perfect example of this is the traditional sit-and-reach test in which a person sits down on the floor with straight legs and reaches forward as far as possible. This test is often used to measure the flexibility of the lower back and hamstrings. A sit-and-reach test, however, doesn't take into consideration limb lengths. Everything else being equal, those with long arms and/or short legs have a distinct anatomical advantage in a sit-and-reach test. These individuals might appear to be quite flexible but may actually be quite inflexible. Conversely, those with short arms and/or long legs have a distinct anatomical disadvantage in a sit-and-reach test. These individuals might appear to be quite inflexible but may actually be quite flexible. In the case of a sit-and-reach test, using a goniometer to measure the angle of flexion between the lumbar spine and upper legs yields an appraisal of flexibility that's more impartial. (A goniometer is a protractor-like instrument with two movable arms that enable you to measure joint angles.)

It should be noted, too, that flexibility is joint-specific; a high degree of flexibility in one joint doesn't necessarily indicate a high degree of flexibility in another joint. Along these lines, it wouldn't be unusual for flexibility to vary from one side of the body to the other.

Therefore, the purpose of assessing flexibility shouldn't be to compare your performance to that of someone else. Assessments of flexibility are much more meaningful when your present flexibility is compared to your past flexibility.

STRETCHING AND INJURIES

For many years, it had been thought that pre-activity stretching reduces the risk of injury. This belief wasn't based on any research but it seemed reasonable to assume such. As it turns out, there's scant research on the effects of pre-activity stretching on the risk of injury. And the relatively few studies that have been conducted on the topic show that pre-activity stretching doesn't reduce injuries.

Two of the studies involved Australian Army recruits. The studies were conducted as they went through 12 weeks of basic training.

In the first study, one group of 549 recruits stretched their calves prior to physical training and another group of 544 recruits didn't stretch their calves. Those who stretched before physical training had 23 injuries to their lower leg while those who didn't stretch had 25 injuries to their lower leg.

In the second study, one group of 735 recruits stretched their lower-body muscles (calves, hamstrings, quadriceps, hip adductors and hip flexors) prior to physical training and another group of 803 recruits didn't stretch their lower-body muscles. Those who stretched before physical training had 158 injuries to their lower body while those who didn't stretch had 175 injuries to their lower body.

To summarize, the 1,284 recruits who stretched prior to physical training had 181 injuries and the 1,347 recruits who didn't stretch had 200 injuries. So in both studies, the incidence of injury was very similar regardless of whether or not stretching was done before an activity. Pooling the data from both studies showed that pre-activity stretching reduced the risk of injury by 5% (which wasn't statistically significant). Over the same period of time, the expected risk of injury was 20%. This means that a reduction in the relative risk of injury by 5% translated into a reduction in the absolute risk of injury by only 1%. Based on these data, the researchers calculated that, on average, about 100 people would need to stretch for 12 weeks to prevent one injury. And one person would need to stretch for 23 years to prevent one injury.

So, pre-activity stretching doesn't prevent injury. But pre-activity stretching doesn't cause injury.

STRETCHING AND PERFORMANCE

Another long-time assumption has been that pre-activity stretching improves performance. Again, this belief has been based more on a "gut feeling" than on scientific research. Most studies have shown that stretching prior to an activity can actually hinder a muscle's ability to produce maximum force, at least temporarily. To date, in fact, no study has shown that pre-activity stretching improves performance. But there's more to the story.

In one study, 13 subjects were exposed to three different conditions of passive stretching (for durations of two, four and eight minutes) and a control (non-stretching) condition. Passive stretching of the calves was performed on a dynamometer for 30 seconds then released for 20 seconds. This stretch-release sequence was repeated until the muscle was stretched for the assigned duration. For example, two minutes of stretching involved four 30-second stretches.

The researchers found that stretching decreased strength by as much as 6%. However, this wasn't significantly different than the control condition in which stretching wasn't done. The decreases were dose dependant in that as the length of the stretching protocol increased so did the reduction in strength.

This dose-response effect has been corroborated by a systematic review of more than 100 studies. According to the review, no detrimental effects on performance occur when stretches are held for up to 30 seconds. Decrements in performance are most likely to occur when stretches are held for more than 60 seconds.

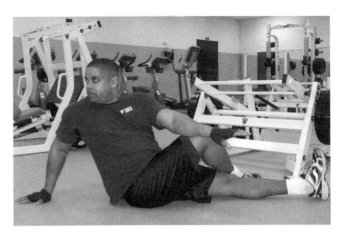

Pre-activity stretching doesn't hurt performance as long as it's not excessive.

So, pre-activity stretching doesn't help performance. But pre-activity stretching doesn't hurt performance as long as it's not excessive.

WARMING UP

The research regarding the need for a warm-up is inconclusive. Some studies have shown that performances with a warm-up are better than those without a warm-up; other studies have shown that performances with a warm-up are worse or no different than those without a warm-up. Nonetheless, a warm-up has both physiological and psychological importance.

For years, warming up was synonymous with stretching. However, warming up and stretching are two separate entities and must be treated as such. Warming up is meant to prepare you for an upcoming session of physical training; stretching is meant to induce a more long-term change in your ROM.

A warm-up should precede flexibility training. Warm-up activities usually consist of low-intensity movements such as light jogging or calisthenics. Regardless of the warm-up activity that you choose, the idea is to systematically increase your body temperature and the blood flow to your muscles. Breaking a light sweat during the warm-up indicates that your body temperature has been raised sufficiently and that you're ready to begin stretching your muscles. As noted previously,

187

muscles and connective tissue that are warmed up have increased flexibility and extensibility. (When the environmental temperature is high, it's likely that your body temperature is already elevated enough for you to start stretching your muscles.)

By the way, there's no need for you to warm-up or stretch prior to strength training, provided that you do a relatively high number of repetitions and lift the weight in a smooth, controlled manner without any explosive or jerking movements. But warming up prior to a physical activity that involves rapid muscular contractions – such as sprinting – is highly advisable to ready your muscles for high-speed movements.

METHODS OF STRETCHING

There are a few methods of stretching that you can employ to improve your flexibility. Here's a thumbnail sketch of four methods of stretching:

Static Stretching

The safest and most effective means of developing a greater ROM is, arguably, static stretching. With this method, the muscles are stretched slowly to the point of slight discomfort and that position is held for a prescribed amount of time.

Static stretching can be active or passive. Active static stretching involves holding the stretched position with one or more agonist muscles. An example of this is contracting the quadriceps (here, an agonist) to stretch the hamstrings. Passive static stretching involves holding the stretched position with help from another individual, gravity or an object such as a towel or stretch band.

Ballistic Stretching

Bouncing and jerking movements are inherent to ballistic stretching. These actions produce momentum which aggressively and erratically forces a muscle beyond its natural ROM.

Obviously, this can increase the potential for injury. Therefore, ballistic stretching is the least preferred method of stretching and shouldn't be considered as a viable option.

Dynamic Stretching

Easily and frequently confused with ballistic stretching is dynamic stretching. The main difference between the two is that dynamic stretching involves a slow and gradual transition from one position to another without the bouncing and jerking movements that are associated with ballistic stretching.

Dynamic stretching often employs specific movements that are involved in a sport or an activity. For instance, sprinters might perform knee pumps and arm swings as part of their preparation for a race or an interval workout on the track. But dynamic stretching can also involve general movements such as arm circles.

Proprioceptive Neuromuscular Facilitation

Another method of stretching is known as proprioceptive neuromuscular facilitation (which, thank goodness, usually goes by the letters PNF). With PNF stretching, an isometric contraction of the targeted muscle is done for a handful of seconds against resistance that's supplied by a partner. This is followed by an assisted stretch for the same muscle in the same position for a period of about 30 seconds with the help of the partner. The contract-relax cycle is repeated several times.

Take heed: An inexperienced partner can unknowingly apply an excessive amount of

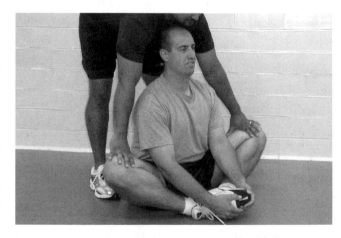

With PNF stretching, an isometric contraction of the targeted muscle is done for a handful of seconds against resistance that's supplied by a partner. (Photo by Peter Silletti.)

resistance which could cause an injury. As a result, this type of stretching should be used only with assistance from a competent individual. Even when done correctly, PNF can be quite uncomfortable. And because it's somewhat complicated and involves the use of another individual, PNF isn't a practical means of stretching.

STRETCHING STRATEGIES

Although your ROM may be limited by the factors that were mentioned previously, it can be improved through flexibility training. Like all other forms of physical training, flexibility training has certain concepts that must be considered in order to make it safe and productive. The concepts can be crafted into strategies that will permit you to maintain or improve your current ROM with a lower risk of injury.

Here are some stretching strategies for your flexibility training:

1. Do a warm-up prior to stretching.

A warm-up in which you break a light sweat will be adequate to elevate your body temperature enough and make your muscles and connective tissue more flexible and extensible.

2. Stretch under control without using any bouncing or jerking movements.

Bouncing or jerking actually makes the stretch more painful and increases your risk of muscular soreness and tissue damage.

3. Inhale and exhale normally during the stretch without holding your breath.

When you hold your breath, it elevates your blood pressure which disrupts your normal breathing pattern and makes it more difficult for you to relax.

4. Stretch comfortably in a pain-free manner.

Since pain is an indication that you're stretching at or near your structural limits, you should only stretch to a point of tightness or slight discomfort.

5. Relax during the stretch.

Relaxing mentally and physically allows you to stretch your muscles throughout a greater ROM.

6. Hold the stretched position for about 10 to 30 seconds.

By gradually stretching your muscles to a point of tightness or slight discomfort, holding that position and then gradually returning them to their pre-stretched length, you can stretch farther with little risk of pain or injury.

7. Attempt to stretch slightly farther than the last time.

In another application of the Overload Principle, progressively increasing your ROM improves your flexibility.

8. Perform stretches on a regular basis.

You should stretch daily and either before or after physical training.

THE STRETCHES

Although your body has roughly 200 joints, it's not necessary to perform a stretch for each one. Your joints range from those that are relatively immovable (such as the sutures of your skull) to those that are freely movable (such as your hips and elbows). You can stretch the muscles of your major joints in a comprehensive manner by performing a little more than a dozen stretches. There are many variations of stretches that involve the same muscle groups. Because of this, your flexibility training can be individualized to meet your personal preferences.

This chapter describes and illustrates the safest and most productive stretches that can be performed. Included in the discussions of each stretch are the muscle(s) stretched, start position, performance description and training tips for making the stretch safer and more productive.

These 16 stretches are described in this chapter: neck forward, neck backward, lateral neck, scratch back, front shoulder, rear shoulder, standing calf, tibia stretch, sit and reach, V-sit, lateral reach, butterfly, spinal twist, knee stack, knee pull and lying quad.

NECK FORWARD

NECK BACKWARD

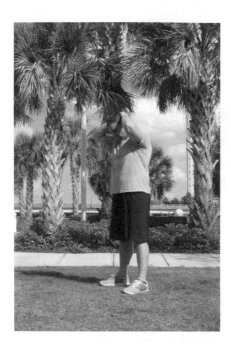

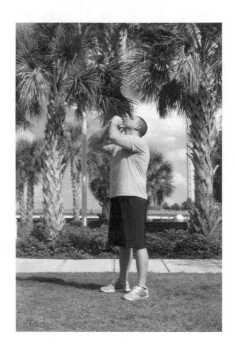

Muscles Stretched: neck extensors and trapezius

Start Position: While standing, spread your feet about shoulder-width apart. Place your hands behind your head and interlock your fingers.

Performance Description: Pull your head to your chest and hold.

Training Tips:

• The stretch must be done carefully since the cervical spine is involved.

• You can also perform this stretch while sitting.

Muscle Stretched: sternocleidomastoideus

Start Position: While standing, spread your feet about shoulder-width apart. Place your thumbs under your chin.

Performance Description: Push your head backward and hold.

Training Tips:

• The stretch must be done carefully since the cervical spine is involved.

• You can also perform this stretch while sitting.

LATERAL NECK

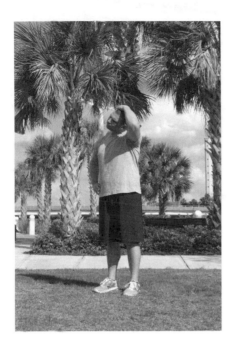

SCRATCH BACK

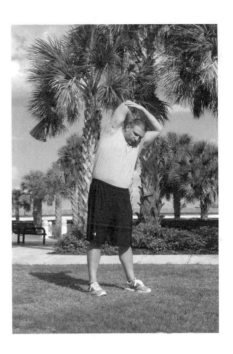

Muscle Stretched: sternocleidomastoideus

Start Position: While standing, spread your feet about shoulder-width apart. Place your left hand on the right side of your head.

Performance Description: Pull your head to your left shoulder and hold. Repeat the stretch for the other side of your body.

Training Tips:

- The stretch must be done carefully since the cervical spine is involved.

- You can also perform this stretch while sitting.

Muscles Stretched: upper back, triceps and obliques

Start Position: While standing, spread your feet about shoulder-width apart. Place your right hand behind your head on the upper part of your back and grab your right elbow with your left hand.

Performance Description: Pull your torso to the left and hold. Repeat the stretch for the other side of your body

Training Tips:

- Avoid moving your hips.

- You can also perform this stretch while sitting.

- This stretch may be contraindicated if you have shoulder-impingement syndrome.

FRONT SHOULDER

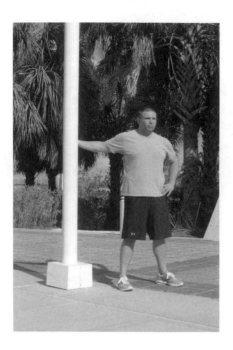

Muscles Stretched: chest and anterior deltoid

Start Position: While standing, spread your feet about shoulder-width apart. Position your right arm so that it's parallel to the floor. Place your right hand on a wall (or something similar that's stable) and your left hand on your hip.

Performance Description: Turn your feet and body to the left and hold. Repeat the stretch for the other side of your body.

Training Tips:

• This stretch may be contraindicated if you have shoulder-impingement syndrome.

REAR SHOULDER

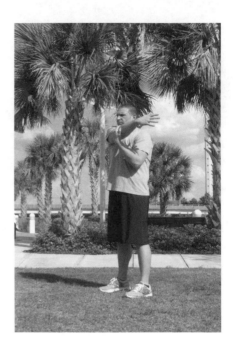

Muscles Stretched: upper back, posterior deltoid, trapezius and rhomboids

Start Position: While standing, spread your feet about shoulder-width apart. Position your right arm so that it's parallel to the floor. Place your left hand above your right elbow.

Performance Description: Pull your upper arm toward your torso and hold. Repeat the stretch for the other side of your body.

Training Tips:

• You can also perform this stretch while sitting.

STANDING CALF

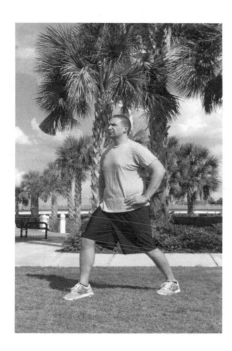

Muscles Stretched: calves and iliopsoas

Start Position: While standing, place your hands on your hips. Step forward with your right foot and bend your right leg. Straighten your left leg and place your left foot flat on the floor. Point your feet straight ahead.

Performance Description: Lean forward and hold. Repeat the stretch for the other side of your body.

Training Tips:

- Keep the heel of your back foot flat on the floor.

- Keep your feet pointed straight ahead.

- Refrain from bending forward at the waist.

TIBIA STRETCH

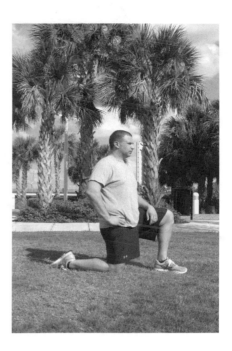

Muscles Stretched: dorsi flexors

Start Position: Kneel down on your right knee. Position your right upper leg so that it's perpendicular to the floor. Point your right toes away from your body. Position your left foot so that your left upper leg is parallel to the floor and your left lower leg is perpendicular to the floor. Place your left foot flat on the floor.

Performance Description: Press your right lower leg and the top part of your right foot flat on the floor and hold. Repeat the stretch for the other side of your body.

Training Tips:

- Keep the top part of the foot that's being stretched flat on the floor.

193

SIT AND REACH

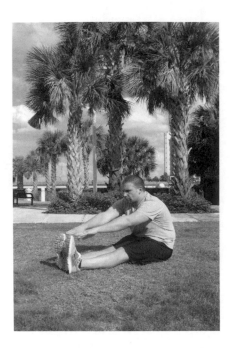

Muscles Stretched: gluteus maximus, hamstrings, calves, upper back and lower back

Start Position: While sitting, straighten your legs and bring them together. Point your toes upward.

Performance Description: Reach forward as far as possible and hold.

Training Tips:

• Keep your legs straight and toes pointed upward.

• A partner can help you obtain a greater stretch by carefully pushing on your upper back.

• You can also perform this stretch while standing (with your torso bent forward at the waist, your legs together and your arms hanging down).

V-SIT

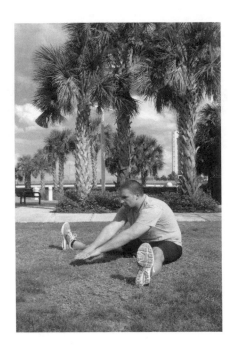

Muscles Stretched: gluteus maximus, hip adductors, hamstrings, calves, upper back and lower back

Start Position: While sitting, straighten your legs and spread them apart as far as possible. Point your toes upward.

Performance Description: Reach forward as far as possible and hold.

Training Tips:

• Keep your legs straight and toes pointed upward.

• A partner can help you obtain a greater stretch by carefully pushing on your upper back.

• You can also perform this stretch while standing (with your torso bent forward at the waist, your legs spread apart and your arms hanging down).

LATERAL REACH

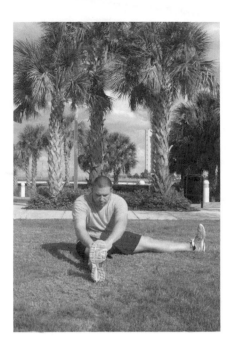

Muscles Stretched: gluteus maximus, hip adductors, hamstrings, calves, upper back, obliques and lower back

Start Position: While sitting, straighten your legs and spread them apart as far as possible. Point your toes upward.

Performance Description: Reach down your right leg as far as possible and hold. Repeat the stretch for the other side of your body.

Training Tips:

- Keep your legs straight and toes pointed upward.

- A partner can help you obtain a greater stretch by carefully pushing on your upper back.

- You can also perform this stretch while standing (with your torso bent laterally at the waist, your legs spread apart and your arms reaching down your leg).

BUTTERFLY

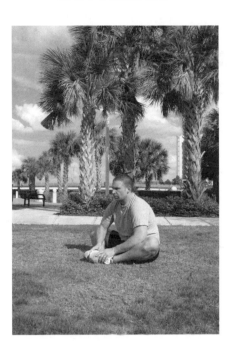

Muscles Stretched: hip adductors and lower back

Start Position: While sitting, place the soles of your feet together. Bring your heels as close to your hips as possible and place your elbows on the insides of your knees.

Performance Description: Push your legs down with your elbows and hold.

Training Tips:

- A partner can help you obtain a greater stretch by carefully pushing on the inside of your knees

195

SPINAL TWIST

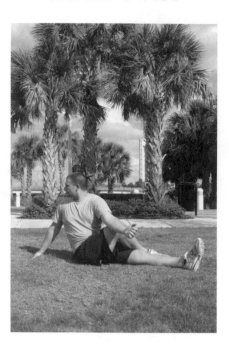

Muscles Stretched: gluteus medius, gluteus minimus, obliques and lower back

Start Position: While sitting, straighten your left leg and position your right foot on the outside of your left knee. Place your left elbow against the outside of your right knee.

Performance Description: Push against the outside of your right knee with your left elbow, look to your right as far as possible and hold. Repeat the stretch for the other side of your body.

Training Tips:

• You can also perform this stretch while lying supine (with your shoulders flat on the floor and rotating one leg to the side).

KNEE STACK

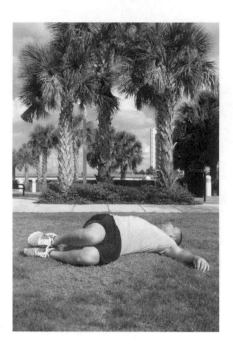

Muscles Stretched: hip abductors, obliques, lower back, chest and shoulders

Start Position: While lying supine, bend your knees. Bring your heels near your hips and position your feet flat on the floor. Keep your shoulders flat on the floor.

Performance Description: Rotate your legs to the left with your right leg "stacked" on top of your left leg and hold. Repeat the stretch for the other side of your body.

Training Tips:

• Keep your shoulders flat on the floor.

KNEE PULL

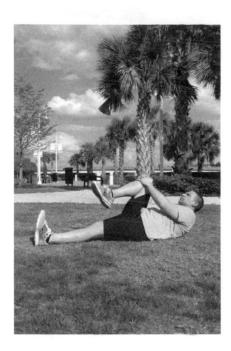

Muscles Stretched: gluteus maximus, hamstrings and lower back

Start Position: While lying supine, straighten your left leg and point your toes upward. Grasp your right leg below your knee.

Performance Description: Pull your right leg toward your chest and hold. Repeat the stretch for the other side of your body.

Training Tips:

- Keep one leg straight and toes pointed upward while the other leg is being stretched.

LYING QUAD

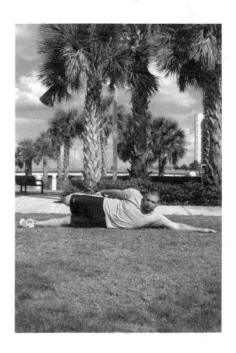

Muscles Stretched: quadriceps, iliopsoas and abdominals

Start Position: Lie down on your left side and grab your right ankle with your right hand.

Performance Description: Pull your right heel toward your hip and hold. Repeat the stretch for the other side of your body.

Training Tips:

- You can also perform this stretch while lying prone.

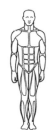

14 Aerobic Training

The most important aspect of your physical profile is your aerobic fitness. Specifically, your aerobic fitness is a measure of how well your body consumes, transports and uses oxygen during physical exertion. The best way for you to improve these physiological mechanisms is through aerobic training.

The energy pathway that's responsible for your aerobic fitness is your Aerobic System (which is vital in efforts that are of low intensity and prolonged duration). It's no surprise, then, that the main purpose of aerobic training is to improve the functional ability of your Aerobic System. By increasing your aerobic fitness, your Aerobic System can operate more efficiently and more effectively. More than any other type of physical training, aerobic training decreases your resting heart rate. A lower resting heart rate means that your heart won't have to work as hard to accomplish a given task.

Aerobic training helps to modify several factors that contribute to the risk of coronary artery disease and heart attack. This includes diabetes, hypertension (high blood pressure), overweight/obesity and physical inactivity.

Besides conferring a variety of health-related benefits, aerobic training also has an impact on performance in sports and activities. A highly conditioned athlete can work at greater levels of intensity for longer periods of time at a lower heart rate than a poorly conditioned athlete. This "aerobic advantage" means that an athlete won't expend as much energy as an opponent and can perform skills and activities with less effort. Not only that but the exercising heart rate returns to normal more quickly, an obvious advantage during athletic endeavors.

Aerobic training is also needed to establish a solid foundation of aerobic support in

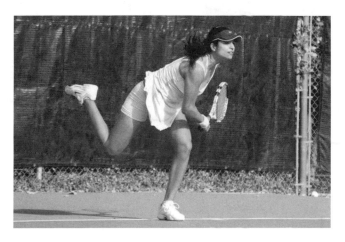

A highly conditioned athlete can work at greater levels of intensity for longer periods of time at a lower heart rate than a poorly conditioned athlete. (Photo provided by Shikha Uberoi.)

preparation for anaerobic training. The more finely tuned your aerobic pathway becomes, the better your anaerobic pathways are able to function. Clearly, your Aerobic System must operate as efficiently and as effectively as possible to provide physiological support for your anaerobic efforts.

In addition to the many physiological adaptations, aerobic training – when used in conjunction with sound nutritional training – helps to maintain your percentage of body fat at an acceptable level. This, of course, will improve your appearance.

There are psychological enhancements, too. This includes increased mental alertness, self-confidence and self-esteem.

AEROBIC GUIDELINES

Your aerobic fitness may be improved and maintained by using several easy-to-follow guidelines that have been adapted from a 2011 position stand by the American College of Sports

Medicine (ACSM) on prescribing exercise for healthy adults. These guidelines can be organized under the acronym FITT which stands for Frequency, Intensity, Time and Type.

Frequency

In order to improve your aerobic fitness, you should do aerobic training three to five days per week. Training less frequently doesn't appear adequate enough to promote any meaningful improvement in your aerobic fitness; training more frequently may produce a greater improvement in your aerobic fitness but the amount is negligible (which usually isn't worth the time spent).

Having said that, doing aerobic training more frequently may be beneficial if you're a highly competitive athlete. And doing aerobic training more frequently can be beneficial when weight (fat) loss is a goal.

Be advised that beginning with too much activity too soon may very well lead to an overuse injury such as tendinitis. This is especially true of certain populations including younger children, older adults and those who are inactive or in poor physical condition. Individuals who are susceptible to overuse injuries should initially perform aerobic training two or three days per week to reduce their potential for overuse injuries. As these individuals adjust and adapt to the unfamiliar demands, their dosage of aerobic training can be increased to a frequency of three to five days per week.

Intensity

Other than your genetic (inherited) profile, the most important aspect of aerobic training is your level of intensity (or effort). Your heart rate increases in direct proportion to the demands of an activity. As such, your exercising heart rate is commonly used to estimate your aerobic intensity.

Since there's a slight but steady decrease in maximum heart rate with aging, estimates of it are made on the basis of age. It's recommended that you maintain a level of 60 to 90% of your age-predicted maximum heart rate to improve your aerobic fitness.

One way to find a rough estimate of your age-predicted maximum heart rate in beats per minute (bpm) is to use a prediction equation. Since 1938, dozens of equations have been proposed as a means to estimate age-predicted maximum heart rates. However, no equation has been more widely used in the fitness industry than "220 - age." Yet, the equation has a murky origin: The data on which it's based doesn't support the equation. And despite its popularity, the accuracy of the equation has been questioned.

Nonetheless, when "220 - age" is compared to other equations, there's really very little difference between them. For nearly all age groups, most of the equations differ by no more than about five beats per minute (which becomes an even smaller difference when multiplied by 60 to 90% to determine a heart-rate training zone).

The fact of the matter is that actual maximum heart rates vary considerably and, thus, are difficult to estimate in a precise manner. So, understand that every equation is only an estimate of an age-predicted maximum heart rate. And most equations offer roughly the same degree of accuracy. But the equation "220 - age" is more convenient and less complicated than others.

To use this equation, simply subtract your age from 220. For instance, the age-predicted maximum heart rate of a 30-year-old individual is 190 bpm [220 - 30 = 190]. To find the recommended heart-rate training zone, multiply 190 bpm by 60% and 90% (or 0.60 and 0.90). This means that a 30-year-old individual needs to maintain an exercising heart rate of about 114 to 171 bpm to improve aerobic fitness [190 bpm x 0.60 = 114 bpm; 190 bpm x 0.90 = 171 bpm].

In the case of maximum heart rate, it's important to note that the equation "220 - age" has a standard deviation of about 11 bpm. Considering all 30-year-old individuals, this means that about 68.26% of them have maximum heart rates of about 179 to 201 bpm, 95.44% of them about 168 to 212 bpm and 99.73% of them about 157 to 223 bpm.

(Note: According to the ACSM, children and adolescents up to the age of about 16 should maintain an exercising heart rate of about 170 to 180 beats per minute. After that age, a prediction equation can be employed to estimate their maximum heart rate.)

Some people may need to maintain their heart rates above the training zone that's recommended for others of the same age. If you're highly active or have an above-average level of fitness, for example, you should train with a higher percentage of your age-predicted maximum heart rate to produce meaningful results; if you're inactive or have a below-average level of fitness, you should train with a lower percentage of your age-predicted maximum heart rate to avoid potential risks. Using a lower level of intensity may also be necessary in the early stages of aerobic training to increase the likelihood of adherence to the program.

Remember, a favorable response to aerobic training requires an appropriate level of intensity. Intensity is a relative term that depends on your level of fitness. For some people, training with a lower percentage of their age-predicted maximum heart rate may actually represent a high level of intensity and an adequate workload for them. Stated otherwise, exercise of low intensity for an active individual may be of high intensity for an inactive individual. Depending on the initial level of fitness, training with a heart rate that's below the recommended threshold can actually produce some improvement in aerobic fitness.

To determine an appropriate level of intensity, you should adjust your effort based on whether the activity feels too easy or too difficult. If it feels too easy, increase your intensity; if it feels too difficult, reduce your intensity. Also keep in mind that your intensity is influenced by many factors including the environmental conditions (altitude, temperature and humidity), your body position (seated or upright) and the amount of muscle mass being used (larger muscles produce a higher exercising heart rate than smaller ones).

Your heart rate can be easily measured at several different sites on your body. Heart-rate

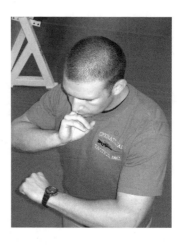

It's recommended that you maintain a level of 60 to 90% of your age-predicted maximum heart rate to improve your aerobic fitness.

monitors can give you an accurate reading of your heart rate. But the easiest and least expensive way to determine your heart rate is to measure it yourself. You can do this by locating your pulse at either the carotid artery (in your neck) or the radial artery (in your wrist). Simply place the tips of your index and middle fingers over one of these sites. (During intense activity, your carotid and radial arteries are easy to find.) Immediately after aerobic training, count your pulse for 10 seconds. Multiplying that number by six yields a good estimate of your exercising heart rate (in beats per minute). You can obtain a similar estimate by counting your pulse for 15 seconds and multiplying that number by four.

Time

To attain improvements in your aerobic fitness, you should do 20 to 60 minutes of aerobic activity. For years, it was thought that aerobic activities had to be continuous in order to improve aerobic fitness. However, research conducted since the mid-1990s has found that similar benefits can also be derived by doing several bouts of discontinuous activity that are accumulated throughout the course of the day.

In a 2009 review of the literature, researchers looked at 16 studies that involved 836 subjects. In general, the subjects exercised for 20 to 40 minutes per day, three to five days per week, for a period of four to 20 weeks. Those who were assigned to perform discontinuous activity did two to four bouts with each bout lasting 10 to 15 minutes. Most of the studies in the review found no significant differences between equal amounts of discontinuous activity and continuous activity with respect to improving aerobic fitness. There wasn't enough evidence to show that discontinuous activity is as good as continuous activity in other measures such as improving body composition, cholesterol and psychological well-being.

So although 20 to 60 minutes of continuous activity is preferred, you can improve your aerobic fitness by doing multiple bouts of at least 10 minutes in duration that add up to 20 to 60 minutes. For instance, two 15-minute bouts would equal 30 minutes of activity.

Keep in mind, too, that the time of an activity is inversely proportional to the intensity of an activity. This means that the length of your effort can be relatively brief as long as your level of intensity is relatively high. Generally speaking, doing a total of 20 minutes of continuous or discontinuous activity with an appropriate level of intensity is enough for most people to improve their aerobic fitness.

It should also be noted that if the length of your aerobic training is too brief, you might not produce a desirable expenditure of calories. This is an important consideration if one of your primary objectives is to lose or maintain weight. Here, you may need to perform aerobic training for at least 30 minutes (but not more than 60).

When your intensity is low – for whatever reason – your activities should be conducted for a longer period of time to improve your aerobic fitness. Take into account, though, that lengthy workouts may be inappropriate for some people in the initial stages of aerobic training. For one thing, performing too much activity too soon increases the risk of incurring an overuse injury. For another, some individuals may initially have such low levels of fitness that they might only be able to tolerate 5 to 10 minutes of aerobic training. In either case, the length of their aerobic training can be gradually increased as they improve their fitness.

Type

The combined application of the guidelines for the frequency, intensity and duration of aerobic training provides a meaningful workload for your Aerobic System. If these three ingredients of aerobic training produce the same expenditure of total calories, your physiological adaptations will be similar regardless of the type of aerobic activity that you perform. Therefore, you can use a wide assortment of activities to achieve improvements in your aerobic fitness.

The preferred types of aerobic activities are those that require a continuous effort, are rhythmic in nature and involve large amounts of muscle mass. Outdoor activities that meet these criteria include cross-country skiing, cycling, hiking/backpacking, ice/in-line/roller skating, jogging/running, rowing and walking; indoor activities include dancing, rope jumping and swimming along with exercising on stationary equipment such as cycles (upright or recumbent), ellipticals, rowers, steppers/stairclimbers and treadmills. Most of these aerobic options are activities that can be performed – and enjoyed – throughout a lifetime.

You can also attain improvements in your aerobic fitness from activities such as basketball, soccer and tennis. Remember, though, that your level of intensity can vary a great deal during these activities due to their intermittent nature. The way that these activities are structured also influences your level of intensity: In basketball, playing a full-court game is generally more demanding than a half-court game; in tennis, playing a singles match is generally more demanding than a doubles match.

To avoid boredom, it's important for you to change your activities from time to time. Fortunately, aerobic training allows a considerable amount of variety in terms of your activity selections.

Each aerobic activity has its advantages and disadvantages. For instance, swimming is desirable since it's a non-impact, non-weightbearing activity: The water supports your bodyweight which eliminates compressive forces on your bones and joints. On the other hand, swimming requires a fairly high degree of proficiency. If you have poor swimming skills, your heart rate may exceed your recommended training zone in a struggle just to keep yourself afloat. And if you're not skilled at swimming, you'll also tire very quickly. As such, swimming is a bad option if your skills are inadequate. But it's a good option if your skills are adequate.

In addition, some aerobic activities aren't advisable if you're prone to certain injuries or likely to complicate an existing orthopedic condition. For example, rope jumping is a high-impact, weightbearing activity that carries a greater risk of orthopedic stress and overuse injuries than a low-impact, non-weightbearing activity. Thus, rope jumping isn't advisable if you're a larger-than-average person – larger due to either fat or muscle – because of the excessive stress that's placed on your ankles, knees and lower back. Furthermore, someone who has chronic low-back pain would be more comfortable cycling in a recumbent position – in which the angle of the seat places the torso in a position that decreases the amount of stress in the lower back – instead of in the traditional upright position. So, the best advice is for you to select suitable aerobic activities that are enjoyable, compatible with your level of skill and orthopedically safe.

If you happen to be a competitive athlete who's preparing for a specific event – such as running or swimming – the best activities to do are the ones that you're going to perform. In one study, for example, 11 subjects did a 10-week program of running and showed significantly greater improvements in their maximum oxygen intake in running than in swimming (an average increase of 6.3% compared to 2.6%). So if you want to become a better runner, you must mainly run; if you want to become a better swimmer, you must mainly swim.

But there's a caveat for runners and other athletes whose sport or activity involves running. As noted, the best activity for them is running. Unfortunately, running is a high-impact activity. In one study, researchers described running as "a series of collisions with the ground." The impact forces that are encountered when running are at least several times bodyweight. (The same holds true for rope jumping, by the way.) What this means is that runners should include at least

some non- or low-impact activities as part of their aerobic training to minimize the impact forces that are associated with running.

As long as it's orthopedically appropriate, the type of activity that you choose to improve your aerobic fitness isn't as critical as the frequency, intensity and duration of the activity. Your Aerobic System doesn't know if you pedaled on a recumbent cycle one day and ran on a treadmill the next. The only thing that really matters is whether or not you applied a meaningful workload to your aerobic pathway.

APPROPRIATE AEROBIC TRAINING

In a nutshell, you should perform your aerobic training with a frequency, intensity and duration that are suitable and safe while using appropriate activities that require a sustained effort. If you're a healthy adult, your specific training prescription is to perform aerobic activities three to five times per week [frequency] at 60 to 90% of your age-predicted maximum heart rate [intensity] for 20 to 60 minutes [time] using preferred activities [type]. Bear in mind that all of these guidelines must be satisfied in order for you to improve your aerobic fitness.

MEANINGFUL AEROBIC TRAINING

Over a period of time, you'll likely find that the same aerobic workout – which was originally difficult – can be performed with less effort. As you improve your aerobic fitness, your exercising heart rate will be lower for a given level of intensity. Because of this, you must increase your intensity as needed so that you're always training with an appropriate percentage of your maximum heart rate. In addition, your ability to maintain a higher exercising heart rate will become easier. As a result, it's important for you to make your aerobic training progressively more challenging in order to produce further improvements in your aerobic fitness.

There are three main ways to overload your Aerobic System. In comparison to a previous workout, you must attempt to (1) complete the

203

same distance in a shorter duration; (2) cover a greater distance in the same duration; or (3) maintain the same pace for a greater distance or duration. As an example, suppose that you cycled 4.0 miles in 20 minutes (a pace of 12.0 miles per hour). In a future workout, you should try to (1) cycle 4.0 miles in less than 20 minutes; (2) cycle more than 4.0 miles in 20 minutes; or (3) cycle at 12.0 miles per hour for more than 4.0 miles or more than 20 minutes. Regardless of which tactic you employ, you made your Aerobic System work harder than it was accustomed to working. (Note: With some stationary equipment, you can increase the resistance which also makes your Aerobic System work harder than in a previous workout.)

For this reason, it's vital that you keep accurate records of your aerobic training. Maintaining records permits you to track your progress thereby making your aerobic workouts more productive and more meaningful. During aerobic training, the key program components to monitor include the date of your workout, the duration of your workout, the distance that you completed and the level of your intensity (your exercising heart rate).

SCHEDULING TRAINING

Essentially, there are two options for scheduling strength training and aerobic training: The activities can be done on the same day or on alternate days.

The advantage of doing both activities on the same day is that it permits a more complete recovery. If strength training is performed on one day and aerobic training the next, your muscles and energy systems will be constantly stressed and your body may not have adequate time to recover sufficiently. After a while, it may also be very difficult for you to perform these activities several days in a row with a high degree of enthusiasm and requisite level of intensity. Therefore, the recommended way of scheduling strength training and aerobic training is to do both activities on the same day.

Nonetheless, there are some instances where it's more appropriate for individuals to do the activities on alternate days. One scenario, of course, is when there isn't enough time to do both activities on the same day. Or it may simply come down to a matter of personal preference.

If strength training and aerobic training are done on the same day, which activity should be done first? You'll obtain better overall results when aerobic training is done before strength training. In a study by Dr. Wayne Westcott, the subjects did strength training, rested for five minutes and then did aerobic training (cycling for 20 minutes). During a subsequent session, the subjects did aerobic training (cycling for 20 minutes), rested for five minutes and then did strength training. Doing strength training before aerobic training resulted in a 1% improvement in strength performance compared to doing strength training after aerobic training; doing aerobic training before strength training resulted in an 8% improvement in aerobic performance compared to doing aerobic training after strength training. These findings also imply that strength training has a greater impact on aerobic training than aerobic training has on strength training.

If you're a competitive athlete, whether you do strength training or aerobic training first depends on the nature of your sport or activity. If a sport or an activity has a greater strength component (such as shot putting and high jumping), then strength training should precede aerobic training; if a sport or an activity has a greater endurance component (such as basketball and soccer), then aerobic training should precede strength training.

In addition to the possibility of doing strength training and aerobic training on the same day, athletes may also be required to do skill training. If these three activities are performed on the same day, better overall results will be obtained if skill training is done first. Of all three activities, the one that's most critical to athletes is skill training. If athletes are exhausted after aerobic training and/or strength training, they'll be drained both physically and mentally. Therefore, they won't practice very hard or work on their technique very well. In fact, they're sure to be inattentive and their performance will probably be quite careless, labored and awkward. Furthermore, athletes are more prone to injury when practicing in a pre-fatigued state. Because of this, it's best

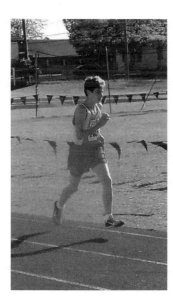

If a sport or activity has a greater endurance component, then aerobic training should precede strength training. (Photo by Greg Fried.)

for athletes to do skill training before aerobic training and/or strength training.

PREDICTING OXYGEN INTAKE

Oxygen intake (aka oxygen consumption) is perhaps the most widely accepted indicator of aerobic fitness. Like virtually all of your other physiological characteristics, your aerobic potential is greatly influenced by your genetic (or inherited) profile (especially as it relates to your predominant muscle fiber type). One of the largest studies on this topic – involving 436 pairs of monozygotic (identical) twins and 622 pairs of dizygotic (fraternal) twins – found that 62% of the differences between individuals in predicted oxygen intake was attributable to genetics. A smaller study – involving 29 pairs of monozygotic twins and 19 pairs of dizygotic twins – found that 66% of the differences between individuals in actual oxygen intake was attributable to genetics.

There are a number of ways to accurately measure oxygen intake in a laboratory. One way is to step up on and down from a bench of a standard height at a fixed rate of stepping. Another way is to pedal a cycle ergometer in an upright or recumbent position using your legs and/or arms. In terms of assessing oxygen intake, the most commonly used laboratory apparatus is probably the treadmill. Using stationary equipment makes it possible for you to perform at different levels of intensity while maintaining your body in a relatively stable position. This allows you to be instrumented in order to measure various physiological responses. For instance, expired gases can be collected and analyzed to determine the exact amount of oxygen that you consumed as well as the response of your heart rate and blood pressure.

Laboratory testing is an excellent means of providing you with accurate data that are reliable and valid. However, it can be expensive, time-consuming and impractical (if it's even available). Fortunately, there's another way to assess your oxygen intake without the inherent drawbacks of laboratory testing. Since these assessments are performed outside the laboratory, they're referred to as field tests. Certain field tests of oxygen intake have a high correlation to laboratory tests.

One of the most popular field tests that can be used to determine oxygen intake is the 1.5-Mile Running Test. The primary objective of this test is to run 1.5 miles in the least amount of time. For this field test to be as accurate as possible, you must run exactly 1.5 miles and it must be on a level (or horizontal) surface. Because of this, running on an indoor or outdoor track is preferred. Generally, the results of the 1.5-Mile Running Test are an excellent predictor of oxygen intake. But it's important to realize that this particular test favors runners since it involves running. (Note: A 1.0-mile run is more appropriate for younger children and older adults.)

Oxygen Intake: Relative

Table 14.1 lists predicted values of oxygen intake based on the time that's taken to complete a 1.5-mile run on a level surface. These values are a relative measure of how much oxygen is consumed in milliliters per kilogram of bodyweight per minute (or mL/kg/min).

Consider a 30-year-old man who weighs 198 pounds and can run 1.5 miles in 12:30. Note in Table 14.1 that his oxygen intake for this particular running time is 42.12 mL/kg/min or, simply, 42.12. In other words, he consumed about 42.12 milliliters of oxygen for every kilogram that he weighed during each minute of his 1.5-mile run.

Table 14.2 shows norms for oxygen intake in relative terms based on age and gender. Note that an oxygen intake of 42.12 mL/kg/min is average for men of his age.

Oxygen intakes of elite endurance athletes typically exceed 80.0 mL/kg/min in men and 70.0 mL/kg/min in women. Among world-class cross-country skiers, for example, average values of 85.6 mL/kg/min for men and 70.1 mL/kg/min for women have been reported. Other endurance athletes with high levels of oxygen intake in relative terms include long-distance runners and cyclists and rowers.

Table 14.1 is only valid for determining oxygen intake during a 1.5-mile run. The ACSM offers this equation for calculating oxygen intake in mL/kg/min for a run of any known distance and duration on a level surface:

oxygen intake = (speed in m/min) x (0.2 mL/kg/min per m/min) + 3.5 mL/kg/min

As an example, suppose that you just completed a 5K (5,000-meter) race in 20:00. In this scenario, your running speed was 250.0 meters per minute [5,000 m ÷ 20.0 min = 250.0 m/min]. Next, multiply your speed [250.0 m/min] by the oxygen cost of horizontal running [0.2 mL/kg/min per m/min] and add the oxygen cost of resting [3.5 mL/kg/min]. This calculation yields a value of 53.5 mL/kg/min [250.0 m/min x 0.2 mL/kg/min per m/min + 3.5 mL/kg/min = 53.5 mL/kg/min].

For this equation to be accurate, you must run on a level surface at a speed of at least 5.0 miles per hour (mph) or 134.0 m/min. (Note: To convert mph to m/min, multiply the mph by 26.8; to convert miles to meters, multiply the miles by 1,609.)

Oxygen intake can also be calculated for walking speeds between 1.9 and 3.7 mph or 50.0 and 100.0 m/min. (For most people, speeds between 100.0 and 134.0 m/min are too fast for walking and too slow for running.) At low speeds, walking is generally a more efficient process than running. In fact, the oxygen cost of

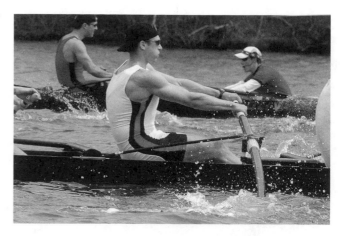

Endurance athletes with high levels of oxygen intake in relative terms include long-distance runners and cyclists and rowers. (Photo by Tom Nowak.)

horizontal walking at a given speed is about one half that of horizontal running. Therefore, the only change to the earlier equation is that the oxygen cost of horizontal walking is used which is 0.1 mL/kg/min per m/min. So if you walked 3,000 meters in 30 minutes, your oxygen intake would be 13.5 mL/kg/min [100.0 m/min x 0.1 mL/kg/min per m/min + 3.5 mL/kg/min = 13.5 mL/kg/min].

Oxygen Intake: Absolute

Oxygen intake can also be expressed in absolute terms in liters per minute (L/min). To determine oxygen intake in L/min, you must first convert bodyweight to kilograms (kg). To do this, divide bodyweight in pounds (lb) by 2.2. Using the earlier example of the 30-year-old male, his 198-pound bodyweight is equal to 90 kg [198 lb ÷ 2.2 kg/lb = 90 kg]. Next, multiply his bodyweight (in kilograms) by his oxygen intake (in mL/kg/min). Staying with the same example as before produces a value of 3,790.8 mL/min [90 kg x 42.12 mL/kg/min = 3,790.8 mL/min]. Finally, divide this number by 1,000 (to convert from milliliters to liters). To divide by 1,000, simply move the decimal point three places to the left. This means that a 198-pound individual who ran 1.5 miles in 12:30 would consume about 3.79 liters of oxygen during every minute of his run.

Table 14.3 shows norms for oxygen intake in absolute terms based on age and gender. Note that an oxygen intake of 3.79 L/min is excellent for men of his age. Recall that when bodyweight wasn't considered, his aerobic fitness was average.

Oxygen intakes of elite endurance athletes typically exceed 6.0 L/min in men and 4.0 L/min in women. Among world-class cross-country skiers, for example, average values of 6.38 L/min for men and 4.28 L/min for women have been reported. Other endurance athletes with high levels of oxygen intake in absolute terms include heavyweight rowers (since their bodyweight is a factor here).

A World-Class Application

It's interesting to calculate the oxygen intake of a world-class runner. In 1996, Daniel Komen of Kenya, at the age of 20, set the world record in the men's 3,000-meter run on an outdoor track with a time of 7:20.67. The ACSM equation can be used since the distance and time are known and the performance was done on a level surface without any inclines or declines.

In setting the world record, his running speed was 408.47 meters per minute. (Note: The decimal equivalent of 7:20.67 is 7.3445 minutes.) Multiplying his speed by 0.2 mL/kg/min per m/min and adding the oxygen cost of resting is an oxygen intake of 85.19 mL/kg/min which is literally "off the charts." Multiplying this number by his bodyweight of 55 kilograms (according to the International Association of Athletics Federations) is 4,685.45 mL. Dividing this number by 1,000 reveals an oxygen intake of about 4.69 L/min which is also off the charts but not as impressive because of his low bodyweight.

Expected Oxygen Intake

According to the ACSM, the following regression equations can be used to predict expected oxygen intake (in mL/kg/min) based on activity level, gender and age:

active men: 69.7 - (0.612 x age)

active women: 42.9 - (0.312 x age)

inactive men: 57.8 - (0.445 x age)

inactive women: 42.3 - (0.356 x age)

For instance, an active 30-year-old man would be expected to have an oxygen intake of about 51.34 mL/kg/min [0.612 x 30 = 18.36; 69.7 - 18.36 = 51.34].

Comparing your expected oxygen intake to your actual oxygen intake determines whether or not you have any Functional Aerobic Impairment (FAI). The FAI can be found by subtracting the actual oxygen intake from the expected oxygen intake. This value is divided by the expected oxygen intake and then multiplied by 100 (to convert the number to a percentage).

If the 30-year-old man in this example was found to have an actual oxygen intake of 42.12 mL/kg/min, he would have an FAI of about 18.0% [51.34 mL/kg/min - 42.12 mL/kg/min ÷ 51.34 mL/kg/min x 100 = 17.96%]. A positive percentage indicates that the actual oxygen intake is worse than expected; a negative percentage indicates that the actual oxygen intake is better than expected. It must be reiterated that your genetic profile plays a major role in determining your level of aerobic fitness.

Finally, the purpose of assessing your aerobic fitness shouldn't be to compare your performance to that of someone else. Assessments of aerobic fitness are much more meaningful when your present level is compared to your past level.

Oxygen Intake and Strength Training

As mentioned earlier, your exercising heart rate is a good indicator of your effort. However, the response that's produced by strength training is different than the response that's produced by aerobic training.

For any given heart rate, strength training generates a lower oxygen intake compared to aerobic training; some research has shown that the difference is about 70%. So, attaining a heart rate of 140 bpm during aerobic training might correspond to an oxygen intake of 20 mL/kg/min but that same heart rate during strength training might correspond to an oxygen intake of 14 mL/kg/min.

Or look at it this way: For any given oxygen intake, strength training requires a higher exercising heart rate compared to aerobic training. So, attaining an oxygen intake of 20 mL/kg/min during aerobic training might require a heart rate of 140 bpm but that same oxygen intake during strength training might require 160 bpm.

ESTIMATING CALORIC EXPENDITURE

Basically, a calorie is a unit of heat. In scientific terms, a calorie is defined as the amount of heat that's required to raise the temperature of one gram of water by one degree Celsius. In practical terms, a calorie is a measure of your energy intake (eating) as well as your energy output (exercising).

The caloric equivalent of one liter of oxygen ranges from 4.7 calories when fat is used as the sole source of energy to 5.0 calories when carbohydrates are used as the sole source of energy. (The caloric equivalent of one liter of oxygen is 4.4 calories when proteins are used as the sole source of energy. Under most circumstances, however, the use of protein is negligible during exercise and, therefore, usually disregarded.) For all practical purposes – and with little loss in precision – about 5.0 calories are used for every liter of oxygen that's consumed.

To determine the rate of caloric expenditure, simply take oxygen intake in L/min and multiply it by 5.0 calories per liter (cal/L). Recall the earlier example of the 198-pound male whose oxygen intake was 3.79 L/min. In this case, his rate of caloric expenditure would be almost 19.0 calories per minute [3.79 L/min x 5.0 cal/L = 18.95 cal/min].

To determine the total number of calories that he used during his 1.5-mile run, multiply his rate of caloric expenditure (in cal/min) by his running time. In this case, multiplying 18.95 cal/min by 12.5 minutes (12:30 in decimal form) indicates that he used about 237.0 calories during his run [18.95 cal/min x 12.5 min = 236.88 cal].

Remember that when Daniel Komen set the world record of 7:20.67 in the 3,000-meter run, his oxygen intake was about 4.69 L/min. Multiplying this by 5.0 cal/L is a caloric expenditure of 23.45 cal/min. Multiplying this

by his time of 7.3445 minutes is about 172.23 calories. Not bad for a little more than seven minutes of exertion.

MET LEVELS

Another way to quantify oxygen intake (and caloric expenditure) is to use a MET or metabolic equivalent. A MET is a multiple of oxygen intake while at rest. Specifically, 1.0 MET is the amount of oxygen that's consumed while resting in a seated position which is about 3.5 mL/kg/min. A value of 2.0 METs is equal to an oxygen intake of 7.0 mL/kg/min [3.5 mL/kg/min x 2.0 = 7.0 mL/kg/min].

An activity that has a value of 2.0 METs requires twice as much oxygen (or energy) as an activity that has a value of 1.0 MET (7.0 mL/kg/min compared to 3.5 mL/kg/min); an activity that has a value of 6.0 METs requires three times as much oxygen as an activity that has a value of 2.0 METs (21.0 mL/kg/min compared to 7.0 mL/kg/min).

It's easy to express oxygen intake in METs. To do so, simply divide oxygen intake in mL/kg/min by 3.5 mL/kg/min. For instance, the 198-pound male in the ongoing example had an oxygen intake of 42.12 mL/kg/min when he ran 1.5 miles in 12:30. In this case, his oxygen intake is equal to about 12.0 METs [42.12 ÷ 3.5 mL/kg/min = 12.03 METs]. Or look at it this way: His effort was about 12 times more demanding than resting in a seated position.

The MET level can also be used to estimate the rate of caloric expenditure in calories per kilogram of bodyweight per minute (cal/kg/min) and calories per minute (cal/min). A value of 1.0 MET is equal to about 0.0175 cal/kg/min. Therefore, caloric expenditure can be estimated in cal/kg/min by multiplying the MET level by 0.0175 cal/kg/min. For example, the 198-pound man who recorded a MET level of 12.03 used about 0.210525 cal/kg/min [12.03 x 0.0175 cal/kg/min = 0.210525 cal/kg/min]. To estimate cal/min, multiply his bodyweight in kilograms [90] by his cal/kg/min [0.210525]. This produces a value of about 18.95 cal/min [90 kg x 0.210525 cal/kg/min = 18.947 cal/min]. (Recall that when a different series of calculations was used in the preceding section, his rate of caloric expenditure was estimated as 18.95 cal/min.)

AEROBIC INTENSITY: HIGH OR LOW?

Energy can be provided by carbohydrates, fat and protein. However, your body doesn't like to use protein as an energy source. In fact, protein is generally used as a last resort. Remember, protein is located in your muscles and if you must rely on it as an energy source, then you're literally cannibalizing yourself.

So that leaves carbohydrates and fat as your main sources of energy. What your body elects to use is dictated by your level of intensity. During activity of lower intensity, your body prefers to use fat; during activity of higher intensity, your body prefers to use carbohydrates. (Carbohydrates are a more efficient source of energy but fat is used because your body doesn't need to be efficient at lower levels of intensity.)

Note that both carbohydrates and fat are used during activity but to different degrees. With low-intensity activity, fat is the main source of energy but carbohydrates are also used; with high-intensity activity, carbohydrates are the main source of energy but fat is also used. So, as an activity becomes more intense, the body shifts to a greater reliance on carbohydrates.

These physiological facts have led to the mistaken belief that low-intensity (or "fat-burning") activity is better than high-intensity (or "carbohydrate-burning") activity when it comes to losing weight, "burning fat" and expending calories. This misconception has also spawned the notion that people should train within their so-called fat-burning zones.

The idea of keeping the intensity low in order to mobilize and selectively use a higher percentage of fat may sound logical but it doesn't hold up mathematically and has never been verified in the laboratory. In truth, even though a greater *percentage* of fat calories are used during low-intensity activity, a greater *number* of fat calories (and total calories) is used during high-intensity activity.

During any activity, the rate of caloric expenditure is directly related to the intensity of effort: The higher the intensity, the greater the rate of caloric expenditure. In the case of running, for example, intensity is directly associated with speed: The faster the running speed, the greater the rate of caloric expenditure. The time of activity is also a factor: The longer that a given activity is performed, the greater the total caloric expenditure.

Based on the ACSM equations for calculating oxygen intake and caloric expenditure during walking and running, a 165-pound man who walks 3.0 miles in 60 minutes on a level surface uses roughly 4.33 cal/min. Over the course of his 60-minute walk, then, he'd use about 260 calories. If that same individual ran those 3.0 miles in 30 minutes, he'd use about 13.38 cal/min. (Note the higher rate of caloric expenditure.) Over the course of his 30-minute run, then, he'd use about 401 calories. So, exercising at a higher level of intensity used significantly more calories than exercising at a lower level of intensity [401 calories compared to 260 calories]. This is true despite the fact that the activity of lower intensity was performed for twice as long as the activity of higher intensity.

These calculations have been corroborated by research performed in the laboratory. In one study, 16 subjects walked on a treadmill at an average speed of 3.8 mph for 30 minutes. In this instance, they used about 8.0 cal/min for a total caloric expenditure of 240 calories. Of these 240 calories, 59% [144 calories] were from carbohydrates and 41% [96 calories] were from fat. As part of the study, the subjects also ran on a treadmill at an average speed of 6.5 mph for 30 minutes. At this relatively higher level of intensity, they used about 15.0 cal/min for a total caloric expenditure of 450 calories. Of these 450 calories, 76% [342 calories] were from carbohydrates and 24% [108 calories] were from fat. In other words, exercising at a higher level of intensity resulted in a greater total caloric expenditure than exercising at a lower level of intensity [450 calories compared to 240 calories] and also used a greater number of calories from fat in the same length of time [108 calories compared to 96 calories]. Other studies have also demonstrated that more calories are expended when running a given distance than walking the same distance. (By the way, this means that walking a mile doesn't use the same number of calories as running a mile as some people have suggested.)

The intent behind advocating low-intensity activity of long duration is to enhance safety and improve adherence, especially in those who are new to training. However, low-intensity activity isn't more effective for fat loss than high-intensity activity. Think about it: The activity that uses the greatest percentage of fat as an energy source is sleeping. And who would recommend sleeping as the best activity to lose fat?

In terms of losing weight, you must expend more calories than you consume in order to produce a caloric deficit. Whether you use carbohydrates or fat to produce this shortfall is immaterial. A caloric deficit that's created by the use of fat as an energy source doesn't necessarily translate into greater loss of fat compared to an equal caloric deficit that's created by the use of carbohydrates as an energy source. The main determinant of fat loss and weight loss is *calories*, not *composition*.

In short, researchers in the area of exercise and weight management generally agree that it probably doesn't matter whether you use carbohydrates or fat while exercising in order to lose weight. (Chapter 22 discusses the subject of weight management in greater detail.) Finally, it should also be noted that low-intensity activity might not elevate the heart rate enough to improve aerobic fitness.

Table 14.1: Predicted values of oxygen intake (in mL/kg/min) based on the time to complete a 1.5-mile run on a level surface

TIME	VALUE	TIME	VALUE	TIME	VALUE	TIME	VALUE
8:00	63.84	10:00	51.77	12:00	43.73	14:00	37.98
8:05	63.22	10:05	51.37	12:05	43.45	14:05	37.77
8:10	62.61	10:10	50.98	12:10	43.17	14:10	37.57
8:15	62.01	10:15	50.59	12:15	42.90	14:15	37.37
8:20	61.42	10:20	50.21	12:20	42.64	14:20	37.18
8:25	60.85	10:25	49.84	12:25	42.38	14:25	36.98
8:30	60.29	10:30	49.47	12:30	42.12	14:30	36.79
8:35	59.74	10:35	49.11	12:35	41.86	14:35	36.60
8:40	59.20	10:40	48.75	12:40	41.61	14:40	36.41
8:45	58.67	10:45	48.40	12:45	41.36	14:45	36.23
8:50	58.15	10:50	48.06	12:50	41.11	14:50	36.04
8:55	57.63	10:55	47.72	12:55	40.87	14:55	35.86
9:00	57.13	11:00	47.38	13:00	40.63	15:00	35.68
9:05	56.64	11:05	47.05	13:05	40.39	15:05	35.50
9:10	56.16	11:10	46.73	13:10	40.16	15:10	35.33
9:15	55.68	11:15	46.41	13:15	39.93	15:15	35.15
9:20	55.21	11:20	46.09	13:20	39.70	15:20	34.98
9:25	54.76	11:25	45.78	13:25	39.48	15:25	34.81
9:30	54.31	11:30	45.47	13:30	39.28	15:30	34.64
9:35	53.87	11:35	45.17	13:35	39.04	15:35	34.48
9:40	53.43	11:40	44.87	13:40	38.82	15:40	34.31
9:45	53.01	11:45	44.58	13:45	38.61	15:45	34.15
9:50	52.59	11:50	44.29	13:50	38.39	15:50	33.99
9:55	52.18	11:55	44.01	13:55	38.19	15:55	33.83

Table 14.2: Norms for oxygen intake in relative terms based on age and gender

MEN					
AGE	LOW	FAIR	AVERAGE	GOOD	HIGH
20 - 29	<38	39 - 43	44 - 51	52 - 56	57+
30 - 39	<34	35 - 39	40 - 47	48 - 51	52+
40 - 49	<30	31 - 35	36 - 43	44 - 47	48+
50 - 59	<25	26 - 31	32 - 39	40 - 43	44+
60 - 69	<21	22 - 26	27 - 35	36 - 39	40+
WOMEN					
AGE	LOW	FAIR	AVERAGE	GOOD	HIGH
20 - 29	<28	29 - 34	35 - 43	44 - 48	49+
30 - 39	<27	28 - 33	34 - 41	42 - 47	48+
40 - 49	<25	26 - 31	32 - 40	41 - 45	46+
50 - 65	<21	22 - 28	29 - 36	37 - 41	42+

Table 14.3: Norms for oxygen intake in absolute terms based on age and gender

MEN					
AGE	LOW	FAIR	AVERAGE	GOOD	HIGH
20 - 29	<2.79	2.80 - 3.09	3.10 - 3.69	3.70 - 3.99	4.00+
30 - 39	<2.49	2.50 - 2.79	2.80 - 3.39	3.40 - 3.69	3.70+
40 - 49	<2.19	2.20 - 2.49	2.50 - 3.09	3.10 - 3.39	3.40+
50 - 59	<1.89	1.90 - 2.19	2.20 - 2.79	2.80 - 3.09	3.10+
60 - 69	<1.59	1.60 - 1.89	1.90 - 2.49	2.50 - 2.79	2.80+
WOMEN					
AGE	LOW	FAIR	AVERAGE	GOOD	HIGH
20 - 29	<1.69	1.70 - 1.99	2.00 - 2.49	2.50 - 2.79	2.80+
30 - 39	<1.59	1.60 - 1.89	1.90 - 2.39	2.40 - 2.69	2.70+
40 - 49	<1.49	1.50 - 1.79	1.80 - 2.29	2.30 - 2.59	2.60+
50 - 65	<1.29	1.30 - 1.59	1.60 - 2.09	2.10 - 2.39	2.40+

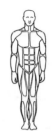

15 Anaerobic Training

Many sports and activities are composed of brief, intense movements that rely heavily on your anaerobic fitness. The best way for you to prepare for these specific physiological demands is through anaerobic training. (Literally, the term anaerobic means in the absence of oxygen.)

The main purpose of anaerobic training is to improve the functional ability of your anaerobic pathways, namely your ATP-PC System and Anaerobic Glycolysis. A second purpose of anaerobic training is to improve your performance potential, especially in sports and activities that require short-term, high-intensity efforts such as basketball, football and soccer.

But anaerobic training also produces some unexpected results. In a 1996 study that was led by Dr. Izumi Tabata, seven subjects did anaerobic training four times per week for six weeks. Each workout consisted of seven to eight repeats of 20 seconds of all-out sprinting on a stationary cycle with 10 seconds of recovery between each sprint. (This became known as the Tabata Protocol.) Once per week, the subjects also did 30 minutes of aerobic training along with four repeats of 20 seconds of all-out sprinting on a stationary cycle with 10 seconds of recovery between each sprint. The subjects not only increased their anaerobic fitness by 28% but also significantly improved their oxygen intake from about 48 mL/kg/min to 55 mL/kg/min. It's likely that the aerobic training had some influence on the improvement in oxygen intake but it's unclear as to what degree. Nonetheless, since this seminal study, additional research has found that anaerobic training can produce benefits that are nothing short of spectacular.

In one of those studies, eight subjects did anaerobic training three times per week for two weeks. Each workout consisted of four to seven repeats of a Wingate Test (30 seconds of all-out sprinting on a stationary cycle) with four minutes of recovery between each sprint. In the two-week period, the subjects did a total of 32 bouts of 30-second sprints, amounting to 16 minutes of sprinting. The longest "workout" involved 3.5 minutes of effort. The subjects improved their time to fatigue while cycling at 80% of their maximum oxygen intake by nearly 100% (from 26 minutes to 51 minutes). The results would have been even more astonishing if the data didn't include one subject who sustained an ankle injury (unrelated to the study) the day before the post-test and whose endurance decreased by 16%.

One other study deserves mention since it directly compared aerobic training to anaerobic training. In this study, researchers assigned 16 subjects to two groups: One group did aerobic training that consisted of 90 to 120 minutes of continuous exertion. The other group did anaerobic training that consisted of four to six repeats of a Wingate Test on a stationary cycle with four minutes of recovery between each sprint. Both groups did their assigned workout six times over a period of two weeks. In a cycling test that equated to about 18.65 miles, the group that did aerobic training decreased (improved) their time by 7.5% while the group that did anaerobic training decreased their time by 10.1%; in a cycling test that equated to about 1.24 miles, the group that did aerobic training decreased their time by 3.5% while the group that did anaerobic training decreased their time by 4.1%. Over the two-week period, the total exercise time of the group that did aerobic training was 630 minutes. Meanwhile, the total exercise time of the group that did anaerobic training was *15 minutes* (135 minutes if you count the recovery taken between sprints).

These studies and others haven't escaped notice by the media. This attention has produced a new-found awareness and appreciation of anaerobic training by the general population.

Note: Before you initiate anaerobic training, you must first establish a solid base of aerobic support through aerobic training. Your anaerobic pathways can't function at optimal levels without assistance from your aerobic pathway.

ANAEROBIC GUIDELINES

Anaerobic training is a bit more complex than aerobic training. The anaerobic pathways play a significant role in activities that last anywhere from a split second to roughly three minutes (assuming, of course, that the intensity of effort is great enough to justify an anaerobic response). Specifically, the ATP-PC System is used for efforts of about 30 seconds or less. The ATP-PC System and Anaerobic Glycolysis are used for efforts of about 30 to 90 seconds. Anaerobic Glycolysis and the Aerobic System are used for efforts of about 1.5 to 3.0 minutes. (The Aerobic System is used for efforts of about three minutes or more.)

Your anaerobic fitness may be improved and maintained by using several easy-to-follow guidelines. These guidelines can be organized under the acronym FITT which stands for Frequency, Intensity, Time and Type.

Frequency

In order to increase anaerobic fitness, anaerobic training should be done one or two days per week. The low frequency is required due to the intense nature of anaerobic training.

Highly active individuals may opt for greater frequency. In this case, the frequency of anaerobic training is dependent on the duration of the efforts. Long- and middle-duration efforts of 1.5 to 3.0 minutes (such as running between about 400 to 800 meters) can be done up to three days per week; short-duration efforts of 90 seconds or less (such as running roughly 400 meters or less) can be done up to four days per week. If you reach a point where you're no longer making improvements, then you're probably doing too much anaerobic training.

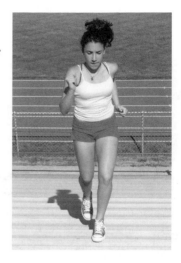

In order to increase anaerobic fitness, anaerobic training should be done one or two days per week. (Photo by Fred Fornicola.)

Intensity

With anaerobic training, your efforts must be done in an aggressive and enthusiastic fashion. To engage your anaerobic pathways, then, your intensity must be great enough such that you can't train continuously for much more than about three minutes at a time (which is the upper limit of the anaerobic domain).

Anaerobic intensity can be measured the same way as aerobic intensity: by monitoring your exercising heart rate. But anaerobic training requires a much higher level of intensity than aerobic training. In order to involve your anaerobic pathways, you must elevate your heart rate to near-maximum levels for brief periods of time. Raising your heart rate to 90% or more of your age-predicted maximum is usually a good indication that you're employing your anaerobic pathways. (Chapter 14 describes how you can determine your age-predicted maximum heart rate.)

If you're very active or have an above-average level of fitness, you should train with a higher percentage of your age-predicted maximum heart rate; if you're inactive or have a below-average level of fitness, you should train with a lower percentage of your age-predicted maximum heart rate.

Remember, the cornerstone of anaerobic training is short-term, high-intensity efforts. Unlike aerobic training – where a decreased level of intensity can be sacrificed for an increased duration of activity – it's an absolute requirement that anaerobic training is performed with a level of effort that's as high as possible.

Time

In determining whether or not an effort is anaerobic, the duration of the activity is more critical than the distance of the activity. As an example, suppose that two individuals who have different levels of fitness each ran 400 meters as fast as possible. The person who has the higher level of fitness may have completed the distance in one minute while the person who has the lower level of fitness may have needed two minutes. So, the distance that was run by the two individuals was the same but the time that was taken by the two individuals was different which means, in this case, that the energy pathways were different: The one-minute, all-out effort involved the ATP-PC System and Anaerobic Glycolysis while the two-minute, all-out effort involved Anaerobic Glycolysis and the Aerobic System.

That said, it's often more practical to consider distance rather than duration when performing anaerobic training. If a handful of seconds to three minutes is used as the range of time for anaerobic training, you can easily determine a range of distances. For example, an all-out effort that lasts a handful of seconds correlates to running about 40 meters (or 40 yards). And an all-out effort that lasts three minutes correlates to running about 800 meters (or one-half mile), at least for people who are in reasonably good condition. (You can determine a precise range of distances for your anaerobic efforts during rowing, running, swimming and other activities based on the energy continuum and your level of fitness.)

For competitive athletes, the distances (times) that are used during their anaerobic training should approximate the distances (times) that are used during their sport or activity. For example, if a sport or an activity involves a series of intense efforts that are 30 meters or less, then these specific distances should receive the most emphasis during anaerobic training. At least some

of the efforts, however, should also consist of distances (times) that are a little beyond those normally encountered in competition.

Type

Most of the same activities that can be used for aerobic training can also be used for anaerobic training. Outdoor activities include cycling, rowing and running; indoor activities include rope jumping and swimming along with exercising on stationary equipment such as cycles (upright or recumbent), ellipticals, rowers, steppers/stairclimbers and treadmills.

If you're a competitive athlete who's training for a specific event – such as cycling or rowing – the best activities to do are the ones that you're going to perform. If you want to become a better cyclist, you must mainly cycle; if you want to become a better rower, you must mainly row.

For runners and other athletes whose sport or activity involves running, the best activity is, of course, running. However, they can – and should – occasionally use non- or low-impact activities to minimize the impact forces that are associated with running.

MEANINGFUL ANAEROBIC TRAINING

Over a period of time, you'll likely find that the same anaerobic workout – which was originally difficult – can be performed with less

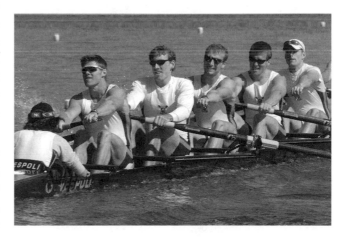

If you want to become a better cyclist, you must mainly cycle; if you want to become a better rower, you must mainly row. (Photo by Tom Nowak.)

effort. As you improve your anaerobic fitness, your exercising heart rate will be lower for a given level of intensity. Because of this, you must increase your intensity as needed so that you're always training with an appropriate percentage of your maximum heart rate. In addition, your ability to maintain a higher exercising heart rate will become easier. As a result, it's important for you to make your anaerobic training progressively more challenging so that you can produce further improvements in your anaerobic fitness.

There are three main ways to overload your anaerobic systems. In comparison to a previous workout, you must attempt to (1) complete the same distances in shorter durations; (2) maintain the same pace for greater distances or durations; or (3) decrease the duration of the recovery between efforts. As an example, suppose that you rowed a series of eight 200-meter sprints in an average time of 1:00 (a pace of 200 meters per minute) and took an average recovery time of 2:30 between your efforts. In a future workout, you should try to (1) row eight 200s in an average time of less than 1:00; (2) row eight sprints of more than 200 meters at an average pace of 200 meters per minute; or (3) take an average recovery time of less than 2:30 between the eight 200s. Regardless of which tactic you employ, you made your anaerobic systems work harder than they were accustomed to working. (Note: With some stationary equipment, you can increase the resistance which also makes your anaerobic systems work harder than in a previous workout.)

For this reason, it's vital that you keep accurate records of your anaerobic training. Maintaining records permits you to track your progress thereby making your anaerobic workouts more productive and more meaningful. During anaerobic training, the key program components to monitor include the date of your workout, the distances that you completed, the durations of your efforts, the durations of your recovery between your efforts and the level of your intensity (your exercising heart rate).

METHODS OF ANAEROBIC TRAINING

Several different methods can be used to develop your anaerobic pathways. Remember that the parameters for time and intensity must be satisfied in order for an activity to be considered anaerobic. Doing an activity with an intense effort in about three minutes or less is necessary to improve your anaerobic pathways.

For the sake of simplicity, most of the ensuing discussions of anaerobic training use running as the example. However, all of the methods that can be used to increase your running performance can be applied to virtually any type of activity as well as any type of equipment. For instance, if your goal in a particular workout is to run six 400-meter sprints in 90 seconds per sprint, you could cycle, row or do another activity with an intense effort for 90 seconds a total of six times.

The most common method of anaerobic training is to perform a series of intense efforts that last for brief periods of time such as repeated sprints. But in order for your anaerobic training to be as productive as possible, it must be done in an organized manner. Performing anaerobic training on an informal basis can certainly produce favorable results but a formal program that's structured and has a scientific foundation is more precise and more productive.

Three popular methods of anaerobic training are interval training, fartlek training and acceleration sprinting.

Interval Training

Structured interval training has been around since the 1930s and remains especially popular for running and swimming. However, the principles of interval training can be applied to just about any type of activity and equipment. In fact, these concepts have been promoted as high-intensity interval training (or HIIT), the basis of which had its genesis in the research of Dr. Tabata.

Essentially, interval training is a series of repeated segments (or intervals) of intense activity (such as sprinting) alternated with periods of recovery that can be either reduced activity (such as walking or jogging) or complete inactivity. As an example, you'd run a given distance at an intended pace or in a specified time, recover and then repeat the run-recovery sequence until your workout is completed.

Interval training allows you to repeatedly reach and sustain a high level of intensity for a cumulative time that's greater than what you could achieve during continuous training with the same intensity. The reason for this is because the recovery periods allow your anaerobic systems the opportunity to partially recover thereby permitting you to make a physiological comeback between your intense efforts. By dividing your workout into short, intense efforts with intervals of recovery interspersed between your efforts, you can perform a greater volume of work with the same intensity. So, with an appropriate amount of recovery between anaerobic efforts, you can run a series of six 400-meter sprints at a pace that might otherwise completely exhaust you after two or three consecutive 400s without a recovery period.

An interval program consists of seven different variables that you can manipulate to effectively overload your anaerobic pathways. These variables are dependent on your level of fitness; someone who has a low level of fitness won't be able to perform as much volume of training as someone who has a high level of fitness. The seven variables are:

1. Number of Repetitions

One variable to consider during interval training is the number of repetitions (or times) that the anaerobic efforts are performed. For example, you might do eight repetitions of a specified distance during your workout.

2. Distance

A second variable during interval training is the distance of the anaerobic efforts such as running 800 meters or swimming 200 meters in a specified time. An interval workout usually begins with longer efforts and tapers down to shorter ones. For instance, you'd complete all of

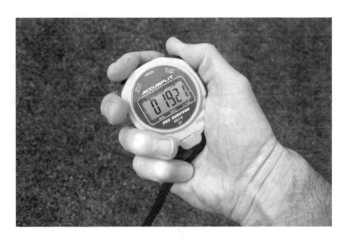

It's important for you to receive a sufficient amount of recovery between your anaerobic efforts.

the 400-meter sprints followed by all of the 200-meter sprints and so on.

If you're an athlete who's interested in improving your anaerobic fitness to better prepare yourself for competition, the distance of your intense efforts should approximate the requirements of your sport or activity. So, a softball player who's looking to get down the base path more quickly should emphasize intense efforts of 20 yards (the distance from home plate to first base).

3. Work Interval

The intended time of the anaerobic effort is the work interval. Your goal, for example, might be to row a specified distance in a work interval of 30 seconds or less.

4. Recovery Interval

The time that's allotted to recuperate between the work intervals is the recovery interval. It's important for you to receive a sufficient amount of recovery between your anaerobic efforts. This allows your depleted anaerobic systems enough time to recover so that you can make another intense effort. As an example, the recovery intervals between your work intervals might provide 90 seconds of recuperation.

The duration of the recovery interval is related to the time that it takes to complete the work interval. You can customize the duration of your recovery intervals by using your heart rate to

Table 15.1: Summary of times, running distances and work:recovery ratios

WORK/TIME (sec)	DISTANCE (m)	WORK:RECOVERY RATIO
0 to 30	0 to 200	1:4 to 1:3
30 to 90	200 to 400	1:3 to 1:2
90 to 180	400 to 800	1:2 to 1:1

Note: The ranges of time apply to both the highly and poorly conditioned; the running distances are for those who are in reasonably good condition.

determine when you're physiologically ready to perform your next work interval. For instance, you might begin your next work interval when your heart rate drops to a predetermined level such as 60% of your age-predicted maximum heart rate. An appropriate decrease in heart rate depends on several factors including the length of the last work interval and your level of fitness.

The recovery interval can consist of either reduced activity (that ranges from light to moderate) or complete inactivity. For anaerobic efforts that last about 30 seconds or less, the recovery interval should consist of complete inactivity. This gives your ATP-PC System the opportunity to replenish much of its stores. Moderate activity hinders this process which places greater demands on your other anaerobic system, Anaerobic Glycolysis. For anaerobic efforts that last about 30 seconds or more, the recovery interval should consist of light activity (such as walking) or moderate activity (such as jogging). This doesn't significantly impact the recovery of your ATP-PC System and allows for the partial removal of blood lactate.

Incidentally, most sports and activities have built-in recovery intervals because of their intermittent nature. Though these inherent respites are unofficial, unscientific and unpredictable, they permit a fairly successful replenishment of your stockpiles of ATP and PC.

5. Work:Recovery Ratio

The recovery interval is usually expressed in relation to the work interval. This is known as the work:recovery ratio and is most often designated as 1:1, 1:2, 1:3 or 1:4. These particular ratios state that the recovery interval should be

one, two, three or four times the duration that it took you to perform the work interval. As a rule of thumb, the shorter the duration of effort – and the higher the intensity of effort – the greater the work:recovery ratio.

Because of the high level of intensity, any anaerobic effort that you complete in 30 seconds or less requires a work:recovery ratio of at least 1:3. As an example, an all-out effort that takes you 15 seconds to perform should be followed by a recovery interval of about 45 seconds or more. An all-out effort that's done in 30 to 90 seconds needs a work:recovery ratio between 1:3 and 1:2. Finally, an all-out effort that's done in 90 to 180 seconds needs a work:recovery ratio between 1:2 and 1:1. Table 15.1 shows a summary of times, running distances and their accompanying work:recovery ratios.

6. Workout Distance

The sum of all the distances that are performed in an interval workout is the workout distance. When performing work intervals that last between about 1.5 and 3.0 minutes, the total distance of your workout shouldn't exceed about 2.0 to 2.5 miles (or 3,200 to 4,000 meters) of running; when performing work intervals that last less than about 90 seconds, the total distance of your workout shouldn't exceed about 1.5 to 2.0 miles (or 2,400 to 3,200 meters) of running. (Note: Swimming distances equate to roughly 20% of running distances.)

7. Frequency of Workouts

A final variable to consider is the frequency of the interval workouts. Except for highly active individuals, interval training shouldn't be done more than once or twice a week because of the high level of intensity that's required.

A prescription for interval training can be written in shorthand. In the language of interval training, for example, "8 x 100 m (0:20/1:00)" indicates that you're to perform eight 100-meter work intervals and that each effort should be done in 20 seconds (or less) with a recovery interval of one minute between each of the eight repetitions. (Note that the work:recovery ratio is 1:3 because each effort is less than 30 seconds in duration.)

Table 15.2 is a detailed example of a nine-week interval program for running that has an anaerobic emphasis. As mentioned earlier, interval training that's designed for running can be easily adapted to virtually any type of activity and equipment.

Fartlek Training

The predecessor of interval training is thought to be fartlek training. Originally developed by the Swedes, fartlek training was introduced to the United States in the 1940s.

The Swedes are famous in physical-education circles for developing systems of training that were basic in structure and used the outdoors as much as possible. It's no surprise, then, that fartlek training is usually performed outside over natural but varied terrain that ranges from flat surfaces to steady inclines and declines. For this reason, fartlek training was probably a precursor of the hill training that's often used by modern runners. Fartlek training can also be done indoors using a wide variety of equipment.

Sometimes referred to as speed play, fartlek training is quite similar to interval training. In structure, fartlek training is less formal and less exact than interval training. Nonetheless, fartlek training improves anaerobic fitness by employing different combinations of effort such as walking, jogging and running. The work and recovery intervals are left entirely up to the individual; you can change your pace and recover at your own discretion. So, there's a clear intent to "play" with speed.

A sample fartlek workout for running that emphasizes your anaerobic pathways might look like this:

1. jog 400 meters

2. walk 200 meters

3. jog 400 meters

4. walk 200 meters

5. sprint 100 meters uphill and walk 100 meters downhill in an alternating fashion for six minutes

6. jog 400 meters

7. walk 400 meters

8. sprint 50 meters and walk 50 meters in an alternating fashion for three minutes

Acceleration Sprinting

An effective technique that's used by many runners to increase their speed is acceleration sprinting. This technique, however, can also be used to increase speed in other activities such as cycling, rowing and swimming.

As the name implies, acceleration sprinting is characterized by a gradual increase in speed until a full, all-out effort is reached. When running, for example, you'd begin by jogging then increase to striding and finally accelerate to sprinting the intended distance or duration. Between work intervals, the recovery intervals can consist of either reduced activity or complete inactivity.

Gradually increasing your speed throughout your effort allows you to concentrate on your technique which is enormously important in speed development. Acceleration sprinting also provides a smooth transition towards an all-out sprint thereby minimizing the potential for a muscle strain or pull.

A series of 100 meter acceleration sprints for running might look like this:

1. jog 20 meters, stride 30 meters and sprint 50 meters

2. walk 50 meters and repeat the series for a total of 10 times

Table 15.2: Sample nine-week interval program for running

WEEK	SPRINT REPS	DISTANCE (m)	WORK: RECOVERY RATIO	WORK TIME	RECOVERY TIME	WORKOUT DISTANCE	WORKOUTS PER WEEK
1	4	800	1:1	3:00	3:00	3,200	1
2	3	800	1:1	3:00	3:00	3,200	1
	2	400	1:2	1:30	3:00		
3	2	800	1:1	2:55	3:00	3,200	1
	4	400	1:2	1:30	3:00		
4	1	800	1:1	2:55	3:00	3,200	1
	6	400	1:2	1:25	2:45		
5	4	400	1:2	1:25	2:45	2,400	2
	4	200	1:3	0:40	2:00		
6	3	400	1:2	1:20	2:45	2,400	2
	4	200	1:3	0:40	2:00		
	4	100	1:3	0:20	1:00		
7	2	400	1:2	1:20	2:45	2,400	2
	6	200	1:3	0:39	2:00		
	4	100	1:3	0:20	1:00		
8	1	400	1:2	1:15	2:30	2,400	2
	6	200	1:3	0:39	2:00		
	8	100	1:3	0:19	1:00		
9	1	400	1:2	1:15	2:30	2,400	2
	4	200	1:3	0:38	1:45		
	8	100	1:3	0:19	1:00		
	8	50	1:4	0:10	0:45		

MEASURING ANAEROBIC FITNESS

Evaluating anaerobic fitness is complicated. The difficulty arises because no single test serves as a reliable indicator of your anaerobic fitness. Remember, the two anaerobic pathways – the ATP-PC System and Anaerobic Glycolysis – contribute in varying ways to a wide range of efforts that last from an instant up to about three minutes. To obtain a true picture of your anaerobic fitness, it's necessary to perform several tests across the anaerobic spectrum. (Needless to say, measuring an instantaneous effort has plenty of room for error.)

There's an inverse relationship between the duration that you can sustain an intense effort and the output of power during the effort: The shorter the duration of an intense effort, the greater the output of power. Therefore, you can estimate your anaerobic fitness by measuring your power output.

In scientific terms, power is defined as the amount of work done per unit of time or, more simply, work divided by time. In this case, work is the application of a force over a distance or force times distance. For example, if you moved 100 pounds [lb] a distance of three feet [ft], you did 300 foot-pounds [ft-lb] of work [100 lb x 3 ft = 300 ft-lb]. If you performed this effort in 0.25 seconds [sec], your power output was 1,200 ft-lb/sec [300 ft-lb ÷ 0.25 sec = 1,200 ft-lb/sec].

In a laboratory setting, a popular test of anaerobic fitness is the Margaria-Kalamen Power Test. The test was developed by Dr. Rodolfo Margaria and two of his colleagues in 1966 at the University of Milan and later modified by Dr. Jerome Kalamen. At the start of this test, you're to stand six meters in front of a staircase. Initiating movement on your own, you'd run up the stairs as fast as possible, contacting every third step (in other words, taking three steps at a time).

Your power output can be calculated by multiplying your bodyweight times the vertical distance between the third and ninth step divided by the time of your effort (to the nearest hundredth of a second). For instance, suppose that you weigh 198 pounds and covered a vertical distance of four feet in 0.75 seconds. In this case, your power output would be 1,056 foot-pounds per second [198 lb x 4 ft ÷ 0.75 seconds = 1,056 ft-lb/sec]. (Values for some heavier athletes can exceed 2,000 ft-lb/sec.)

Several field tests have a high correlation with anaerobic fitness. Field tests evaluating all-out efforts that last a mere instant include the vertical jump, standing long jump and medicine-ball put. (Think of this as doing the shot put with a medicine ball.) A test of anaerobic fitness that's a little farther up the energy continuum is running a 40-yard dash.

Of slightly longer duration – though still in the anaerobic realm – is a highly popular laboratory assessment that's known as the Wingate Anaerobic Test or, simply, the Wingate Test. The test is named after the Wingate Institute for Physical Education and Sport in Netanya, Israel where it was developed in 1974. As mentioned earlier, this test is 30 seconds of all-out sprinting on a stationary cycle. Finally, your overall anaerobic fitness – the effectiveness of your ATP-PC System and Anaerobic Glycolysis – can be inferred from intense efforts that last about 30 to 90 seconds such as sprinting 200 to 400 meters as fast as possible.

As noted previously, the upper edge of the anaerobic spectrum is actually about three minutes. Keep in mind, though, that your Aerobic System begins providing help for intense efforts that are beyond roughly 90 seconds in duration. Therefore, a valid measurement of your unassisted anaerobic fitness should involve efforts of less than about 90 seconds.

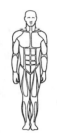

16 Metabolic Training

Most people typically perform their strength training separate from their aerobic training. Yet, many people – especially athletes – are required to integrate their muscular strength with their aerobic fitness. Good examples of this are basketball, football and soccer in which athletes must do brief, intense efforts that are spread out over a lengthy period of time. Being able to merge your muscular (or anaerobic) fitness with your aerobic fitness is a true measure of your metabolic fitness.

Essentially, metabolic training is a marriage of strength training (or other anaerobic efforts) and aerobic training. The physiological demands of metabolic training are shared by your musculoskeletal, respiratory and circulatory systems.

Unfortunately, metabolic training is rarely emphasized or even addressed. However, a thorough understanding of metabolic training and an application of specific methods can enhance your performance in activities that involve the collective efforts of your muscular strength and aerobic fitness.

PROJECT TOTAL CONDITIONING

In the spring of 1975, research designated as Project Total Conditioning was conducted at the United States Military Academy in West Point, New York. The subjects were drawn from the Corps of Cadets who were athletes at the academy. Project Total Conditioning actually consisted of several different studies. For instance, one study examined the effects of a strength program on the neck size and strength of rugby players; another study examined the effects of two different training protocols on the vertical jump of volleyball players.

However, the main portion of Project Total Conditioning was a study that investigated metabolic training. In this study, 19 football players did strength training three times per week for six weeks. The workouts were done on non-consecutive days with two days of recovery after the third workout of the week. (The subjects did 17 workouts during the six-week period.) Each workout consisted of 10 exercises; six exercises for the neck were also performed twice per week. One set of each exercise was done to the point of muscular fatigue within a repetition range of 5 to 12. The subjects took a minimum amount of recovery between exercises.

Prior to the study, the subjects followed the training protocol for two weeks in order to reduce the influence of the learning effect. Pre-testing was done after those first two weeks to collect baseline data. (Note: The learning effect refers to the dramatic increases that are often attained by individuals in the initial stages of a training program that are attributable to improvements in neurological function rather than muscular function.)

The study produced very compelling results. After six weeks of training, the subjects increased the resistance that they used by 58.54%. The minimum improvement in strength was 45.61% while the maximum improvement was 69.70%. The subjects also increased the number of repetitions that they performed by 6.59%.

Interestingly, the time that the subjects needed to complete their workouts decreased substantially. The subjects reduced the duration of their workouts by 24.09% – from 37.73 minutes to 28.64 minutes. Two subjects almost literally cut their workout times in half – one from 49 minutes to 25 minutes and the other from 43 minutes to 22 minutes – yet they increased their strength by 68.32% and 65.59%, respectively. A third subject reduced his workout time from 42 minutes to 27 minutes and increased his strength by 66.32%.

Besides the tremendous improvements in strength, the subjects also decreased their time in the two-mile run by 88 seconds, from 13:18 to 11:50. This represented an improvement of 11.03% . . . without having performed any running except during the course of spring football practice (which occurred during the first four weeks of training). The subjects also had lower resting heart rates and lower exercising heart rates at various workloads on a stationary cycle. Moreover, they were able to perform more work before reaching heart rates of 170 beats per minute.

The subjects decreased their time in the 40-yard dash from 5.1467 seconds to 5.0933 seconds, an improvement of 1.04%. Their vertical jump increased from 22.600 inches to 24.067 inches, an improvement of 6.49%. And they improved their range of motion in torso flexion by 5.57%, shoulder flexion by 11.62% and torso extension by 15.58%.

The results are even more startling when you consider the fact that they were accomplished in such a time-efficient manner: The total amount of actual training time performed by each subject during the six-week study was less than 8.5 hours which is less than 30 minutes per workout. It should be noted, too, that the subjects were highly conditioned football players who were already quite strong and fit at the start of the study. Nonetheless, this study demonstrated the far-reaching effects of short-duration, high-intensity strength training on metabolic fitness.

TYPES OF METABOLIC TRAINING

You can improve your metabolic fitness by simply doing your strength training with a high level of intensity while taking very little recovery between exercises/sets (à la Project Total Conditioning). When performed in this fashion, the shared demands that are placed on your major biological systems create metabolic

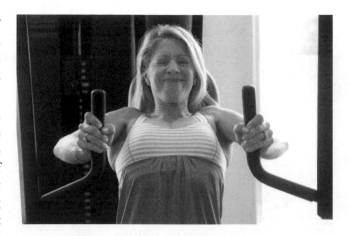

A form of metabolic training that has seen continued interest is high-intensity training or, simply, HIT. (Photo provided by Luke Carlson.)

improvements that can't be approached by traditional methods of strength training.

Two of the most popular types of metabolic training are high-intensity training and circuit training.

High-Intensity Training

A form of metabolic training that has seen continued interest is high-intensity training or, simply, HIT. The term high-intensity training appears in trade publications as early as 1973. (The acronym HIT became fashionable in 1988 with the publication of the *HIT Newsletter*.) HIT can be effective for anyone – regardless of lifting experience or aspiration – as long as it encourages progressive overload and allows sufficient recovery between workouts. The past four decades have provided literally tens of thousands of examples of individuals – both male and female with various levels of experience ranging from untrained beginners to highly trained athletes – as empirical evidence that HIT can be extremely productive.

Since it was first popularized in the early 1970s, there have been endless interpretations, variations and applications of HIT. Nevertheless, most versions of HIT have a number of common denominators. As the name implies, HIT is characterized by intense, aggressive efforts. Each set is typically performed to the point of muscular fatigue. Another characteristic of HIT is the emphasis on progressive overload. Whenever possible, an attempt is made to increase either the resistance that's used or the repetitions that are performed in comparison to a previous workout. A minimum number of sets are performed, often only one set of each exercise but sometimes several sets. With safety and efficiency in mind, the repetitions are done with a smooth, controlled speed of movement so that momentum doesn't play a significant role in raising the resistance. Additionally, HIT is comprehensive; addressing all of the major muscles is a priority.

HIT involves very brief workouts with a minimum amount of recovery between exercises/sets. The abbreviated recovery interval enables you to maintain a fairly high exercising heart rate for the duration of your workout. Like other types of metabolic training, the length of the recovery interval that's taken between exercises/sets depends on your level of fitness. The recovery interval isn't usually structured, timed or predetermined. Initially, however, a recovery interval of perhaps several minutes may be necessary between efforts; with improved fitness, your pace should be quickened to the point where you're moving as rapidly as possible between exercises/sets. (To be clear: The pace should be quickened, not the speed of repetitions.)

In short, HIT can place an incredible workload on every major muscle in your body and, at the same time, stress your respiratory and circulatory systems. Furthermore, HIT can be used to improve your metabolic fitness in a safe and time-efficient manner.

The 3x3 Workout. A simple but effective type of HIT workout that deserves special note is a 3x3 Workout or, for short, a 3x3 (pronounced "three by three"). A 3x3 Workout involves a series of three multiple-joint movements: one for the hips, one for the chest and one for the upper back. This series of three exercises is done a total of three times (thus the moniker 3x3). Virtually every major muscle in your body is addressed in a 3x3 Workout including your hips, hamstrings, quadriceps, chest, upper back, shoulders, biceps, triceps and forearms.

There are numerous options for multiple-joint movements that can be used in a 3x3 Workout. The safest and most effective multiple-joint movements for your hips are the deadlift, leg press and ball squat. Any multiple-joint movement that involves a pushing motion – such as the bench press, incline press, decline press, dip and push-up – can be used to target the muscles of your chest (as well as those of your shoulders and triceps); any multiple-joint movement that involves a pulling motion – such as the bench row, seated row, underhand lat pulldown, chin-up and pull-up – can be used to target the muscles of your upper back (along with your biceps and forearms).

The first time that the series of three exercises is done, you should reach muscular fatigue by about 20 repetitions for the hip exercise and 10 for the chest and upper-back exercises. The second time through the series, you should reach muscular fatigue by about 15 repetitions for the hip exercise and 8 for the chest and upper-back exercises. And the third time though the series, you should reach muscular fatigue by about 12 repetitions for the hip exercise and 6 for the chest and upper-back exercises. In summary, the target number of repetitions for each of the three sets should be 20, 15 and 12 for the hip exercise and 10, 8 and 6 for the chest and upper-back exercises.

As you might imagine, there are countless variations of a 3x3 Workout. Perhaps the most demanding series of exercises is the deadlift, dip and chin-up. Another version is a series of the leg press, bench press and seated row. Not to belabor a point but in both examples, the series of three exercises would be done three times (for a total of nine sets in the workout). As a side note, each of the three series can contain different exercises. For instance, a 3x3 Workout could be the deadlift, incline press, pull-up, leg press, bench press, seated row, ball squat, decline press and underhand lat pulldown.

In doing a 3x3 Workout, you should take as little recovery as possible between exercises/sets. This will yield excellent improvements in your metabolic fitness. Plus, it makes a 3x3 Workout extremely time-efficient; most variations can be performed in about 20 minutes or less.

225

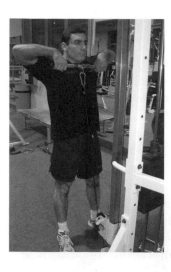

A popular way of doing CST is on a multi-station machine. (Photo by Peter Silletti.)

The simplicity of this type of HIT workout can be deceptive. Though it may not appear so, a 3x3 Workout – if done as outlined here – can be incredibly challenging and demanding. Remember, you're doing exercises that engage a large amount of muscle mass while training to the point of muscular fatigue and taking as little recovery as possible between each of the nine sets.

Circuit Training

One of the oldest and most popular types of metabolic training is circuit training. The birth of circuit training can be traced back to Ronald Morgan and Graham Adamson who developed the system at the University of Leeds in the early 1950s. It wasn't long before circuit training made its way across the Atlantic where it became all the rage in the United States, especially in high schools and colleges.

With circuit training, the idea is to perform a series of exercises (or activities) in a sequence (or circuit) with a very brief recovery interval between each station. In a sense, therefore, circuit training is a form of interval training.

Circuit Strength Training. The traditional version of circuit training is essentially strength training with a fast pace between exercises/sets. This can be referred to as circuit strength training (CST).

A popular way of doing CST is on a multi-station machine (aka multi-station gym). This offers several advantages. First of all, the exercises of a multi-station gym are in close proximity to

each other which allows you to move quickly around the circuit. Secondly, the selectorized weight stacks of a multi-station gym enable you to make quick and easy adjustments in the resistance. But CST can also be performed with single-station equipment and/or free weights provided that the distance between the exercises isn't too great.

CST is very versatile; you can manipulate the number of exercises in the circuit, the number of repetitions for each exercise and the amount of recovery that's taken between the exercises. The number of exercises that you do in the circuit and the amount of recovery that you take between the exercises are a function of your level of fitness. However, a comprehensive workout of CST involves a series of about 12 to 14 exercises that address your major muscles.

Many multi-station gyms don't offer exercises for the hips, legs and mid-section. In this case, a multi-station gym would need to be augmented with some single-station machines and/or free weights in order to target all of the major muscles. An example of a total-body circuit that incorporates a multi-station gym and a few supplemental exercises is the ball squat, leg curl, leg extension, bench press, push-up, chin-up, overhand lat pulldown, upright row, scapulae adduction, bicep curl, tricep extension, wrist flexion, side bend and back extension.

At each station, you can either perform a given number of repetitions or do as many repetitions as possible during a specified time frame (with a smooth, controlled speed of movement). Using a pace of 60 seconds per exercise (the work interval) with 30 seconds of recovery between stations including the set-up for the next exercise (the recovery interval), a circuit of 12 to 14 exercises can be completed in as little as 18 to 21 minutes. It should be noted that the resistance you use at each station should permit you to reach muscular fatigue by the end of the allotted work interval.

With CST, there are three main ways of overload. In comparison to a previous workout, you must attempt to (1) increase the resistance that you use at a given station; (2) increase the length of the work interval (thereby doing more repetitions); or (3) decrease the length of the recovery interval that's taken between stations. Though well intended, you shouldn't try to increase the number of repetitions that you do in a certain amount of time since this encourages poor technique.

To summarize CST: You begin at a particular station and complete one set of an exercise. After this, you move to the next station in the circuit where you set up for your next exercise and recuperate for the remainder of the recovery interval. This process is repeated until the entire circuit is completed.

Circuit Strength and Anaerobic Training. A second version of circuit training is to integrate strength training with another form of anaerobic training. For instance, you might do the chest press, pedal a stationary cycle for one to two minutes, do the underhand lat pulldown, pedal a stationary cycle for another one to two minutes and so on. The goal is to perform the equivalent of about 20 to 30 minutes of total activity.

Along these lines, you can do a basic but brutal form of metabolic training by alternating dips and chin-ups with sprinting. In other words, you might do a set of dips, sprint a specified distance, do a set of chin-ups, sprint a specified distance and repeat this circuit several times. (If performed indoors, you can run on a treadmill provided that its location is convenient.)

Circuit Aerobic Training. Since the term cross training came into vogue in the mid-1990s, there has been a growing interest in circuit aerobic training (CAT). Although the emphasis of CAT is more on aerobic fitness than metabolic fitness, it's a version of circuit training and, thus, merits note here.

CAT involves a series of aerobic activities or stations. It can be designed many different ways; you can vary the number of activities, the duration and intensity of each activity and the amount of recovery that's taken between activities.

As with all other types of physical training, most of these variables are dependent on your level of fitness. Your goal, however, is to perform

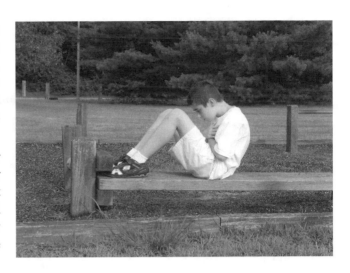

A typical fitness trail consists of numerous stations that are positioned at various points along a circuitous route.

the equivalent of about 20 to 60 minutes of aerobic activity with an appropriate level of intensity. Keep in mind that 30 minutes of activity can be done as two 15-minute bouts, three 10-minute bouts or even six 5-minute bouts. So, you can exercise for 10 minutes on a stationary cycle, 10 minutes on a rower and 10 minutes on a stepper/ stairclimber for a total of 30 minutes of activity. Or, you might perform each of those same three activities for five minutes but repeat the circuit twice for a total of 30 minutes of activity. Regardless, your level of intensity should be as high as possible during each of your efforts.

The Fitness Trail. Originating in several of the Scandinavian countries, the so-called fitness trail is a type of circuit training that's performed outdoors in a natural environment such as a park. A typical fitness trail consists of numerous stations that are positioned at various points along a circuitous route. You'd run or sprint to a station, stop and perform some kind of exercise or activity that may be for agility (such as hurdles, log walks or vaults), strength (such as push-ups, abdominal crunches, dips or chin-ups) or flexibility (such as a calf stretch) and then proceed to the next station.

METABOLIC DYNAMICS

Metabolic training presents an enormous physiological challenge to your musculoskeletal, respiratory and circulatory systems. In response to the demands, these three systems make a number of sudden – and sometimes dramatic – adjustments that gradually return to resting levels once the activity is completed.

Detailing your specific responses to metabolic training is impossible. Your responses can vary a great deal based on your intensity and the duration of the activity as well as the type of metabolic training that was done. Other factors that determine your response include your size, gender and level of fitness. Therefore, what follows is an overview of your general responses to metabolic training.

In going from rest to intense activity, these metabolic responses occur:

- An increase in the rate and depth of breathing. Labored breathing is an unmistakable indicator of intense activity. This leads to a heightened sense of respiratory distress, general discomfort and widespread fatigue.

- An increase in tidal volume (the amount of air that you inhale or exhale in a single breath, measured in liters per breath).

- An increase in minute ventilation (the amount of air that you inhale or exhale each minute, measured in liters per minute). Minute ventilation is calculated by multiplying the rate of your breathing by your tidal volume.

- An increase in oxygen intake and the rate of caloric expenditure.

- An increase in the involvement of the respiratory muscles, specifically the abdominals and internal intercostals (which lie between your ribs). During intense activity, your respiratory muscles may require 25% or more of your oxygen intake.

- An increase in heart rate. During intense activity, your heart beats faster to meet the demands for more blood and oxygen. (Your heart rate actually increases above resting levels *prior* to your effort due to the so-called anticipatory response.)

- An increase in stroke volume (the amount of blood that's pumped by your heart, measured in milliliters per beat).

- An increase in cardiac output (the amount of blood that's pumped by your heart in a given amount of time). Cardiac output is calculated by multiplying your heart rate by your stroke volume. Once your stroke volume reaches your physiological limit, further increases in your cardiac output are only possible through increases in your heart rate.

- An increase in blood flow to more active muscles and organs and a decrease in blood flow to less active muscles and organs. At rest, about 20% of your blood flow goes to your muscles; the majority of the blood goes to your digestive organs, kidneys and brain. During intense activity, about 70% or more of your blood flow goes to your exercising muscles. In addition, there's an increase in the volume of blood flow to your heart as well as to your skin in order to dissipate heat. (The volume of blood flow to your brain is unchanged.)

- An increase in systolic blood pressure and no change or a slight decrease in diastolic blood pressure (measured in millimeters of mercury). Maximum blood pressure usually occurs at maximum heart rate.

- An increase in body temperature, especially in hot, humid conditions. Your body has a temperature-regulatory mechanism that acts in the same manner as a thermostat, trying to maintain its temperature at a relatively constant value of roughly 98.6 degrees Fahrenheit (about 37 degrees Celsius).

- An increase in the production of carbon dioxide and lactic acid. This, in turn, decreases your muscle pH. The lactic acid spreads from your muscles into the surrounding tissues and eventually spills into your blood. This causes your blood pH to decrease. As the lactic acid begins to accumulate, it irritates your nerve endings and causes feelings of pain, discomfort, distress and fatigue. It also causes your breathing to become labored.

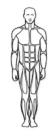

17 Power Training

An important aspect of athletic performance is power. It's no surprise, then, that coaches and athletes are continually looking for ways to improve this valuable physical commodity.

It has long been thought that the so-called quick lifts – such as the power clean, push press, snatch and/or their derivatives – and high-speed repetitions must be done to improve power. But power training doesn't have to incorporate these methods.

POWER DEFINED

Before discussing how you can improve your power, it's important for you to understand the meaning of the term. In physics, a mathematical definition of power is work divided by time. Since work is defined as force times distance, it follows that power is also force times distance divided by time.

Another definition of power is force times velocity. The term velocity is defined as distance divided by time. Once again, it follows that power is force times distance divided by time.

So power has three variables: force, distance and time. Manipulating any of these three variables will affect power.

METHODS FOR IMPROVEMENT

Based on the equation "power equals force times distance divided by time," you can improve your power output three different ways: (1) increase the amount of force; (2) increase the distance of application; and (3) decrease the time of application.

Increase the Amount of Force

If you increase the amount of force that you apply and keep the other two variables in the equation the same – namely, the distance over which you apply the force and the time that it takes you to apply the force – you'll produce more power. Example: If you can bench press 160 pounds a distance of 18 inches (1.5 feet) in two seconds, your power output is 120 foot-pounds per second [160 lb x 1.5 ft ÷ 2.0 sec = 120 ft-lb/sec]. Suppose that at some point in the future, you increased your bench press to 180 pounds. Assuming that the distance you moved the resistance (18 inches) and the time it took you to move the resistance (two seconds) remained the same, your power output is now 135 foot-pounds per second. So by increasing the amount of force that you applied, you've improved your power output.

How do you increase the amount of force that you apply? One way is to increase the strength of your muscles. If you increase the strength of your muscles, they can produce more force; if your muscles produce more force, you'll have the potential to produce more power.

How do you improve your strength so that you can produce more force? While there's no shortage of opinions, any strength program will be productive if – and only if – it incorporates the Overload Principle. Arguably, this principle is the most important underlying construct for improving physical performance, whether it's training for strength, aerobic fitness or even flexibility. As far as strength training is concerned, the principle states that in order for a muscle to increase in strength (and size) it must be stressed or overloaded – with a workload that's beyond its present capacity.

You can overload your muscles by using a double-progressive technique. When employing this technique, overload is accomplished by two means: Increasing the resistance that you use and/or the repetitions that you do in comparison to a previous workout. Your muscles will adapt

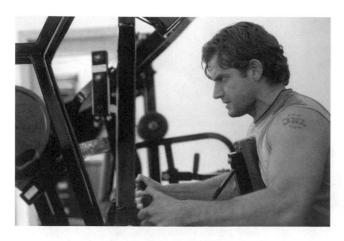

If you increase the strength of your muscles, they can produce more force; if your muscles produce more force, you'll have the potential to produce more power. (Photo provided by Luke Carlson.)

to the overload – from using a heavier amount of resistance or performing a greater number of repetitions – by increasing in strength (and size). Without imposing greater demands, there won't be any compensatory adaptation because your muscles will literally have no reason to get stronger. Stated otherwise, your muscles must be exposed to demands that they haven't previously encountered.

Also remember that it matters little whether your muscles are loaded with resistance from machines, barbells, dumbbells, resistance bands, sandbags, bricks or even other human beings. Your muscles don't possess the ability to distinguish between different types of resistance; they simply respond to being loaded.

Increase the Distance of Application

If you increase the distance over which you apply the force and keep the other two variables in the equation the same – namely, the amount of force that you apply and the time that it takes you to apply the force – you'll produce more power. Example: If you can squat 300 pounds a distance of 21 inches (1.75 feet) in two seconds, your power output is 262.5 foot-pounds per second [300 lb x 1.75 ft ÷ 2.0 sec = 262.5 ft-lb/sec]. Suppose that at some point in the future, you increased your range of motion in the squat so that you're now moving the resistance a

distance of 24 inches. Assuming that the resistance you lifted (300 pounds) and the time it took you to move the resistance (two seconds) remained the same, your power output is now 300 foot-pounds per second. So by increasing the distance over which you applied the force, you've improved your power output.

How do you increase the distance over which you apply force? One way is to become more flexible. If you become more flexible, you can increase the range of motion of your joints; if you increase the range of motion of your joints, you'll have the potential to produce more power.

How do you improve your flexibility so that you can apply force over a greater distance? Like strength training, there's no one optimal way to improve flexibility. But different types of flexibility training that are effective have several commonalities. To reduce your risk of injury, you should stretch under control without using any bouncing or jerking movements. Moreover, you should hold the stretched position for about 10 to 30 seconds. Similar to strength training, you must make your flexibility training progressively more challenging. You can do this by attempting to stretch slightly farther than the last time. Finally, it's important to stretch daily either before or after physical training.

Decrease the Time of Application

If you decrease the time that it takes you to apply the force and keep the other two variables in the equation the same – namely, the amount of force that you apply and the distance over which you apply the force – you'll produce more power. Example: If you can deadlift 400 pounds a distance of 18 inches (1.5 feet) in two seconds, your power output is 300 foot-pounds per second [400 lb x 1.5 ft ÷ 2.0 sec = 300 ft-lb/sec]. Suppose that at some point in the future, you increased your speed of movement in the deadlift to 1.5 seconds (you did the repetition faster). Assuming that the resistance you lifted (400 pounds) and the distance you moved the resistance (18 inches) remained the same, your power output is now 400 foot-pounds per second. So by increasing the speed at which you applied the force, you've improved your power output.

How do you decrease the time that it takes you to apply force? One way is to perfect your technique in a given skill. If you perfect your technique, you can perform the skill more quickly; if you perform the skill more quickly, you'll have the potential to produce more power.

How do you improve your technique so that you can decrease the time that it takes you to apply force? The scientific literature is in general agreement as to how this can best be achieved. First, it's important that you learn how to do the skill correctly. Second, you must perform the skill over and over again until you can execute it with little or no conscious effort. The skill must be practiced perfectly and exactly as it would be used during a sport or an activity. Remember, practice makes perfect . . . but only if your practice is perfect.

PRACTICAL APPLICATIONS

Examples were given to show how the three variables in the power equation – force, distance and time – can be manipulated to improve power output in the bench press, squat and deadlift. Applications of these three variables can also be illustrated during sports. Consider these applications in baseball or softball:

Force: If you apply more force over the same distance in the same amount of time, you'll have the potential to throw with more power.

Distance: If you move a greater distance with the same amount of force in the same amount of time, you'll have the potential to swing with more power.

Time: If you move in less time with the same amount of force over the same distance, you'll have the potential to run with more power.

POWER TO YOU!

So, an individual who's powerful can apply a large force over a long distance in a short time.

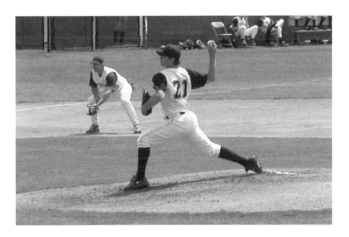

If you apply more force over the same distance in the same amount of time, you'll have the potential to throw with more power. (Photo by Melanie Silletti.)

As demonstrated earlier, your power output can be improved by three different means: (1) increase the amount of force that you apply; (2) increase the distance over which you apply the force; and (3) decrease the amount of time that it takes you to apply the force. This can be accomplished by improving your strength, flexibility and technique.

Be forewarned, however, that just because you can produce more power during a given exercise inside the fitness center (or weight room) doesn't mean that you'll automatically produce more power during a given skill outside the fitness center. Despite an abundance of anecdotal claims, there's no legitimate, scientific evidence to suggest that producing power can transfer from one activity to another.

Think about it: If doing the power clean (or another quick lift) improves your performance in the vertical jump, for example, then doing the vertical jump should improve your performance in the power clean. But it doesn't. The bottom line is that producing power inside the fitness center is one thing and producing power outside the fitness center is another.

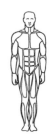

18 Skill Training

Motor learning is the study of how motor skills are acquired, applied and refined. Motor control is the study of how the neuromuscular system works to coordinate the nerves, muscles and limbs that are involved in motor skills. Together, motor learning and motor control investigate the improvement and performance of skills.

Naturally, this information is highly important for those who are trying to learn skills. With skill training, however, there are a number of practices that are well meaning but are often unsupported by the scientific literature.

SKILLS AND ABILITIES

The terms skill and ability are often used interchangeably and are somewhat related. However, skills are much different than abilities.

A skill refers to the level of performance in one specific action. Examples of skills include hitting a baseball, shooting a basketball, throwing a football and kicking a soccer ball. Skills can be improved through practice and experience.

An ability, on the other hand, refers to a general trait. Based on the work of Dr. Edwin Fleishman, there are two different types of abilities: perceptual and physical.

Perceptual abilities include multi-limb coordination, response orientation, reaction time and speed of limb movement. Physical abilities include static flexibility, dynamic flexibility, static balance, dynamic balance, static strength, dynamic strength, explosive strength and stamina.

Although abilities aren't specific skills, they establish the foundation for specific skills. Doing a specific skill such as a handstand, for instance, requires the general abilities of static balance and static strength. Abilities are thought to be genetically determined and, as a result, can be improved but only within inherited limits. Physical abilities likely have a greater potential for improvement than perceptual abilities.

Different skills – no matter how alike they seem – require different abilities. For instance, throwing two balls of different size, shape and/or weight – say, a baseball and football – would involve different abilities. Furthermore, abilities are thought to be independent of each other; the quality of one ability isn't dependent on the quality of another. So, an individual who can perform well in some skills doesn't necessarily perform well in others.

A perfect example of this is when Michael Jordan – perhaps the greatest basketball player of all time – took his world-class abilities from the basketball court to the baseball diamond. In 1994, while playing for the Class AA Birmingham Barons of the Southern League, he stole 30 bases (in 48 attempts) and drove in 51 runs. But Jordan only hit .202 – the lowest batting average of any regular player in the league – and whiffed 114

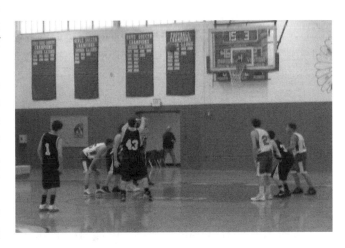

An example of a skill is shooting a basketball. (Photo by Mark Brzycki.)

233

times in 436 at bats. On defense, he led all outfielders in the league with 11 errors. He couldn't return to the basketball court fast enough.

Quickness and Balance Exercises

Athletes often do drills for quickness and balance. The expectation, of course, is that executing drills that involve quickness or balance will transfer to skills that require quickness or balance and, thus, improve athletic performance.

Numerous studies have investigated this possibility. According to Dr. Richard Schmidt, a leading researcher in motor learning, there's little evidence that practicing a skill that requires a certain ability will improve another skill that requires the same ability.

Being quick is advantageous in most sports and activities. Dr. Schmidt notes that at least three abilities are used to be quick: (1) reaction time (the interval of time between an unanticipated stimulus and the start of the response); (2) response orientation (where one of many stimuli is presented, each of which requires its own response); and (3) speed of limb movement (the interval of time between the start of a movement and its completion). These three abilities are separate and independent of each other. For example, studies have shown that reaction time and speed of limb movement have essentially no correlation; the two abilities have very little in common. Additional studies have reported no transfer from quickening exercises to other tasks that require quickness. Therefore, being quick depends on the circumstances under which quickness is required.

Having balance is also advantageous in most sports and activities. As with quickness, the balance that's required for one activity isn't related to the balance that's required in another. In a classic study that involved 320 subjects, two balance tasks were found to be contingent on separate and independent abilities. The researcher concluded that the correlation between the two balance tasks was "little more than zero." In another study, researchers examined six tests of static and dynamic balance and found that the abilities supporting one test of balance were separate from those supporting another. Therefore, having balance depends on the circumstances under which balance is required.

Open and Closed Skills

Skills can be classified as either open or closed. Both types of skills differ in several areas that pertain to the context of the environment (which consists of the playing field or surface, objects and other individuals).

Open skills occur in an environment that's variable and unpredictable. An individual reacts to a situation and initiates a response that can match the constantly changing environmental conditions. Since the conditions may vary from one response to another, the individual must have a variety of responses available to accomplish the skill. Examples of open skills are hitting a pitched baseball, rebounding a basketball and heading a soccer ball. Baseball, basketball and soccer are sports in which open skills dominate. In fact, this is true of most team sports.

Closed skills occur in an environment that's stable and predictable. Because the environment doesn't fluctuate, an individual can plan or predict a response well in advance. The individual initiates movement and isn't required to begin until ready to do so. With a closed skill, an object waits to be acted upon by the performer. Examples of closed skills are putting a golf ball, doing a cartwheel and throwing a discus. Golf, gymnastics and track and field are sports in which closed skills dominate. By the way, weightlifting – whether it's competitive or recreational – is an activity in which closed skills dominate.

Designations of open and closed actually mark the extreme points on a continuum. Skills that have assorted degrees of environmental variability and predictability reside between the two extremes.

Open and closed skills demand entirely different strategies for learning. With open skills, diversification is required. This means that open skills should be practiced in a variable environment to learn adaptability. With closed

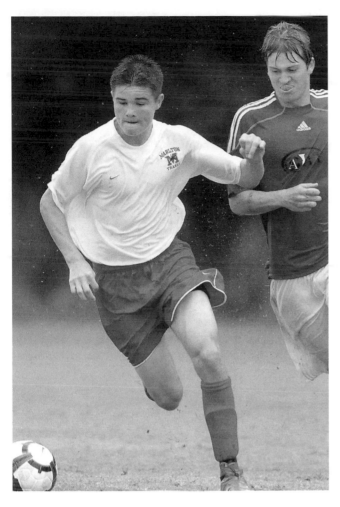

Soccer is a sport in which open skills dominate. (Photo by Karl Wright.)

THE TRANSFER OF LEARNING

The transfer of learning refers to the effects of past learning on the acquisition of a new skill. Many individuals take the transfer of learning for granted. They assume that the learning of one skill always and automatically transfers or "carries over" to the learning of another.

Types of Transfer

The acquisition of skills depends on the correct use of the transfer of learning principles. In reality, the transfer of learning from one skill to another may be positive, negative or neutral (absent altogether).

Positive transfer occurs when the learning of one skill facilitates the learning of another skill. Example: Learning to position yourself to field a baseball would probably facilitate learning to position yourself to field a softball.

Negative transfer occurs when the learning of one skill inhibits the learning of another skill. Example: Learning to shoot free throws on either a nine-foot rim or an 11-foot rim would probably inhibit learning to shoot free throws on a 10-foot rim, at least initially.

Neutral (no) transfer occurs when the learning of one skill has a negligible influence on the learning of another skill. Example: Learning to swim would have no effect on learning to accurately tap a volleyball (as was demonstrated in one study).

THE USE OF WEIGHTED OBJECTS

It's widely believed that using weighted objects contributes to the learning of specific movement patterns and sport skills. This has led to the practice of trying to simulate skills in the fitness center (or weight room) using a variety of implements. In the scientific literature, practicing a skill with a weighted object or additional resistance is known as overload training. Barbells, dumbbells, medicine balls and other weighted objects are used during overload training with the expectation of improving performance.

skills, fixation is required. This means that closed skills should be practiced in a stable environment to learn consistency.

Interestingly, the National Football League (NFL) "combine" – the world's best-known evaluation of athletic ability – includes the 225-pound bench press, 40-yard dash, 20-yard shuttle, 60-yard shuttle, three-cone drill, vertical jump and standing broad jump, all of which are closed skills. This, despite the fact that football is a sport in which open skills dominate. It's no surprise, then, that the usefulness of these tests in predicting success as a football player has been questioned for many years.

The basis for mimicking skills with weighted objects is mostly anecdotal, having very little support from the scientific literature. In one study, for instance, 37 subjects were assigned to two groups: One group threw a weighted softball and the other group threw a regulation softball. (The weighted softball was two ounces heavier than the regulation softball.) Both groups performed a series of lob throws from various distances ranging from 30 to 70 feet with their assigned softball. After six weeks of training, there were no significant differences between the groups in throwing velocity. The researchers concluded: "Training with a weighted ball resulted in essentially the same effect as training with the regulation ball."

Along these lines, many individuals insist that certain weightlifting skills transfer to other skills. If there were a correlation between weightlifting skills and other skills, then highly successful weightlifters would excel at literally every skill that they attempted. And we know that this isn't true.

The Kinesthetic Aftereffect

Research in motor control refers to a kinesthetic aftereffect which is defined by Dr. George Sage as "a perceived modification in the shape, size, or weight of an object . . . as a result of experience with a previous object." Individuals experience the kinesthetic aftereffect during overload training. This phenomenon is exemplified by a person who runs with a weighted vest and after removing it, has the perceived ability to run faster. Essentially, the kinesthetic aftereffect is nothing more than a sensory illusion.

So after doing a skill with a weighted object, an individual might "feel" faster or more powerful but research indicates that there's no measurable improvement in those areas. One study had subjects do elbow flexion with and without resistance. There was no change in the speed of movement shortly after the overload (although the subjects reported "feeling faster"). Another study had subjects perform vertical jumps with a weighted vest followed by jumps without the extra weight. There were no improvements in the vertical jump shortly after the overload. Yet another study had groups sprint with a weighted sled, sprint with a weighted vest or sprint without any additional resistance. After seven weeks of training, those who ran with added resistance performed no better in sprinting than those who ran without added resistance. Many other studies have reported similar results from the use of weighted objects.

Dr. Sage states, "Any attempt to improve performance by utilizing objects that are slightly heavier than normal while practicing gross motor skills that will be later used in sports competition seems to be hardly worth the time spent and the money paid for the weighted objects." Dr. Schmidt adds, "Teaching a particular Skill A simply because you would like it to transfer to Skill B, which is of major interest, is not very effective, especially if you consider the time spent on Skill A that could have been spent on Skill B instead."

Problems with Using Weighted Objects

According to Dr. Wayne Westcott, four problems occur when practicing sport skills with weighted objects. The problem areas relate to neuromuscular confusion, incorrect movement speed, orthopedic stress and insufficient workload.

1. **Neuromuscular confusion.** Every skill involves a movement pattern that's specific to that skill alone. Introducing anything foreign to the pattern – such as a sled, weighted vest, barbell, dumbbell, medicine ball or ankle weights – will only serve to confuse the neuromuscular pathways and produce negative transfer. Watch someone swing a weighted racquet or shoot a weighted basketball and you'll quickly notice that the effort used to direct the unfamiliar weight results in a movement pattern that's labored and awkward; in reality, it's a very different motion altogether. Studies of competitive swimmers consistently show that their stroke mechanics are altered as a result of resisted swimming.

2. **Incorrect movement speed.** To facilitate learning, a skill should be practiced with the speed at which it will be performed. Practicing a skill at a slower or a faster speed than actually would be used in performing the skill will produce negative transfer. In addition, doing a skill at slower speeds – which would occur when doing it with a weighted object – may train the neuromuscular system to function at slower speeds.

3. **Orthopedic stress.** Another problem is the added stress that a weighted object places on the joints. Practicing a skill with an object that's heavier than normal puts orthopedic stress on the joints that's greater than normal. Structural stress is most evident in the shoulder, elbow and wrist.

4. **Insufficient workload.** A weighted object doesn't increase the strength of the involved musculature. The reason is that the extra resistance provided by a weighted object isn't sufficient enough to surpass the threshold for strength development; it's a fraction of what's necessary to overload the muscles.

SPECIFICITY VERSUS GENERALITY

In the early part of the 20th century, Edward Thorndike and Robert Woodworth proposed their Identical Elements Theory of Transfer. Later, Franklin Henry advanced his Specificity Hypothesis. Both theories are forerunners of what's widely known as the Principle of Specificity. The underlying fundamentals of this principle are documented extensively in the scientific literature. Even so, the Principle of Specificity continues to be misinterpreted and misused almost as often as it's referenced.

The Principle of Specificity states that activities must be specific to an intended skill in order for a maximum transfer of learning – or carryover – to occur. Specific means exact or identical, not similar or just like. Indeed, Dr. Sage states, "Transfer is highly specific and occurs only when the practiced movements are identical."

Movement patterns for different skills are never identical. According to Dr. Schmidt, two movement patterns – although outwardly appearing to use the same muscular actions – are actually quite different and require learning and practicing each skill separately. Performing an overhead smash with a tennis racket involves a different movement pattern than performing an overhead smash with a badminton racket. Swinging a golf club involves a different movement pattern than swinging a hockey stick. And throwing a baseball involves a different movement pattern than throwing a javelin.

Case in point: In the summer of 1996, the Olympic Games were held in Atlanta. Shortly thereafter, the Atlanta Braves hosted a tryout for Jan Zelezny, an athlete from the Czech Republic who was a two-time Olympic champion (1992 and 1996) and world-record holder in the javelin. (He would later win an unprecedented third gold medal in the javelin at the 2000 Olympics in Sydney and still owns the top five throws of all time.) According to one account, the international scouting director for the Braves reasoned that "the motions of throwing a javelin and a baseball were not all that different." No doubt, he also felt that the strength of Zelezny's arm and shoulder coupled with his capacity to throw a javelin farther than anyone on the planet – having tossed the spear 323 feet a few months before the tryout – made him a great candidate for pitching in the major leagues. After a few warm up throws, Zelezny took the mound. His third pitch reportedly sailed over the head of the catcher . . . and also over the eight-foot backstop. He threw some additional pitches but the results weren't impressive. Several of his pitches were clocked at around 80 miles per hour which isn't bad but not major-league stuff. At the end of the tryout, Zelezny uncorked a throw for distance that was estimated to be 275 feet but he took a running start. Unfortunately, pitchers don't throw for distance. And they don't take a running start. Don't forget, too, that differences in the weight and shape of a javelin and baseball require different throwing motions; a javelin is a 28.22-ounce spear while a baseball is a five-ounce sphere. The moral of the story: Skills are highly specific and not necessarily transferable.

Exercises that are very similar don't even transfer to each other. In one study, 24 subjects performed three sets of five repetitions of the bicep curl in the standing position three times per week for six weeks. Their strength increased by 14.38 pounds when the bicep curl was measured in the standing position. But their strength increased by only 3.37 pounds when the bicep curl was measured in the supine position. In other words, the strength gained from doing a standing bicep curl didn't transfer to a supine bicep curl, an exercise that's very similar . . . but not identical. Exercises that are performed in the fitness center are even less similar to other skills and, therefore, won't transfer to other skills.

One exercise that has been thought to be specific to a wide range of skills is the power clean. Over the span of about five years, a variety of articles that were published in a "journal" for strength coaches stated that the power clean was specific to the following skills (and others): shooting a basketball; long-snapping a football; spiking a volleyball; rowing a boat; fore-handing a tennis ball; pedaling a bicycle; tackling a football player; hitting a golf ball; swimming the backstroke, butterfly and breaststroke; throwing a javelin, discus and hammer; putting a shot; sprinting; playing baseball; Nordic skiing; pole vaulting; and sled racing. Really? In which of those skills does an athlete grasp an inanimate object that's resting on the ground and then pull it to shoulder level and drop under it all in one motion?

Obviously, it's impossible for the power clean – or any other exercise, for that matter – to be specific to such a broad range of differing skills. In fact, there's no exercise done in the fitness center – with free weights or machines – that will expedite the learning of a skill. So, doing power cleans may be similar to driving off the line of scrimmage and doing lunges may be just like going for a layup but the truth is that power cleans will only help you get better at doing power cleans and lunges will only help you get better at doing lunges. Likewise, heaving medicine balls around is great for improving your skill at heaving medicine balls around and nothing else. And jumping off boxes will only perfect your skill at jumping off boxes. Remember, it's the Principle of *Specificity*, not the Principle of *Similarity*.

On a related note, if Skill A is specific to Skill B, then Skill B should be specific to Skill A. So if the power clean is specific to the pole vault, then the pole vault should be specific to the power clean. In other words, if doing the power clean helps your performance in the pole vault, then doing the pole vault should help your performance in the power clean. But it doesn't.

Elements of Specificity

There are four elements of specificity that define the rules for determining whether or not an exercise is specific to a skill:

1. **Muscle specificity.** The muscles used in the exercise must be exactly the same as in the skill.

2. **Movement specificity.** The movement pattern used in the exercise must be exactly the same as in the skill.

3. **Speed specificity.** The speed of movement used in the exercise must be exactly the same as in the skill.

4. **Resistance specificity.** The resistance used in the exercise must be exactly the same as in the skill.

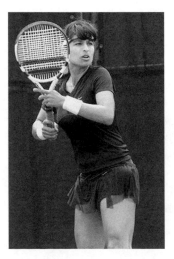

Performing an overhead smash with a tennis racket involves a different movement pattern than performing an overhead smash with a badminton racket. (Photo provided by Shikha Uberoi.)

In order for an exercise to be specific to a skill, all four of these elements would have to be true. An exercise may resemble a skill in terms of exact muscles, movement pattern, speed of movement and resistance. However, at best an exercise can only *approximate* a skill, not *duplicate* it.

Refer back to the laundry list of skills for which the power clean is thought to be specific. Those skills involve different muscles, different movement patterns, different speeds of movement and different resistances. Indeed, just consider the obvious differences between hitting a golf ball and rowing a boat. How, then, can the power clean be specific to such vastly different skills? Answer: It can't.

By the way, specificity doesn't only apply to the learning of sport skills. A guitar and banjo are stringed instruments but if you want to get better at plucking a guitar, don't practice with a banjo. An M16 and AK-47 are assault rifles but if you want to get better at shooting an M16, don't practice with an AK-47.

THE STAGES OF MOTOR LEARNING

Skill development is accomplished in stages or phases of learning. It's important to understand that the learning of a skill is a continuous process. Therefore, the stages don't have a distinct beginning or end and shouldn't be viewed as being separate or unconnected elements.

In the mid-1960s, Paul Fitts and Michael Posner identified three phases of motor learning: an early or Cognitive Phase, an intermediate or Associative Phase and a final or Autonomous Phase.

The Cognitive Phase

In the first phase of motor learning, the skill is completely new to the performer. The performer seeks an understanding of the skill and its demands. During this phase, the attention requirements are high and movements are jerky and fragmented. Gains in proficiency are very rapid but performance is usually very inconsistent. Good strategies are retained and poor ones are discarded. The Cognitive Phase may last anywhere from several moments to several weeks, depending on the complexity of the skill, the frequency of practice and so on.

The Associative Phase

During the second phase of motor learning, the performer organizes more effective and efficient movement patterns that are more coordinated and consistent. The enhanced movement efficiency reduces the energy costs of the skill. Performance improvements in the Associative Phase are rapid, though not as rapid as in the Cognitive Phase. The length of this phase varies considerably and may last several weeks or months.

The Autonomous Phase

In the third phase of motor learning, after many months and possibly years of painstaking practice, the skill becomes highly organized and well-developed. Now, the skills are performed with little or no conscious effort. In other words, the skill becomes automatic. For learning an open skill, the emphasis is on adapting the movement to a variety of environmental conditions and possibilities; for learning a closed skill, the emphasis is on refinement of technique. Because of the high degree of skill, performance improvements are slowest in the Autonomous Phase. At this point, there's simply "not much room for improvement."

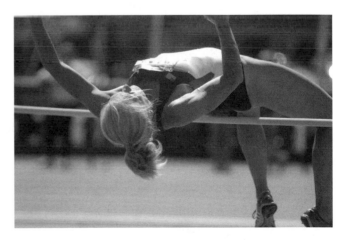

The first requirement for improving a skill is to literally practice the intended skill for thousands and thousands of task-specific repetitions. (Photo by Ken Stone.)

239

IMPROVING SKILLS

The improvement of skills is a process in which an individual develops a set of responses into an integrated and organized movement pattern. In order for you to improve a skill, there are two requirements: Practice the skill and strengthen the muscles that are used to perform the skill.

Practice the Skill

The first requirement for improving a skill is to literally practice the skill for thousands and thousands of task-specific repetitions. Each repetition must be done with perfect technique so that its specific movement pattern becomes firmly ingrained in your "motor memory." The skill must be practiced perfectly and exactly as it would be used during a sport or an activity. Remember, practice makes perfect . . . but only if your practice is perfect. And as noted earlier, the skill shouldn't be practiced with weighted objects.

Strengthen the Muscles

The second requirement for improving a skill is to strengthen the major muscles that are used during the performance of the skill. Remember, strength training shouldn't be done in a manner that tries to mimic or replicate the skill so as not to confuse the neuromuscular pathways or impair the intended movement pattern. A stronger muscle can produce more force; if you can produce more force, you'll require less effort and be able to perform the skill more quickly, more accurately and more efficiently. But again, this is provided that you've practiced enough in a correct manner so that you'll be more skillful in applying that force.

SPORT-SPECIFIC EXERCISES

Are there sport-specific exercises or even position-specific exercises? Should a basketball player do different exercises than a football player or a swimmer? Should a pitcher do different exercises than a catcher or an outfielder?

All athletes have the same muscles that are used in the same manner. For example, the main

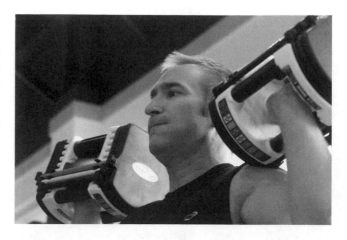

Skill training is specific to a sport or an activity but strength training is general. (Photo provided by Luke Carlson.)

function of the quadriceps is knee extension (straightening the legs). This is true for a diver, shot putter, quarterback, point guard and softball player. It follows, then, that there's no such thing as sport-specific exercises or position-specific exercises. For that matter, there's no such thing as gender-specific exercises, either.

Some athletes need to perform certain exercises as a precautionary measure against injury to a joint that receives a great deal of stress in their particular sport such as wrestlers who do exercises for their neck which other athletes might not need to perform. Some athletes need to perform certain exercises to focus on a muscle that's essential to their sport such as golfers who do exercises for their grip which other athletes might not need to perform.

Aside from that, you should select exercises that train your muscles in the safest and most efficient way possible. Skill training is specific to a sport or an activity but strength training is general. In other words, the development of strength is general but the application of strength is specific.

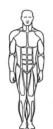

19 Nutrional Training

Nutrition is the process by which you select, consume, digest, absorb and utilize food. Unfortunately, this important aspect of a fitness program is either inadequately addressed or entirely overlooked.

Nutritional training includes being able to recognize and choose desirable foods and understanding the recommended intakes of those foods. This is essential for several reasons.

In general, nutritional training promotes good health. Moreover, becoming familiar with the caloric contributions of the various nutrients and knowing your caloric needs can assist in weight management.

From an athletic perspective, nutritional training plays a crucial part in your capacity to perform at optimal levels and assists in the improvement of your strength, endurance and fitness. Consuming the right foods/fluids before and after an activity allows you to maximize your performance. Pre-activity foods/fluids affect your ensuing performance; post-activity foods/fluids affect your recovery from that performance. And because so many meals are eaten away from home – especially at fast-food

(aka quick-serve) restaurants – it's important to be aware of healthy options.

THE SIX NUTRIENTS

Everything that you do requires energy. The energy is obtained through the food that you consume and is measured in calories (which, technically, are units of heat). Essentially, the food that you eat is fuel for your body. Food is also necessary for the ongoing growth, maintenance and repair of your biological tissues such as muscle and bone.

In order to be considered nutritious, your food intake must contain the recommended amounts of nutrients. No single food satisfies this requirement. As a result, variety is the key to a healthy diet. (Here and in other discussions that follow, the term diet simply refers to a normal food intake, not a specialized regimen of eating.)

Foods have varying proportions of six nutrients. These nutrients can be divided into macronutrients and micronutrients based on the relative amounts that you should consume. Macronutrients are needed in relatively large amounts and include carbohydrates, protein, fat and water; micronutrients are needed in relatively small amounts and include vitamins and minerals.

Carbohydrates

The primary function of carbohydrates (or carbs) is to furnish you with energy, especially during intense activity. Your body breaks down carbohydrates into glucose (blood sugar). Glucose can be used as an immediate form of energy during activity or stored as glycogen in your liver and muscles for future use. Highly conditioned muscles can stockpile more glycogen than poorly conditioned muscles. If your glycogen stores are depleted, you'll feel overwhelmingly exhausted.

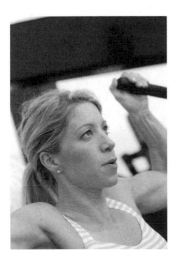

Nutritional training plays a crucial part in your capacity to perform at optimal levels and assists in the improvement of your strength, endurance and fitness. (Photo provided by Luke Carlson.)

Having greater glycogen stores can give you a significant physiological advantage thus the enormous importance of carbohydrates.

But all carbohydrates aren't created equal. Indeed, carbohydrates run the gamut from potatoes to pastries, from corn to cola and from peas to pies. Most nutritional authorities recognize two types of carbohydrates: simple and complex.

Simple carbohydrates – made of one or two sugars – are digested more quickly than complex carbohydrates. This means that simple carbohydrates enter your bloodstream more quickly and raise your blood glucose more quickly.

Foods and beverages that are high in simple carbohydrates – including cake, candy, cookies and soda – use refined ingredients such as white sugar, white flour and high fructose corn syrup and have no nutritional value. Consequently, these products are considered sources of "empty calories." Simple carbohydrates are also found in milk and milk products, fruits, vegetables, honey and yogurt. These foods and beverages have a greater nutritional value, making them more favorable sources of carbohydrates.

Complex carbohydrates – made of three or more sugars though usually referred to as starches – are digested more slowly than simple carbohydrates. This means that complex carbohydrates enter your bloodstream more slowly and raise your blood sugar more slowly (providing you with a sustained level of energy throughout the day). Complex carbohydrates also offer you a wealth of vitamins and minerals.

Foods that are high in complex carbohydrates include certain vegetables (broccoli, corn and potatoes), breads, cereals, grains, legumes (beans, lentils and peas), yams, rice, spaghetti and macaroni.

Fiber – a category of complex carbohydrates – only comes from plant-based foods and passes through your system undigested. There are two types of fiber: soluble and insoluble.

Soluble fiber can be dissolved in water. It binds to fatty substances and escorts them out of your body as waste. Soluble fiber is found in legumes, nuts, oat bran and various fruits and vegetables. Insoluble fiber can't be dissolved in water. It ushers food through your intestinal tract and promotes regular bowel movements. Insoluble fiber is found in brown rice, wheat bread, whole wheat, whole grains and certain fruits and vegetables.

About 50 to 65% of your daily calories should be from carbohydrates. (Active individuals should be at the higher end of this range.) It's preferable that your intake is comprised of more complex carbohydrates and less simple carbohydrates.

Protein

The term protein is derived from the Greek word protos which means first. That's an apt description since protein is the major functional and structural component of every cell in your body; it's necessary for the growth, maintenance and repair of your biological tissues, particularly muscle tissue. Additionally, protein regulates water balance and transports other nutrients. Protein can also be used as an energy source in the event that adequate carbohydrates and fat aren't available (although this is generally as a last resort).

The "building blocks" of protein are amino acids. Nine amino acids must be provided in your diet and are considered essential (or indispensable) amino acids. Five amino acids can be synthesized by the body and are considered non-essential (or dispensable) amino acids. And six amino acids can be synthesized by the body but this process may be limited by certain diseases or conditions (such as severe stress on the body from a burn injury) and are considered "conditionally indispensable" amino acids.

Like carbohydrates, not all proteins are created equal. There are two types of protein: complete and incomplete.

A complete protein contains all of the essential amino acids in amounts that facilitate the growth, maintenance and repair of biological tissues. Proteins that are found in animal sources – such as meat, poultry, fish, eggs, milk, cheese and yogurt – are complete proteins. (Soy is also regarded as a complete protein.) An incomplete protein lacks at least one of the essential amino acids. Proteins that are found in plants, legumes, grains, nuts, seeds and vegetables are incomplete proteins.

Another term that's used in the discussion of protein is biological value. This is an index in which all protein sources are compared to egg whites which are the most complete protein. (Egg whites have a biological value of 100.) Animal sources (complete proteins) have a high biological value, meaning that a large portion of the protein is absorbed and retained. (An exception is gelatin.) Vegetable sources (incomplete proteins) have a low biological value, meaning that a small portion of the protein is absorbed and retained. White potatoes, for instance, have a biological value of 34.

About 15 to 20% of your daily calories should be from protein. It's preferable that your intake is comprised of protein from quality sources such as lean or low-fat meat and poultry.

Fat

It may be difficult to believe but fat is actually essential to a balanced diet. First, fat serves as the major source of energy during low-intensity activities such as sleeping, reading and walking. Second, fat helps in the transportation and the absorption of certain vitamins. Third, fat adds considerable flavor to foods. This makes food more appetizing . . . and also explains why fat is craved so much.

Like carbohydrates and protein, not all fats are created equal. There are several types of fat: saturated, unsaturated, trans and essential fatty acids.

Saturated fat is found in red meats, certain oils (such as coconut and palm oils), high-fat dairy products (such as butter and lard) and many processed foods. Unsaturated fat – which can be subdivided into monounsaturated and polyunsaturated fats – is found in fish (such as halibut, mackerel, salmon and trout), nuts, olives, seeds and a variety of oils (such as canola, corn, olive, soybean and sunflower oils).

There are at least two ways that unsaturated fat can be distinguished from saturated fat. For one thing, unsaturated fats are vegetable fats and saturated fats are animal fats. And at room temperature, unsaturated fats tend to be liquid and saturated fats tend to be solid.

Trans fat – or trans fatty acids – is formed when liquid oils are made more solid in a chemical process called hydrogenation. Most trans fat is found in shortenings, stick margarine, cookies, crackers, snack foods, fried foods, doughnuts, pastries, baked goods and other processed foods that are made with or fried in partially hydrogenated oils.

Unsaturated fat is less harmful than saturated fat and trans fat. It's well known that saturated fat and trans fat increase low-density lipoprotein (the "bad" cholesterol) and decrease high-density lipoprotein (the "good" cholesterol). This clogs arteries and raises the risk of heart disease in later life.

There are two types of essential fatty acids (EFAs): omega-3 and omega-6 fatty acids. The main omega-3 fat is alpha-linolenic acid and the main omega-6 fat is linoleic acid. These fats are deemed essential because the body can't produce them and, therefore, need to be obtained from outside sources.

EFAs are found in polyunsaturated fats. The best sources of omega-3 fats are fish (such as cod, flounder, halibut, pollock, salmon, sardines, scallops, swordfish and trout). Other sources include walnuts, flaxseeds, flax oil and eggs that are fortified with omega-3s. Omega-6 fats are found in seeds and nuts – and the oils extracted from them – but the main sources are refined vegetable oils which are used in most snack foods, cookies and crackers.

In general, omega-6 fats increase inflammation and blood clotting while omega-3 fats decrease those responses. It becomes apparent, then, that an emphasis should be put on eating foods that are high in omega-3s.

Some studies have found that consuming omega-3 fats can decrease the risk of heart disease but other studies have found no benefit. These contradictory findings might be best

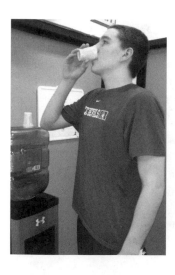

Water regulates your body temperature which is especially critical when exercising in hot, humid conditions. (Photo by Fred Fornicola.)

summed up by the US Food and Drug Administration which notes that there's "supportive but not conclusive research" that omega-3 fats "may reduce the risk of coronary heart disease."

About 20 to 25% of your daily calories should be from fat. This includes about 10 to 15% from unsaturated fat and no more than about 10% from saturated fat and trans fat combined. It's preferable that your intake is comprised of unsaturated fat and food sources that provide high levels of omega-3 fats.

Water

Since it's needed in rather large quantities, water is classified as a macronutrient. Incredibly, almost two thirds of your bodyweight is water.

Unlike the other three macronutrients, water doesn't have any calories and, thus, doesn't provide you with any energy. However, water does have significant roles in your body. For one thing, it regulates your body temperature. This is especially critical when exercising in hot, humid conditions. Also, water helps to lubricate your joints. And water helps to carry nutrients to your cells and waste products from your cells.

Water can be obtained from a variety of sources including fruits, fruit juices, vegetables, vegetable juices, milk, soup and, of course, drinking water. Caffeinated beverages – including coffee, tea, soda and energy drinks – are sources of water, of course, but aren't good

ones because of their diuretic effects which can, ironically, cause a loss of water.

The volume of water that's needed can vary greatly from one person to the next based on such factors as age, size, level of fitness and the duration and intensity of activity as well as the environment. (Cold, heat, humidity and altitude all increase the need for water.) You should consume about 16 ounces of water for every pound of bodyweight that you lose while training or competing.

Vitamins

The term vitamine was coined in 1912 by Casimir Funk, a Polish chemist. Vitamins are potent compounds that are required in very small amounts. They're found in a wide assortment of foods, especially in fruits and vegetables. You can get an adequate intake of vitamins from a balanced diet that contains a variety of healthy foods.

Even though vitamins have no calories and, therefore, aren't a source of energy, they perform many different functions that are vital to an active lifestyle. There are two types of vitamins: fat soluble and water soluble.

Vitamins A, D, E and K are considered fat-soluble vitamins because they require the presence of adequate amounts of fat before transportation and absorption can take place. Excessive amounts of fat-soluble vitamins are stored in your body. Table 19.1 lists the fat-soluble vitamins along with their functions and sources.

The eight B vitamins (biotin, cobalamin, folate, niacin, pantothenic acid, pyridoxine, riboflavin and thiamine) and vitamin C are considered water-soluble vitamins because they're found in foods that have a naturally high content of water. There's minimal storage of water-soluble vitamins in your body; excess amounts are generally excreted in your urine. Table 19.2 lists the water-soluble vitamins along with their functions and sources.

Minerals

Minerals are required in very small amounts, too. Like vitamins, all of the minerals that you need can be obtained from an ordinary intake of healthy foods. Also like vitamins, minerals have no calories but have many important functions. There are two types of minerals: macrominerals and microminerals.

As the name implies, macrominerals are needed in larger amounts than microminerals specifically, more than 250 milligrams per day. The macrominerals are calcium, chloride, magnesium, phosphorus, potassium, sodium and sulfur. Table 19.3 lists the macrominerals along with their functions and sources.

As you might suspect, microminerals are needed in smaller amounts than macrominerals specifically, less than 20 milligrams per day. The microminerals are chromium, copper, fluoride, iodine, iron, manganese, molybdenum, selenium and zinc. (A number of other minerals – including arsenic, boron, cobalt, lithium, nickel, silicon, tin and vanadium – are probably essential in very small amounts but their roles in the human body are unclear and recommended intakes haven't been established.) Table 19.4 lists the microminerals along with their functions and sources.

THE PYRAMID AND THE PLATE

After nearly 20 years of service as a tool to educate people about a healthy diet, the Food Pyramid was retired in 2011. Introduced jointly in 1992 by the US Department of Agriculture and US Department of Health and Human Services, the Food Pyramid showed four food groups in the shape of a pyramid – thus the name – with the number of recommended servings that should be eaten from each group. Residing at the widest part – the base – were breads, cereals, rice and pasta (6 to 11 servings per day); at the narrowest part – the tip – were fats, oils and sweets ("use sparingly"). In 2005, a revision added two more food groups, renamed some food groups and depicted a person walking up steps on the left side of the pyramid to symbolize the need for exercise.

The Food Pyramid has been replaced with a much simpler concept known as MyPlate or the Food Plate. At the present time, the US

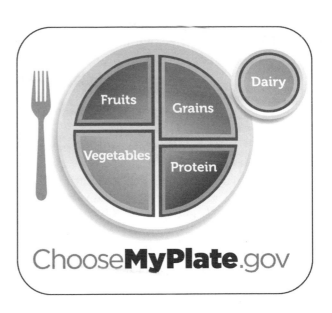

The current recommendations for a healthy diet are to fill 50% of your plate with fruits and vegetables, 25% with grains and 25% with protein. (Icon provided by the US Department of Agriculture.)

Department of Agriculture recognizes five food groups. MyPlate has four colored sections that represent four of the food groups: fruits (red), grains (orange), protein (purple) and vegetables (green). Think of a circle that's divided into four parts of equal size. In other words, the current recommendations for a healthy diet are to fill 50% of your plate with fruits and vegetables, 25% with grains and 25% with protein. (An "athletic" food plate should have more carbohydrates and less protein.) Near the plate is a smaller circle that represents the fifth food group: dairy (blue).

THE FIVE FOOD GROUPS

Since the basis of the Food Plate is the five food groups, it's important to discuss them in greater detail.

The Grain Group

This group consists of foods that are made from wheat, rice, oats, cornmeal, barley or another cereal grain. Examples include bread, pasta, oatmeal and breakfast cereals.

There are two sub-groups of grains: whole grains and refined grains. Whole grains contain the entire grain kernel. Examples include whole-wheat flour, oatmeal and brown rice. Refined grains have been milled which eliminates parts of the grain kernel (the bran, germ and endosperm). This process removes dietary fiber, iron and many B vitamins. Examples include white flour, white bread and white rice.

The Vegetable Group

Any vegetable and any 100% vegetable juice is included in this group. The vegetables can be raw, cooked, fresh, frozen, canned, dried/dehydrated, whole, cut or mashed. There are five categories of vegetables (examples in parentheses): dark green (broccoli, spinach and romaine lettuce); red and orange (carrots, sweet potatoes and tomatoes); beans and peas (black beans, kidney beans and split peas); starchy (corn, green peas and potatoes); and other (beets, celery and cucumbers).

The Fruit Group

Any fruit and any 100% fruit juice is included in this group. The fruits can be fresh, frozen, dried/dehydrated, canned, whole, cut or pureed. Examples include apples, berries, grapes, melons, peaches and pears.

The Dairy Group

This group consists of all fluid milk products and foods that are made from milk that retain their calcium content. (For this reason, cream cheese and butter are excluded from the Dairy Group.) Examples include milk, milk-based desserts, calcium-fortified soy milk, cheese and yogurt.

The Protein Foods Group

This group consists of a wide range of foods in six different sub-groups (examples in parentheses): meats (beef, ham and liver); poultry (chicken, duck and turkey); eggs; beans and peas; nuts and seeds (almonds, peanut butter and sesame seeds); and seafood (salmon, lobster and sardines). Note that beans and peas are also part of the Vegetable Group.

DIETARY REFERENCE INTAKES

The most recent approach for assessing and planning diets is the use of the Dietary Reference Intake (DRI). The DRIs include these four "reference values":

Estimated Average Requirement (EAR): The average daily nutrient intake level estimated to meet the needs of 50% of all healthy individuals for a particular age or gender.

Recommended Dietary Allowance (RDA): The average daily nutrient intake level estimated to meet the needs of 97.5% of all healthy individuals for a particular age or gender.

Adequate Intake (AI): The average daily nutrient intake level based on observed or experimentally determined approximations or estimates by a group of healthy individuals.

Tolerable Upper Intake Level (UL): The highest average daily nutrient intake level that's unlikely to produce any adverse effects in almost all individuals in the general population.

The RDA is the recommended goal for everyone. First published in 1943 and updated regularly, the RDAs were developed by the Food and Nutrition Board of the National Academy of Sciences/National Research Council. The RDAs are set by first determining the floor below which deficiency occurs and then the ceiling above which harm occurs. A margin of safety is included to meet the needs of nearly all healthy people. In other words, the RDAs exceed what most people require in order to meet the needs of those who have the highest requirements. So, the RDAs aren't minimum standards. And failing to consume the recommended amounts doesn't necessarily indicate that you have a dietary deficiency. (Note: The AI is used when the RDA for a nutrient can't be determined.)

FOOD LABELS

If you purchase your own food in a supermarket or convenience store, do you examine the food label? Most people do.

Nutrition Facts

Serving Size 1 cup (228g)
Servings Per Container about 2

Amount Per Serving	
Calories 250	Calories from Fat 110

	% Daily Value*
Total Fat 12g	18%
Saturated Fat 3g	15%
Trans Fat 3g	
Cholesterol 30mg	10%
Sodium 470mg	20%
Total Carbohydrate 31g	10%
Dietary Fiber 0g	0%
Sugars 5g	
Proteins 5g	
Vitamin A	4%
Vitamin C	2%
Calcium	20%
Iron	4%

* Percent Daily Values are based on a 2,000 calorie diet. Your Daily Values may be higher or lower depending on your calorie needs:

	Calories:	2,000	2,500
Total Fat	Less than	65g	80g
Saturated Fat	Less than	20g	25g
Cholesterol	Less than	300mg	300mg
Sodium	Less than	2,400mg	2,400mg
Total Carbohydrate		300g	375g
Dietary Fiber		25g	30g

Figure 19.1: Sample Nutrition Facts panel (Image provided by the U.S. Food and Drug Administration.)

According to one survey, about 79% of Americans said that they frequently or occasionally check food labels. Nevertheless, about 44% of Americans said that they buy foods that are bad for them even after they read the labels.

Clearly, then, simply reading food labels isn't good enough. In order to make healthy choices, it's important for you to understand the information that's on food labels.

Thanks to the Nutrition Labeling and Education Act of 1990 – which amended the 1938 Federal Food, Drug and Cosmetic Act – food labels are required for most packaged foods. This includes breads, cereals, canned/frozen foods, snacks, desserts and beverages. Food labels aren't required for fruits, vegetables and fish. In addition, any health claims that are made on food labels must comply with specific regulations.

The Nutrition Facts Panel

Located on the food label is an area that's known as the Nutrition Facts panel. (For the ensuing discussions, refer to Figure 19.1.) Near the top of the facts panel are the serving size and servings per container. Unfortunately, this information is often ignored – especially the servings per container – and, as a result, can cause you to unknowingly consume an excessive amount of calories.

In order to compare similar foods, serving sizes are standardized in an amount of food "customarily consumed" and use a "common household measure that is appropriate to the food" (such as cups, ounces, pieces, tablespoons and teaspoons) followed by metric amounts in parentheses (such as grams and milliliters). What's more, some of the measures incorporate fractions (such as 1/2, 1/3 and 1/4). Do you know the difference between a tablespoon and a teaspoon? Or what 1/2 cup of potatoes actually looks like? How about three ounces of chicken? Most people don't know the answers to these questions. (For the record, one tablespoon equals three teaspoons; 1/2 cup of potatoes looks like half of a tennis ball; and three ounces of chicken are about the size of a deck of cards.)

Remember, the serving size and servings per container influence the quantity of the ingredients that are listed on the facts panel. Key point: Unless it's a single-serving package, the amount of each ingredient is only for a portion of the contents. If a food has two servings per container, then eating the entire contents literally doubles the amount of calories as well as fat and other nutrients.

After the information on the serving size and servings per container is a section on calories and calories from fat. If you want to determine the percentage of fat in a food, simply divide the calories from fat by the total calories. In Figure 19.1, for example, one serving of the food has 250 calories of which 110 are from fat, meaning that it's 44% fat.

Directly below the information on calories is a section on nutrients. The top of this section provides details about total fat which is subdivided into saturated fat and, as of January 2006, trans fat.

Appearing next on the facts panel is an area that's devoted to cholesterol and sodium. Cholesterol is linked to heart disease and sodium is linked to high blood pressure. Your intake of cholesterol should be less than 300 milligrams per day; your intake of sodium should be less than 2,400 milligrams per day.

Information on total carbohydrate and protein follows this section. Total carbohydrate is sub-divided into dietary fiber and sugars.

The final nutrients that are listed on the facts panel are vitamins and minerals. Information on vitamin A, vitamin C, calcium and iron is required on the facts panel. This isn't to say that all other vitamins and minerals are unimportant; rather, these four micronutrients aren't typically consumed in sufficient amounts and, thus, demand greater awareness.

Percent Daily Value

An important term that's used on the facts panel is Percent Daily Value or % Daily Value (%DV). It appears on the right-hand side of the facts panel and at the bottom of the panel as a footnote (provided that the label is large enough). Essentially, the %DV is your allowable intake of a particular nutrient for the day.

The %DVs that are on the right-hand side of the facts panel are representative of a 2,000-calorie diet. If you consume less calories or more calories, you can still employ this information. For instance, you can determine at a glance if a serving of a food is low or high in a given nutrient. As a rule of thumb, a DV that's 5% or less is low; a DV that's 20% or more is high.

To see the usefulness of %DVs, consider Figure 19.1 in which the food has 12 grams of fat per serving. For a 2,000-calorie diet, the facts panel recommends an intake of 65 grams of fat per day. In this case, the %DV is 18% which isn't high but it's close. Now remember, this applies to one serving. If you ate two servings of this food, you'd consume 24 grams of fat. Here, the %DV is 36% which is considered high. Or look at it this way: You just consumed 36% of your daily allowance for fat (assuming a 2,000-calorie diet, of course). Does this mean that you should toss this particular food into someone else's shopping cart? No. It simply means that for the remainder of the day, you have to examine the fat content of foods a little more carefully and make better choices.

The DVs in the footnote are based on intakes of 2,000 and 2,500 calories. If the full footnote is used, the information is the same for all products. It should be noted that total fat, saturated fat, cholesterol and sodium have upper limits, meaning that this is the maximum amount that you should consume; carbohydrates and dietary fiber have lower limits, meaning that this is the minimum amount that you should consume.

For a 2,000-calorie diet, note that the facts panel recommends DVs for total fat and total carbohydrate of 65 grams and 300 grams, respectively. Since there are nine calories in one gram of fat and four calories in one gram of carbohydrates, some quick math reveals that this equates to 585 calories from fat and 1,200 calories from carbohydrates. With an intake of 2,000 calories, this means that the recommendations on the facts panel are for a caloric intake that's comprised of 29.25% fat, 60% carbohydrates and, by default, 10.75% protein. A better guideline for active individuals, however, is a caloric intake that's comprised of about 20% fat, 65% carbohydrates and 15% protein.

Note that %DVs haven't been established for trans fat and sugars. Also, a %DV isn't listed for protein unless a claim is made such as "high in protein."

Ingredient Lists

If a food has more than one ingredient, they must be listed on the food label. What many individuals don't realize is that the ingredients on the food label are listed in "descending order of predominance by weight." In other words, the first ingredient weighs the most and the last ingredient weighs the least. So, a food or beverage that has some form of sugar among its first few ingredients has low or no nutritional value and, for that reason, does nothing to improve health.

And while on the subject, understand that sugar can take several forms. Ingredients that end in "ose" – such as dextrose, lactose and sucrose – are sugars but not all sugars end in these letters. Ingredients that are sugar or sugar-based include corn sweetener, high fructose corn syrup, honey, malt syrup, molasses and nectars.

CALORIC CONTRIBUTIONS

As mentioned earlier, three macronutrients furnish you with calories, albeit in different amounts. Carbohydrates and protein yield four calories per gram (cal/g) while fat yields nine cal/g, making it the most concentrated form of energy. (By the way, alcohol yields seven cal/g.) Armed with this information, you can determine the caloric contributions for each of the three energy-providing macronutrients in any food, provided that you know how many grams of each macronutrient are in a serving.

As an example, consider a snack food such as LAYS® Classic Potato Chips (Frito-Lay, Incorporated). Examining the facts panel reveals that a one-ounce serving of this food has 15 grams of carbohydrates, 2 grams of protein and 10 grams of fat. To find the exact number of calories that are supplied by each macronutrient, simply multiply its number of grams per serving by its corresponding energy yield. Therefore, each serving has 60 calories from carbohydrates [15 g x 4 cal/g], 8 calories from protein [2 g x 4 cal/g] and 90 calories from fat [10 g x 9 cal/g]. So, this food has a total of 158 calories per serving (which is rounded to 160 on the facts panel). In this product, then, nearly 57% of the calories (90 of the 158) are supplied by fat. (Note that consuming the entire contents of a 2.875-ounce bag would contribute a whopping 29 grams of fat – or 261 calories from fat – to your daily budget of calories.)

Compare this to Baked! LAYS® Original Potato Crisps, another snack food by the same manufacturer. A one-ounce serving of this food has 23 grams of carbohydrates, 2 grams of protein and 2 grams of fat. Therefore, each serving has 92 calories from carbohydrates [23 g x 4 cal/g], 8 calories from protein [2 g x 4 cal/g] and 18 calories from fat [2 g x 9 cal/g]. So, this food has a total of 118 calories per serving (which is rounded to 120 on the facts panel). In this product, then, only 15.25% of the calories (18 of the 118) are supplied by fat.

On a related note, some products carry a statement on the packaging that they're a certain percent fat free. It's important for you to determine the exact fat content of these foods so that this statement isn't misinterpreted. Case in point: A package that proclaims a product to be 99% fat free leads many consumers to believe that only 1% of its calories come from fat. But the designation of 99% fat free means that it's 99% fat free by *weight*, not by *calories*. How critical is this distinction? Very. Placing one gram of fat in 99 grams of water forms a product that, in terms of weight, is 99% fat free. Since water has no calories, however, this particular 99% fat free product, in terms of calories, is actually *100% fat*.

The preceding example is hypothetical. But if you think that this doesn't occur with real products, think again. Here are three examples:

A can of College Inn® Chicken Broth (H. J. Heinz Company) states that it's "99% fat free." But one serving of this product (8.12 ounces) has 13 calories of which 9 are from fat, meaning that it's 69.23% fat. (The numbers on the facts panel are rounded to 15 calories per serving with 0 calories from fat. No typo, the facts panel says that "0" calories are from fat even though it also says that there's one gram of fat per serving.)

A package of Hershey®'s Chocolate Drink (Hershey® Foods Corporation) states that it's "99% fat free." But one serving of this product (eight ounces) has 133 calories of which 9 are from fat, meaning that it's 6.77% fat. (The numbers on the facts panel are rounded to 130 calories per serving with 10 calories from fat.)

The designation 99% fat free means that a product is 99% fat free by weight, not by calories.

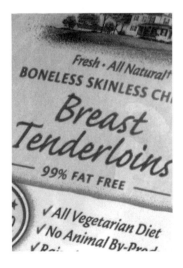

A package of Black Bear of the Black Forest™ Maple Glazed Ham (Black Bear Enterprises, Incorporated) states that it's "97% fat free." But one serving of this product (two ounces) has 61.5 calories of which 13.5 are from fat, meaning that it's 21.95% fat. (The numbers on the facts panel are rounded to 60 calories per serving with 15 calories from fat.)

While the percentage of fat in these three products isn't terribly bad, it's certainly a far cry from how the statements on the package can be interpreted.

ESTIMATING YOUR CALORIC BUDGET

Your caloric needs are determined by several factors including your age, gender, size, body composition, metabolic rate and level of activity. During a resting state, your caloric requirements can be established precisely by both direct and indirect calorimetry. Direct calorimetry measures the heat that's given off by the body in a small, insulated chamber; indirect calorimetry calculates the heat that's given off by the body based on the amount of oxygen that's consumed and carbon dioxide that's produced. But both of these methods can be expensive and impractical for most people.

For a quick and reasonably accurate estimate of your daily caloric needs, you can multiply your bodyweight by a number that corresponds to your gender and approximate level of activity. Essentially, this number represents your energy requirements in calories per pound of bodyweight (cal/lb). For a woman, the values are 14 if she's sedentary, 18 if moderately active and 22 if very active; for a man, the values are 16, 21 and 26, respectively. To illustrate, a 200-pound man who's very active requires approximately 5,200 calories per day (cal/day) to meet his energy needs [200 lb x 26 cal/lb/day]. Although this calculation has gray areas – such as the characterization of the term moderately active – it still results in a fairly good approximation.

Once you've estimated your caloric budget, you can determine how many of these calories should come from carbohydrates, protein and fat. For a diet that consists of 65% carbohydrates, 15% protein and 20% fat, someone who requires about 5,200 cal/day should consume roughly 845 grams of carbohydrates [5,200 cal/day x 0.65 ÷ 4 cal/g = 780 g], 195 grams of protein [5,200 cal/day x 0.15 ÷ 4 cal/g = 195 g] and 115 grams of fat [5,200 cal/day x 0.20 ÷ 9 cal/g = 115.56 g].

GLYCEMIC INDEX AND GLYCEMIC LOAD

A 1981 study by a group of Canadian and British researchers determined the glycemic index (GI) of 62 foods and sugars. The research was done to determine the effects that different foods have on blood glucose to assist people with diabetes. The first table of GI was published in 1995 and had 565 entries that were collected from the scientific literature. The most recent table was published in 2002 and has almost 1,300 entries.

The GI is a system of quantifying the carbohydrates in foods based on how they affect blood glucose compared to a reference food (either glucose or white bread). A value is assigned to a food that correlates to the magnitude of the increase in blood glucose. For instance, a food with a GI of 50 means that it elevates blood glucose to a level that's 50% as great as consuming the same amount of pure glucose which has a GI of 100. (Note: In the subsequent discussions of GI, glucose is used as the reference food.)

A limitation of the GI is that it's not related to portion size. So, the GI is the same whether an individual consumes 50 grams of a particular food or 150 grams. And that's where the glycemic load enters the picture.

The concept of glycemic load (GL) was introduced in 1997 by researchers at the Harvard School of Public Health. It's a measure of the quality *and* quantity of carbohydrates. The GL is the carbohydrate content in grams multiplied by the GI divided by 100. For example, eating a food that has 20 grams of carbohydrates and a GI of 50 yields a GL of 10 [20 x 50 ÷ 100 = 10]; eating a food that has 10 grams of carbohydrates and a GI of 80 yields a GL of 8 [10 x 80 ÷ 100 = 8]. So in this example, the food with the lower GI would actually raise blood glucose more than the food with the higher GI because a larger portion size was consumed. (Note: A GL of 10 or less is considered low, 11 to 19 is medium and 20 or more is high.)

PRE-ACTIVITY FOODS/FUELS

A meal that's consumed prior to an activity – whether it's some type of physical training or a competition – has several purposes. This includes removing your hunger pangs, readying your body with fuel for the upcoming activity, putting you in a relaxed state and easing any anxiety that you might have. There's no food that you can consume before an activity that will improve your performance. But there are some foods that you can consume before an activity that can impair your performance and, for this reason, should be avoided. For instance, foods that are high in fiber, protein and fat are digested slowly and, therefore, shouldn't be eaten prior to training or competing. Other foods to omit include those that are greasy, highly seasoned and flatulent (gas-forming) along with any specific foods that you may personally find distressful to your digestive system. If anything, what you select for your pre-activity meal should be almost bland yet appetizing enough so that you want to eat it.

Prior to an activity, you should also avoid eating foods that cause a sharp increase in your blood glucose. Here's why: In response to heightened levels of blood glucose, your pancreas releases a hormone known as insulin to maintain a stable internal environment (referred to as homeostasis). As a result of this biochemical balancing, your blood glucose is sharply reduced. This leads to hypoglycemia (low blood sugar) which decreases the availability of blood glucose as a fuel and causes you to feel severely fatigued. Although this condition is usually temporary, it remains an important consideration.

The idea, then, is to consume foods that elevate or maintain blood glucose without triggering a dramatic response by the pancreas. At one time, it was believed that simple carbohydrates (sugars) increase blood glucose more rapidly than complex carbohydrates (starches). A more recent trend of thought has been to take into account the GI of a food.

Before an activity, it's best to consume foods that are easy to digest and rich in carbohydrates that have a low GI. These foods help to keep your blood glucose within a desirable range.

Don't simply assume that a sugary food raises blood glucose more than a starchy food. Indeed, an apple (40) has a lower GI than a white bagel (72) and, given these two options, would be a better choice for a pre-activity food.

Foods with a relatively low GI include peanuts (13), cherries (22), plums (24), grapefruit (25), peaches (28), low-fat yogurt (33), pears (33), low-fat chocolate milk (34), tomato juice (38), apples (40), apple juice (40), oranges (40), grapes (43), white spaghetti (44), macaroni (45), orange juice (46) and bananas (51).

Water is perhaps the best liquid for you to drink before training or competing. Your fluid intake should be enough to guarantee optimal hydration during the activity.

The timing of your pre-activity meal is also crucial. To ensure that your digestive process doesn't impair your performance, you should eat your pre-activity meal at least three hours prior to training or competing. (Closer to an activity, you can eat a small snack such as fruit.) In short, your pre-activity meal should include foods that are familiar to you and well tolerated, preferably carbohydrates with a low GI.

POST-ACTIVITY FOODS/FLUIDS

Following an intense activity, proper nutrition accelerates your recovery and better prepares you for your next physical challenge. The idea is to replenish your depleted glycogen stores and to expedite the recovery process as soon as possible.

After an activity, it's best to consume foods that are rich in carbohydrates that have a high GI. These foods will help to restore your muscle glycogen in the quickest fashion.

In one study, seven men ran on a treadmill at a constant speed for 90 minutes on two separate occasions. This was followed by a four-hour recovery period during which they were fed a meal. (The meal came 20 minutes into the recovery period.) One time the meal had a high GI (77) and the other time the meal had a low GI (37). After the four-hour recovery, they ran to exhaustion at the same speed as in the 90-minute run. The subjects ran 15.2% longer after consuming the high GI meal than after consuming the low GI meal (86.6 minutes compared to 75.2 minutes). In other words, the subjects recovered more quickly from 90 minutes of running after they ate foods with a high GI.

Foods with a relatively high GI include whole-grain bread (59), Kellogg's Raisin Bran® (61), raisins (64), pineapples (66), white bread (71), watermelon (72), white bagels (72), waffles (76), Gatorade® (78), jelly beans (80), pizza (80), Kellogg's® Rice Krispies® (82), puffed rice cakes (82), pretzels (83), Kellogg's Corn Flakes® (92), baked russet potatoes (94), buckwheat pancakes (102) and dates (103).

It seems logical to think that after an intense workout, appetite would be stimulated. But after an intense workout, appetite is suppressed, at least initially. (This phenomenon has been dubbed exercise-induced anorexia.) As a result, it may be more practical for you to first consume cold fluids that are high in carbohydrates rather than solid food or a meal. Cold fluids also help to cool your body.

Commercial sports drinks can be excellent post-activity fluids. In terms of recovery, there are two important components of a sports drink: carbohydrates and electrolytes (sodium and potassium). Since all sports drinks are different, you should read the facts panel to be sure of their exact contents.

A good rule of thumb is to consume about 0.5 grams of carbohydrates per pound of your bodyweight (g/lb) within 30 minutes after an activity. This should be repeated again within two hours after the activity. Say, for instance, that the 200-pound man in the continuing example finished training at 8:00am. He should consume about 100 grams of carbohydrates – or 400 calories of carbohydrates – by 8:30am and

another 100 grams of carbohydrates by 10:00am [0.5 g/lb x 200 lb = 100 g].

Delaying the consumption of carbohydrates for a longer period of time significantly reduces the rate at which the glycogen stores are replenished. This will impede the recovery process and impact your future performance.

There's some evidence to suggest that combining carbohydrates with a small amount of protein can expedite recovery by improving the rate at which your glycogen stores are replenished. However, it appears that simply increasing the quantity of post-activity carbohydrates will have the same results. Nonetheless, consuming a small amount of protein following an intense activity may aid in the repair of muscle tissue. If carbohydrates and protein are consumed in combination after an activity, it should be in a 4:1 ratio, meaning that 80% of the calories should be from carbohydrates and 20% of the calories should be from protein. So instead of consuming a total of 200 grams of carbohydrates, the man in our example would consume 160 grams of carbohydrates and 40 grams of protein. (Note: An excellent, easy and inexpensive way to get some protein after training or competing is by drinking low-fat chocolate milk.)

Finally, it's also important to rehydrate after an activity. You should consume about 16 ounces of water for every pound of bodyweight that you lose while training or competing.

FAST FOODS, SLOW CHOICES

If you eat at fast-food restaurants on a regular basis, you're not alone. It has been said that each day, one out of every four Americans eats fast food. No wonder: According to the National Restaurant Association, there were 195,000 fast-food restaurants in the United States in 2007 (and another 80,000 casual-dining restaurants). Sales at fast-food restaurants were projected to reach $167.7 billion in 2011. And Americans spend 49% of their food money eating away from home.

The good news is that fast food is inexpensive, convenient and, of course, fast. But the bad news is that, for the most part, it's not very healthy or nutritious. Fast food tends to be high in calories, fat and sodium. In fact, research has shown that on the days that people eat fast food, they tend to consume more calories and fat than on other days.

Healthy Tactics

Believe it or not, there are healthy tactics that you can employ when eating fast food. Since fast foods are so widespread and can vary so much from one restaurant to another, it's well beyond the scope of this chapter to offer you a detailed list of specific suggestions. However, here are some general suggestions that you'll find useful in your quest to make healthy choices at fast-food restaurants (and, in many cases, full-service restaurants as well):

1. Reduce fat.

Fast food is often synonymous with fat food. In general, you should limit your intake of fat, especially saturated fat and trans fat.

Perhaps the most popular item on a fast-food menu is an order of French fries. Indeed, it's estimated that the average American eats 28 pounds of French fries per year. Unfortunately, French fries are very high in fat. A medium serving can have 18 grams of fat of which 5 grams are saturated fat and 4.5 grams are trans fat. Do you still want fries with that burger?

Onion rings aren't much better. A medium serving can have 16 grams of fat of which 4 grams are saturated fat and 3.5 grams are trans fat. A

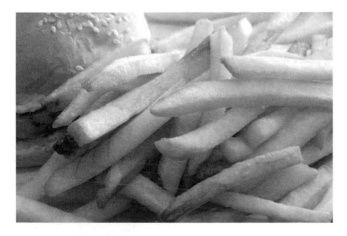

It's estimated that the average American eats 28 pounds of French fries per year.

better choice to accompany your meal is a baked potato which has no fat whatsoever.

Here's another helpful hint to reduce your intake of fat: If you like to eat toast with your breakfast, use jelly or jam instead of butter.

2. Watch sodium.

As noted earlier, your intake of sodium should be less than 2,400 milligrams per day. This is the equivalent of about one teaspoon of table salt per day.

Fast food is notorious for being high in sodium. If you're not careful, you can easily get more than an entire day's worth of sodium in just one meal. An example of this is eating a ham-and-cheese omelet, two pancakes, sausage, bacon, hash browns and a biscuit for breakfast. Eat a cheeseburger, medium fries and a medium milkshake for lunch and a few slices of pizza for dinner and you have a great head start on establishing your very own salt mine (as well as clogging your arterial pipeline).

Most people know that French fries are high in sodium; a medium serving can have 640 milligrams. But a medium serving of onion rings can have 460 milligrams. How about a side order of chili? One serving can have more than 1,000 milligrams of sodium.

The fact of the matter is that sodium shows up in a number of startling places. For instance, a medium vanilla milkshake can have about 300 milligrams or more. Another unexpected surprise is that squirt of ketchup on your burger; a small packet can have as much as 180 milligrams. And those seemingly harmless dill pickles check in at about 200 milligrams. Salad dressings can be loaded with sodium: Fat-free Italian dressing has a whopping 770 milligrams. Cole slaw, surprisingly, is also high in sodium.

3. Think green.

Many fast-food restaurants now offer salads and some even have salad bars. However, just because it's salad doesn't automatically mean that it's healthy. You can't go wrong with ingredients such as lettuce, tomatoes, cucumbers and carrots. But you can sabotage an otherwise excellent choice of food with the dressing.

In general, salad dressings are almost all fat and quite high in sodium. So rather than drown your salad in dressing, order it on the side. Or better yet, use a fat-free or reduced-fat dressing. Remember, though, that using a reduced-fat dressing doesn't give you the license to pour it on *ad libitum*. Be aware, for example, that a packet of reduced-fat creamy ranch dressing still has 100 calories of which 70 are from fat (along with 550 milligrams of sodium).

Something else to avoid on salads are croutons which are 30% fat or more and high in sodium. Along these lines, skip the bacon bits. Also, a garden salad is much healthier than a Caesar salad.

4. Limit toppings/sauces.

A traditional topping for a sandwich is mayonnaise. Choosing to "hold the mayo" could save you 150 calories or more . . . and they're all from fat. If you need to put something on a sandwich, try using mustard instead of mayonnaise.

As noted earlier, a baked potato is a better choice than French fries or onion rings. But get it sans butter, sour cream or other toppings/ stuffings. Having a baked potato "stuffed" with bacon and cheese can increase the calories from about 300 to 580, the fat calories from 0 to 200 and the milligrams of sodium from 25 to 950. Yikes!

Few foods are as inextricably linked with toppings more than the ever-popular pizza. It's important to understand that a cheese pizza has more calories from fat than you might think. One medium slice of cheese pizza can have 240 calories of which 10 grams are from fat, including 5 grams of saturated fat (plus 650 milligrams of sodium). And seriously, who eats just one slice? Add meat toppings and it only gets worse. Consider this: One medium slice of sausage pizza can have 340 calories of which 18 grams are from fat, including 8 grams of saturated fat (plus 910 milligrams of sodium). All in one slice! So if you're going to have pizza, order it plain or with vegetable toppings. An even healthier option is get pizza with whole-wheat dough.

Ketchup is a popular condiment but, again, it's high in sodium. Sauces, too, are usually high in sodium. Get tarter, barbeque and other sauces on the side. The same is true of gravy: If you want it with mashed potatoes, order it on the side.

5. Go grilled.

A good rule of thumb when eating at fast-food restaurants – or anywhere else, actually – is to limit your intake of fried foods. Everything else being equal, grilled food is *always* healthier than fried (or breaded) food. Other healthier ways to prepare food are to have it baked, broiled, charbroiled, roasted or steamed. In addition to avoiding foods that are fried or breaded, steer clear of foods that are dubbed crispy.

6. Choose poultry/fish.

Here's another good rule of thumb: Lighter meats are healthier than darker meats. So instead of ordering beef, choose chicken, turkey or fish. For breakfast, ham is a healthier choice than bacon or sausage.

As mentioned previously, the way that a food is prepared has an enormous impact on its nutritional content. Grilled chicken is a better choice than fried chicken. If the chicken that you ordered has skin, remove it; the skin has plenty of calories and fat. Interestingly, some parts of a chicken are healthier than others. A drumstick, for instance, has much less calories and fat than a thigh.

Like vegetables, fruits are very low in calories and fat and packed with nutrients.

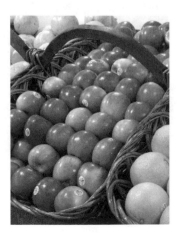

7. Eat fruit.

Like vegetables, fruits are very low in calories and fat and packed with nutrients. In an effort to provide healthier choices, many fast-food restaurants have begun to offer choices of fruit. Hint: Apple pies, blueberry muffins, cherry turnovers and strawberry shakes aren't charter members of the Fruit Group.

Besides a garden salad, you might be able to get a fruit salad. Another healthy option is yogurt.

8. Drink responsibly.

What do you drink at fast-food restaurants? Two beverages to avoid are milkshakes and sodas. Besides being high in sodium, milkshakes are high in calories and fat: A medium vanilla shake can have 41 grams of fat of which 27 grams are saturated fat. Gulp. A better choice is low-fat milk. Sodas are very high in sugar which has virtually no nutritional value. Couple that with free, unlimited, help-yourself refills and you have a recipe for dietary disaster. If you simply have to drink soda, choose a diet version.

Of course, an excellent choice for a beverage is water which has no calories. Another healthy option for a beverage is some type of juice.

9. Get substitutes.

When you order your food, you have the right to ask for substitutes. Just because a value meal comes with soda doesn't mean that you can't ask for low-fat milk; just because a value meal comes with French fries doesn't mean that you can't ask for a baked potato (plain, of course); just because the sandwich comes with a sesame-seed bun doesn't mean that you can't ask for a whole-grain bread/roll. Remember, you can "have it your way."

10. Control portions.

Value meals sure sound tempting, right? But remember, the "value" is *economical*, not *nutritional*. Yeah, you do get a lot of food for your money but what you usually get is a lot of bad food for your money: more calories, more fat and more sodium. Some bargain.

One of the most important things that you can do when eating fast food is to exercise portion control. Get the smallest burger, not the largest one (and get it minus cheese). Get the smallest order of fries, not the largest one. In short, you'd be very wise *not* to "supersize." Also keep in mind that there are no standards for portion sizes. So a small size at one restaurant can be larger than a small size at another restaurant.

11. Share food.

Just because you sprung for a value meal, there's nothing that says that you have to eat it by yourself. You can save some calories by getting a large-size value meal and then splitting it with another individual. Or, you can get part of it wrapped and eat it later.

12. Become knowledgeable.

A food at one restaurant can be dramatically different from the same food at another. For example, researchers from the Consumer Union – the non-profit publishers of *Consumer Reports* magazine – compared the nutritional profiles of 36 chicken sandwiches from 16 fast-food chains. They found that a chicken sandwich at one fast-food restaurant had 360 calories of which 7 grams were from fat, including 2 grams of saturated fat. And a chicken sandwich at another fast-food restaurant had 950 calories of which 56 grams were from fat, including 10 grams of saturated fat. For that matter, a restaurant can offer different types of chicken sandwiches with vastly different nutrients.

You should become familiar with the menus and nutritional information of the fast-food restaurants at which you typically visit. At this point in time, all of the major fast-food chains have their own websites that contain very detailed information about the nutritional content of their foods. Sometimes, you can even find nutritional information conveniently posted right on menu boards in restaurants.

RECIPE FOR SUCCESS

Nutrition is a critical part of a fitness program. The proper application of nutritional training will help you to maximize your performance.

Table 19.1: Summary of fat-soluble vitamins and their functions and sources

FAT-SOLUBLE VITAMIN	FUNCTIONS	SOURCES
Vitamin A (retinol)	is required for normal vision (especially at night) and promotes bone growth, healthy hair, skin and teeth	organ meats, dairy products, fish, eggs, carrots, spinach and sweet potatoes
Vitamin D (calciferol)	enhances calcium absorption and is vital for strong bones and teeth	fish, fortified milk products and cereals, dairy products and egg yolks
Vitamin E (tocopherol)	acts as an antioxidant, aids in the formation of red blood cells and helps to maintain muscles and other biological tissues	poultry, seafood, eggs, vegetable oils, nuts, fruits, vegetables and meats
Vitamin K	assists in blood clotting and bone metabolism	green leafy vegetables, Brussels sprouts, cabbage, potatoes, plant oils, oats, margarine and organ meats

Table 19.1: Summary of fat-soluble vitamins and their functions and sources

Table 19.2: Summary of water-soluble vitamins and their functions and sources

WATER-SOLUBLE VITAMIN	FUNCTIONS	SOURCES
biotin	helps to synthesize glycogen, amino acids and fat	liver, fruits, vegetables, nuts, eggs, poultry and meats
cobalamin (B_{12})	forms and regulates red blood cells, prevents anemia and maintains a healthy nervous system	fortified cereals, meats, fish, poultry and dairy products
folate (folic acid and folacin)	is needed to manufacture red blood cells and aids in the metabolism of amino acids	enriched cereal grains, fruits, dark green leafy vegetables, meats, fish, liver, poultry, enriched and whole-grain breads and fortified cereals
niacin (B_3)	promotes normal appetite, digestion and proper nerve function and is required for energy metabolism	meats, fish, poultry, eggs, potatoes, enriched and whole-grain breads and bread products, orange juice, peanuts and fortified cereals
pantothenic acid (B_5)	helps in the metabolism of carbohydrates, protein and fat	chicken, beef, potatoes, oats, cereals, tomato products, liver, kidney, yeast, egg yolks, broccoli and whole grains
pyridoxine (B_6)	assists in the formation of red blood cells and the metabolism of carbohydrates, protein and fat	fortified cereals, organ meats, lean meats, poultry, fish, eggs, milk, vegetables, nuts and bananas
riboflavin (B_2)	aids in the maintenance of skin, mucous membranes and nervous structures	organ meats, poultry, beef, lamb, fish, milk, dark green leafy vegetables, bread products and fortified cereals
thiamine (B_1)	maintains a healthy nervous system and heart and helps to metabolize carbohydrates and amino acids	enriched, fortified and whole-grain products, bread and bread products, ready-to-eat cereals, meats, poultry, fish, liver and eggs
Vitamin C (ascorbic acid)	promotes healing, helps in the absorption of iron and the maintenance and repair of connective tissues, bones, teeth and cartilage	citrus fruits, tomatoes, tomato juice, potatoes, Brussels sprouts, cauliflower, broccoli, strawberries, watermelon, cabbage and spinach

Table 19.3: Summary of macrominerals and their functions and sources

MACROMINERAL	FUNCTIONS	SOURCES
calcium	is essential in blood clotting, muscle contraction, nerve transmission and the formation of bones and teeth	milk, cheese, yogurt, oysters, broccoli and spinach
chloride	is an electrolyte that regulates body fluids in to and out of cells and helps to maintain a proper acid-base (pH) balance	table salt, milk, canned vegetables and animal foods
magnesium	is essential for healthy nerve and muscle function and bone formation	green leafy vegetables, nuts, meats, poultry, fish, oysters, starches, milk and beans
phosphorus	maintains pH, helps in energy production and is essential for every metabolic process in the body	milk, yogurt, ice cream, cheese, peas, meats, poultry, fish and eggs
potassium	is an electrolyte that regulates body fluids in to and out of cells and promotes proper muscular contraction and the transmission of nerve impulses	citrus fruits, bananas, deep yellow vegetables and potatoes
sodium	is an electrolyte that regulates body fluids in to and out of cells, transmits nerve impulses, maintains normal blood pressure and is involved in muscle contraction	table salt, milk, canned vegetables and animal foods
sulfur	is needed to make hair and nails	beef, peanuts, clams and wheat germ

Table 19.4: Summary of microminerals and their functions and sources

MICROMINERAL	FUNCTIONS	SOURCES
chromium	functions in the metabolism of carbohydrates and fat and helps to maintain blood-glucose levels	meats, poultry, fish and peanuts
copper	stimulates the absorption of iron and has a role in the formation of red blood cells, connective tissues and nerve fibers	organ meats, seafood, nuts, beans, whole-grain products and cocoa products
fluoride	prevents dental caries and stimulates the formation of new bones	fluoridated water, teas and marine fish
iodine	is necessary for proper functioning of the thyroid gland and prevents goiter and cretinism	seafood, processed foods and iodized salt
iron	is involved in the manufacture of hemoglobin and myoglobin (two proteins that transport oxygen to the tissues) and has a role in normal immune function	liver, fruits, vegetables, fortified bread and grain products, meats, poultry and shellfish
manganese	is involved in the formation of bones and the metabolism of carbohydrates	nuts, legumes, coffee, tea and whole grains
molybdenum	helps to regulate the storage of iron	dark green leafy vegetables, legumes, grain products, nuts and organ meats
selenium	protects cell membranes	organ meats, chicken, seafood, whole-grain cereals and milk
zinc	has a role in the repair and growth of the biological tissues	fortified cereals, meats, poultry, eggs and seafood

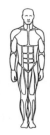

20 Nutritional Supplements

Research has shown that 54% of American adults report taking at least one nutritional supplement; 10% report taking more than five. Because their use is so widespread, no detailed discussion of nutrition would be complete without an examination of nutritional supplements.

The most popular nutritional supplements include protein and vitamins/minerals. But many people also use herbal supplements and a wide variety of other nutritional supplements. As a result, it's important to know what the research says about the safety and effectiveness of some of these nutritional supplements.

PROTEIN AND VITAMIN/ MINERAL SUPPLEMENTS

As noted, protein and vitamin/mineral supplements are highly popular. There are many misconceptions about these products, however.

Protein Supplements

Many individuals think that they need to consume large amounts of protein in order to increase their muscular size and strength and, for that reason, take protein supplements. A number of studies have shown that the protein needs of active individuals are higher than those of their inactive counterparts. But this need has been drastically exaggerated and overrated by the manufacturers of protein supplements.

The fact of the matter is that individuals who consume adequate calories generally obtain adequate protein. Remember, your caloric requirements are determined by several factors, including your size and level of activity. Larger, more active individuals require and consume more calories than the average person. With these additional calories comes additional protein. In

other words, the increased protein need of active individuals is met by an increased caloric intake.

For adults, the Recommended Dietary Allowance (RDA) for protein is 0.8 grams per kilogram of bodyweight per day (g/kg/day) or about 0.36 grams per pound of bodyweight per day. Assuming a sufficient caloric intake, 1.2 to 2.0 g/kg/day – about 150 to 250% of the RDA for adults – is present in any normal diet that contains 15% of its calories as protein. In Chapter 19, it was calculated that a 200-pound man who's very active requires approximately 5,200 calories per day (cal/day) to meet his energy needs. If 15% of these calories came from protein, he'd be receiving 780 calories from protein or 195 grams [780 cal ÷ 4 cal/g]. Based on the RDA of 0.8 g/kg/day, he'd be consuming enough protein to meet the daily needs of a man who weighed *a little more than 536 pounds* [195 g/day ÷ 0.8 g/kg/day x 2.2 lb/kg = 536.25 lb]. This amount of protein is actually about 2.15 g/kg/day . . . or about 2.5 times the RDA. And don't forget, this is without the person making any effort to consume extra protein. So even if the requirement for active individuals is greater, it's likely that they're already consuming enough protein to ensure proper levels of consumption. If you're concerned that you're not getting enough protein in your diet, you can obtain adequate amounts by simply consuming more foods that are high in protein such as lean or low-fat meat and poultry.

It must be understood that an excessive intake of protein carries the potential for many adverse effects. An intake of protein that's greater than the needs for the growth, maintenance and repair of biological tissues is either stored as fat or excreted in the urine. When a large amount of protein is urinated, it places a heavy burden on the liver and kidneys and the

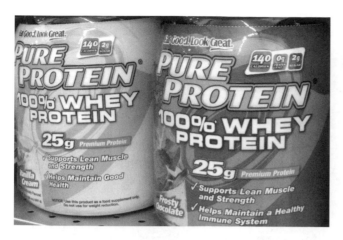

The increased protein need of active individuals is met by an increased caloric intake.

stress may damage those organs. A high intake of protein also increases the risk of dehydration which, in turn, increases the risk of developing a heat-related disorder such as heat exhaustion, heat stroke or heat cramps. Other potential adverse effects from a high intake of protein include diarrhea, cramps, gastrointestinal upset and an excessive loss of calcium in the urine.

Vitamin/Mineral Supplements

Many people believe that their foods don't provide sufficient micronutrients and, therefore, take vitamin/mineral supplements. There's no unbiased, scientific evidence to suggest that those who consume a balanced diet need vitamins and minerals in excess of the RDA. And there's no unbiased, scientific evidence to suggest that an intake of vitamins and minerals that's in excess of the RDA confers any extra benefits or improves performance.

As noted earlier, active individuals require and consume more calories than the average person. With these additional calories come additional vitamins and minerals. In truth, even a marginal diet provides adequate vitamins and minerals. Understand, too, that your liver is a storehouse for vitamins and minerals. This organ can quickly compensate for a temporary dietary shortfall by releasing its stored nutrients as needed and then replenishing its reservoirs when the opportunity arises.

That being said, some individuals may need a multi-vitamin/mineral supplement. For example, a nutritional supplement may be warranted for vegetarians and women who are pregnant or lactating. A nutritional supplement may also be appropriate for athletes who restrict their caloric intake in order to "make weight" to compete in sports such as competitive weightlifting, boxing, judo, wrestling and lightweight crew. And since women are at an increased risk for iron and calcium deficiency, nutritional supplements may be justified for those two minerals.

Whenever possible, though, it's better to get vitamins and minerals from foods rather than pills because the high concentration of these micronutrients in pill form may interfere with the absorption of other nutrients. Also keep in mind that nutritional supplements containing more than 150% of the RDA are for disease treatment and should never be used unless a physician has diagnosed their need.

There's nothing wrong with taking a low-dose multi-vitamin/mineral supplement on a daily basis. When consumed in reasonable doses, vitamins and minerals pose no health or safety risks. The Academy of Nutrition and Dietetics – formerly known as the American Dietetic Association – is the largest organization of food and nutrition professionals in the world. According to this group, high doses of vitamins and minerals pose a risk of toxicity that can lead to serious medical complications. When taken in megadoses – defined as any dose that's greater than 10 times the RDA – vitamins that are in excess of those needed to saturate the enzyme systems function as free-floating drugs instead of receptor-bound nutrients. Like all drugs, high doses of vitamins and minerals have the potential for adverse effects.

Of greatest concern is an excessive intake of the fat-soluble vitamins – particularly vitamins A and D – which can be extremely toxic. Consuming large doses of vitamin A can result in decalcification of bones (resulting in fragile bones), an increased susceptibility to disease, enlargement of the liver and spleen, muscle and joint soreness, nausea, vomiting, diarrhea, drowsiness, headaches, double vision, irritability, amenorrhea (cessation of menstruation), stunted growth, loss of appetite, loss of hair and skin rashes; consuming large doses of vitamin D can result in decalcification of bones, nausea, vomiting, diarrhea, drowsiness, headaches, loss of appetite, loss of hair, loss of weight, hypertension and elevated cholesterol.

Excessive amounts of the B vitamins and vitamin C are generally excreted in the urine (which prompts some authorities to suggest that consuming a high amount of water-soluble vitamins leaves a person with nothing more than expensive urine). This action places an inordinate amount of stress on the liver and kidneys. Though mainly excreted, large amounts of water-soluble vitamins can still produce adverse effects while in the body. For example, a high intake of vitamin C can produce nausea, diarrhea, stomach cramps, kidney stones, bladder irritation, intestinal problems, destruction of red blood cells, elevated cholesterol, ulceration of the gastric wall, leaching of calcium from bones and gout.

HERBAL SUPPLEMENTS

Many herbal and other botanical (plant-derived) supplements are marketed for specific medical purposes for which there often isn't any valid proof. The truth is that a large number of herbal supplements have no recognized role in nutrition.

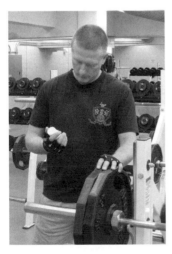

There's no unbiased, scientific evidence to suggest that those who consume a balanced diet need vitamins and minerals in excess of the RDA.

Additionally, there are concerns about the safety of many herbal supplements. For instance, chaparral, comfrey, germander, kava, ma huang (ephedra), pennyroyal and sassafras have been linked to liver toxicity; germander, kava and mistletoe to hepatitis; ma huang to seizures, heart attacks and stroke; ginseng to hypertension, insomnia, depression and skin blemishes; and yohimbine to kidney failure, seizures and death. There are similar fears with high-potency enzymes and glandular extracts from dried animal organs such as the pituitary gland, thyroid gland and testicles.

MISCELLANEOUS SUPPLEMENTS

A host of nutritional supplements have been publicized as ergogenic aids (or performance enhancers). Others have been touted for a variety of reasons, including fat loss, weight reduction, muscle gain and strength improvement. Here's a critical look at some of the notable nutritional supplements that have been promoted in recent years:

Aspartate

Aspartate is a non-essential amino acid. Like most amino acids, aspartate has been investigated as an ergogenic aid. In fact, the first known study on aspartate was conducted more than 50 years ago.

The majority of the research on aspartate has examined its effect on aerobic endurance, almost all of which involved rats swimming to exhaustion. This has yielded a mixed bag of results with some studies showing a positive effect and roughly an equal number of studies showing no effect. Even then, results from animal studies have little relevance to humans. A handful of studies have been conducted on humans, most of which involved cycling to exhaustion. Again, the findings are inconsistent. Research has shown that aspartate has no effect on muscular endurance or strength.

Several studies have looked at the effects of aspartate in combination with other nutritional supplements, most often arginine (another amino acid). These studies offer no direct support for the use of aspartate as an ergogenic aid.

Take note: Researchers caution that adverse effects are possible when aspartate is used alone or with other amino acids.

Beta-alanine

Beta-alanine is a precursor of carnosine, a molecule that's highly concentrated in skeletal muscle. It's thought that beta-alanine can buffer the buildup of lactic acid thereby delaying fatigue and, in theory, improve performance.

In one study, 55 men were randomly assigned to groups that received either beta-alanine, creatine, beta-alanine and creatine or a placebo for 28 days. The researchers examined eight indices of cardiorespiratory endurance. The group that received beta-alanine improved significantly in just one of the eight indices. (The group that received beta-alanine and creatine improved significantly in five of the eight indices.) There were no significant differences between the groups in their improvements. A caveat is that the study was sponsored by a manufacturer of nutritional supplements.

In another study, 15 400-meter sprinters – who had an average personal best time of 50.45 seconds – were randomly assigned to groups that received either beta-alanine or a placebo for four weeks. Both groups significantly decreased their time to run 400 meters and their improvements were similar.

Boron

Individuals have used boron thinking that it will improve their size and strength. However, there's little or no proof to support this belief.

In one study, 12 subjects who received boron for a period of 48 days increased their level of testosterone. But these subjects were postmenopausal women whose testosterone was normally low. What's more, as part of the study, the women had been fed a diet that was deficient in boron for the previous 119 days. The men who were in the study experienced no significant increase in their level of testosterone.

In another study, 19 male bodybuilders were randomly assigned to groups that received either boron or a placebo. After seven weeks of strength

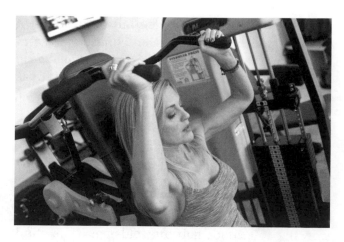

There's no scientific evidence that calcium promotes weight loss or has any ergogenic value. (Photo provided by Luke Carlson.)

training, boron had no significant effect on total testosterone, lean-body mass or strength.

Low doses of boron are generally safe. But high intakes can cause nausea, vomiting, diarrhea and a loss of appetite.

Calcium

Many nutritional supplements have been promoted as an effective means to lose weight. One of the latest to garner attention as a weight-loss product is calcium.

In one study, 340 overweight/obese subjects were randomly assigned to groups that received either calcium or a placebo. After two years, calcium didn't produce significantly better results than the placebo in any measure, including changes in bodyweight, body fat and Body-Mass Index. Nor did calcium yield any significantly better improvements than the placebo in abdominal circumference, hip circumference and tricep skinfold thickness.

Calcium is an important macromineral that's essential in blood clotting, muscle contraction, nerve transmission and the formation of bones and teeth. But there's no evidence that it promotes weight loss. And there's no scientific evidence that it has any ergogenic value.

Chromium

As a micromineral, chromium functions in the metabolism of carbohydrates and fat and helps to maintain blood-glucose levels. It's believed that chromium can promote fat loss and muscle gain.

Most of the claims regarding the benefits of chromium are based on two poorly designed, unpublished studies. These two studies were referenced in a review article that was written by a chemist who was consulting for a manufacturer of nutritional supplements. In 1996, the Federal Trade Commission ordered the manufacturer (and two others) to stop making unsubstantiated claims that chromium decreases body fat and increases muscle mass. Nevertheless, misconceptions about chromium still persist.

The vast majority of studies on chromium have been conducted on animals. Most of the studies on humans have shown that the use of chromium doesn't decrease body fat or promote fat loss in any way. In one study, 95 Navy personnel were alternately assigned to groups that received either chromium or a placebo. After 16 weeks of aerobic training, chromium didn't significantly reduce body fat or increase lean-body mass more than the placebo. A meta-analysis of 10 studies found that chromium produced a weight loss of about 2.4 to 2.6 pounds over the course of 6 to 14 weeks which isn't very impressive.

To date, only one study has reported that chromium increases muscle mass. And in that study, muscle mass was estimated from anthropometric measurements which can be unreliable.

It appears as if chromium doesn't increase strength, either. In one study, 16 men were randomly assigned to groups that received either chromium or a placebo. After 12 weeks of strength training, the placebo actually increased strength more than chromium. No improvements in percentage of body fat, lean-body mass or skinfold thickness were made by either group. Interestingly, another study found that those who received chromium had urinary chromium excretions that were *60 times higher* than those who received a placebo.

Cobalamin (Vitamin B_{12})

Largely because many athletes have said that they've received B_{12} injections (or "shots") – perhaps most famously, Roger Clemens – it's thought that this vitamin has some ergogenic value. But there's no research to support this contention.

In one study, 16 marksmen were randomly assigned to groups that received a combination of three B vitamins (thiamin, pyridoxine and B_{12}) or no treatment for eight weeks. Those who were given the B vitamins significantly improved shooting accuracy with a pistol more than those who were given nothing. The study was repeated the next year in which 19 marksmen were randomly assigned to groups that received the B vitamins or a placebo for eight weeks. The results of the second study were similar to the first study. However, since the subjects used vitamin B_{12} in combination with two other B vitamins, it's impossible to tell if their performance was enhanced by the B_{12}. In other words, these studies offer no direct support for the use of vitamin B_{12} as an ergogenic aid. Although a case could be made that the three B vitamins had an ergogenic benefit, improvements in pistol marksmanship have no relevance to other sports.

Conjugated Linoleic Acid

In studies of animals, conjugated linoleic acid (CLA) has been shown to decrease body fat and increase lean-body mass. But studies of humans have found conflicting results. Some studies have shown that CLA decreases body fat and/or increases lean-body mass while others have shown no effect. Many of the studies that found positive effects had small numbers of subjects and were of short duration which makes it difficult to draw any meaningful conclusions.

In one study, 180 obese subjects were randomly assigned to three groups: Two groups received different types of CLA and another group received a placebo. In comparison to the placebo group, the CLA groups significantly decreased body fat and increased lean-body mass. One CLA group lost 3.74 pounds of fat and gained 1.54 pounds of lean-body mass; the other lost 5.28 pounds of fat and gained 1.32 pounds of lean-body mass. So the results weren't exactly breathtaking, especially considering that this was after taking CLA for 12 months.

Also worth mentioning is that all three groups reduced their caloric intake over the course of the study. By the 12th month, the CLA groups were consuming at least 105 calories per day less than the placebo group. This, of course, could easily account for much of the difference in the results.

Creatine

For many years, creatine has received a great deal of attention within the athletic, scientific and medical communities. It may very well be the most studied nutritional supplement in history.

There are many anecdotal reports that creatine is effective but scientific research is, at best, inconclusive. Much of the research that has investigated creatine has been conducted in a laboratory. In this controlled setting, the best evidence for performance enhancement from the use of creatine is in repeated, maximal, short-term sprints on a stationary cycle. And even then, some studies have shown no improvements. Of the research that has been conducted outside a laboratory, very few studies have shown that creatine improves performance in realistic activities such as running and swimming. In one study that involved nine highly trained sprinters – all were among the top 10 men and women in their country in the 100- and/or 200-meter dash – creatine proved no better than a placebo on single or repeated 40-meter sprint times. In two studies that involved a total of 52 elite male and female swimmers, creatine didn't improve performance in 25-, 50- and 100-meter swim sprints more than a placebo. In some studies, creatine actually *worsened* performance. In short, research has found that any improvements that may occur in laboratory settings don't translate into improvements in realistic activities.

It appears as if using creatine in the recommended dose is safe. However, many individuals – thinking that more is better – typically exceed the recommended dose,

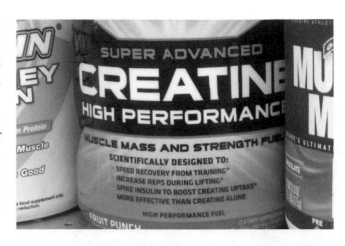

There are many anecdotal reports that creatine is effective but scientific research is, at best, inconclusive.

undoubtedly putting them at greater risk for incurring adverse effects. At this point in time, the long-term effects of creatine are unknown.

Adverse effects are rarely reported in studies. But most studies don't include any formal way of assessing adverse effects. While few adverse effects have been reported in studies that were done in a laboratory, there have been endless accounts from individuals who have experienced adverse effects. Although these observations are anecdotal, their sheer volume is such that they can't be ignored. In a study that surveyed 52 collegiate athletes who voluntarily took creatine, 38 (73.1%) reported at least one adverse effect. There are numerous reports of water retention, muscle cramping, dehydration/heat-related disorder, muscle strains/dysfunction, gastro-intestinal distress (such as an upset stomach, gastrointestinal pain, nausea and vomiting) and liver and kidney dysfunction.

Dehydroepiandrosterone

As a prohormone, dehydroepiandrosterone (DHEA) is a precursor to many hormones, including testosterone. Because of this, it's believed that using DHEA can increase the production of testosterone in the body which could yield the same effects as anabolic steroids. This hasn't been corroborated by research, however.

In one study, 20 male soccer players were randomly assigned to groups that received either

DHEA or a placebo for four weeks. DHEA increased total testosterone more than the placebo but no significant improvements in body composition were made by either group.

Since DHEA is a precursor to steroids, it's no surprise that it has the potential for similar adverse effects. Hair loss, growth of facial hair and a deepening of the voice have been reported in women and gynecomastia (the appearance of female-like breasts on the male physique) in men. DHEA may also increase the risk of uterine and prostate cancer. Understand that this or any other steroid precursor could cause an individual to fail a test for steroids.

Of no small importance is that many DHEA products have been shown to contain inaccurate doses. Independent testing of 16 DHEA products found that only eight (50%) had the exact amount of DHEA that was stated on the labels; the actual levels varied *as much as 150%*. Amazingly, three (18.75%) of the products didn't contain any DHEA whatsoever.

Ecdysterone

A plant sterol, ecdysterone has been promoted as a nutritional supplement to enhance protein synthesis, increase muscle mass and decrease body fat. But there's no evidence that ecdysterone is effective.

Most of the studies on ecdysterone have been conducted on animals. With one exception, all of the studies on humans were published in obscure journals. In the lone study on humans that's legitimate, 45 subjects were randomly assigned to receive either methoxyisoflavone, ecdysterone, sulfo-polysaccharide or a placebo. After eight weeks of strength training, there were no significant differences between any of the three supplements and the placebo in percentage of body fat, maximum strength (the bench press and leg press), power and level of testosterone.

Glutamine

Glutamine is a non-essential amino acid. Like other amino acids, glutamine plays a role in protein synthesis. As a result, it's billed as an ergogenic aid.

In one study, 31 subjects were randomly assigned to groups that received either glutamine or a placebo. After six weeks of strength training, both groups increased their strength and lean-body mass. But there were no significant differences between glutamine and the placebo in those two measures.

Hydroxy Methylbutyrate

A relative newcomer to the ranks of nutritional supplements is hydroxy methylbutyrate which, thankfully, goes by the letters HMB; it's a metabolite of leucine, an essential amino acid.

HMB has been promoted as a nutritional supplement that increases strength and lean-body mass, supposedly by preventing the breakdown of muscle tissue. This has no scientific merit, however. One study did support the theory that HMB may prevent muscle damage. But the study didn't examine whether or not HMB had any effect on strength or lean-body mass. In a study that did look at this aspect, 35 collegiate football players were randomly assigned to groups that received either HMB or a placebo for four weeks. After a one-week washout period, the subjects were switched to the other treatment for four weeks. There were no significant differences between HMB and the placebo in strength and body composition.

Research on HMB has found minimal improvements in performance in untrained individuals and almost none in trained individuals. One meta-analysis pooled data from nine studies that involved 394 subjects. In untrained subjects, HMB produced small improvements in lower-body strength and negligible improvements in upper-body strength; in trained subjects, HMB produced "trivial" improvements in lower-body and upper-body strength. In both untrained and trained subjects, the effect on body composition was also described as trivial.

Nitric Oxide

Recently, nitric oxide has been promoted as an ergogenic aid. Nitric oxide is actually a gas, though not to be confused with nitrous oxide (aka "laughing gas"). Years ago, strange as it may seem, nitric oxide was best known as an air pollutant (formed when nitrogen and oxygen react with each other during combustion and are emitted into the air à la car exhaust). Needless to say, it came as quite a shock when the biological functions of nitric oxide were discovered in the 1980s. In fact, *Science* magazine named it Molecule of the Year in 1992. And three pharmacologists from the United States were awarded the 1998 Nobel Prize in Physiology or Medicine for discovering the role of nitric oxide as a "signaling molecule in the cardiovascular system."

In the body, nitric oxide has numerous roles. For one thing, it signals the body to dilate blood vessels thereby increasing blood flow. (Though at first it sounds bizarre, heart conditions are often treated with nitroglycerin – yes, the active ingredient in dynamite. Nitroglycerin releases nitric oxide which widens the arteries and veins that supply the heart, making it easier for the organ to pump blood.) In addition, nitric oxide is an important neurotransmitter that relays messages between nerve cells.

Be that as it may, this doesn't mean that there are any benefits in taking nitric oxide as a nutritional supplement. At the present time, no studies have shown that nitric oxide improves physical performance or any of the aforementioned biological functions.

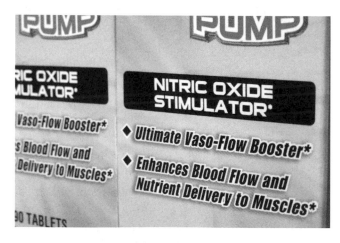

At the present time, no studies have shown that nitric oxide taken as a nutritional supplement improves physical performance or any biological functions.

Pangamic Acid

The use of pangamic acid (aka calcium pangamate and vitamin B_{15}) dates back to at least the mid-1970s. In that Cold War era, there was an enormous fascination with the Soviet sport system, especially as it pertained to training. It was said that Soviet athletes used pangamic acid to reduce fatigue and improve stamina. However, there's no legitimate scientific evidence to support those claims or any others about pangamic acid. In fact, much of the research is from the 1960s and hails from the former Soviet Union. Besides being poorly designed, most of those studies involved animals which, of course, have little relevance to humans.

In one study that was well designed, 16 track athletes were randomly assigned to groups that received either pangamic acid or a placebo for three weeks. There were no significant differences between pangamic acid and the placebo in endurance and recovery heart rate when the subjects ran to exhaustion on a treadmill.

If you look in any nutrition textbook, you'll discover that there's no RDA for pangamic acid. That's because pangamic acid hasn't been shown to be essential in the diet and isn't associated with any deficiency diseases. Actually, there's little or no mention whatsoever of pangamic acid in nutrition textbooks. And for the record, vitamin B_{15} isn't even officially recognized as a vitamin.

Final point: The Food and Drug Administration has ruled that it's illegal to sell pangamic acid as a nutritional supplement in the United States.

Ribose

As noted in Chapter 2, the breakdown of adenosine triphosphate (ATP) is the primary and immediate source of energy that's used to perform muscular work. Since a limited amount of ATP can be stored, it must be rebuilt over and over again. In the body, ribose is a sugar that helps to resynthesize ATP. In theory, then, ribose supplements could increase the levels of ATP and improve performance.

In one study, 11 cyclists and strength-trained individuals were randomly assigned to groups that received either ribose or a placebo 30 minutes prior to a bout of exercise. Each session consisted of three Wingate Tests (30 seconds of all-out sprinting) on a stationary cycle with two minutes of recovery between each test. After a one-week washout period, the subjects were switched to the other treatment and repeated the same protocol. There were no significant differences between ribose and the placebo in any measure, including peak power, average power and percent decrease in power.

In fact, the majority of research hasn't found any significant ergogenic benefits from ribose; in at least one study, ribose produced less improvement than a placebo. In this study, 31 collegiate rowers were randomly assigned to receive either ribose or a placebo. After eight weeks of training, the placebo produced significantly greater improvement in rowing 2,000 meters than ribose.

Sodium Bicarbonate

Sodium bicarbonate (aka baking soda) has a wide range of applications such as treating acid indigestion, whitening teeth and absorbing odors in refrigerators. But it's also been promoted as a substance that delays the onset of fatigue by buffering the buildup of lactic acid. Sodium bicarbonate is one of the few nutritional supplements that seem to be effective as an ergogenic aid.

A great deal of research has shown that sodium bicarbonate improves performance. In one study, 16 female subjects were randomly assigned to groups that received either sodium bicarbonate or a placebo (sodium chloride) prior to a bout of exercise. After eight weeks of interval training on a stationary cycle, sodium bicarbonate had significantly greater improvements in lactate threshold and endurance than the placebo.

Adverse effects from sodium bicarbonate include gastrointestinal disturbances such as nausea, vomiting, diarrhea and flatulence. Sodium citrate is thought to have the same ergogenic value as sodium bicarbonate without the adverse effects. But in one study, eight of nine subjects (elite athletes) who received sodium citrate experienced gastrointestinal distress.

Vanadyl Sulfate

A micro-mineral that's also known as vanadium, vanadyl sulfate has been investigated as an ergogenic aid. There's no proof that it has any effect on muscle mass or strength.

In one study, 40 subjects were paired together based on gender, age, bodyweight, height and training program. One subject from each pair was randomly assigned to receive either vanadyl sulfate or a placebo. After 12 weeks of strength training, there were no significant differences between vanadyl sulfate and the placebo in bodyweight, body composition and muscle girth. Both groups had significant improvements in strength and muscular endurance. However, were no significant differences between the groups in their improvements. (Those who consumed vanadyl sulfate had a significantly better increase in their maximum strength in the leg extension than those who consumed the placebo but this was attributed to their lower level of strength during the pre-testing.)

TAINTED PRODUCTS

There's no shortage of athletes who have tested positive for banned substances. Many of the athletes who have been in this predicament blame it on tainted products and, therefore, assert that the banned substance was taken unknowingly. Nonetheless, they're still held responsible for their actions.

You don't have to be an athlete for this to be a concern; other jobs often require drug testing. Case in point: According to *The New England Journal of Medicine*, a police sergeant who worked "in one of the most dangerous cities in the United States" was fired after a drug test showed the presence of amphetamines. He had been taking a weight-loss product that contained fenproporex, a Schedule IV controlled substance that's used as an appetite suppressant. Inside the body, fenproporex is converted into amphetamines, thus the positive drug test.

Numerous studies have discovered a large number of tainted products. In one study, researchers bought 634 nutritional supplements from 215 companies in 13 countries. The products were purchased in stores, from the Internet and over the phone. The researchers found that 94 of the 634 nutritional supplements (14.8%) contained anabolic steroids. Some of the nutritional supplements contained enough steroids to result in a positive drug test.

In another study, researchers bought 58 nutritional supplements from retail outlets and the Internet. A total of 54 nutritional supplements were successfully analyzed of which 13 (25%) had low levels of steroids and six (11%) had banned stimulants. Of note, 67% of the products that were categorized as testosterone boosters contained steroids and/or stimulants; 29% of the products that were categorized as weight loss contained steroids and/or stimulants.

In yet another study, researchers examined 64 nutritional supplements. They found that eight (12.5%) of the nutritional supplements contained steroids and/or ephedrine, a banned stimulant.

Even products that are as seemingly innocuous as vitamin/mineral supplements can contain banned substances; one study found stanozolol, a steroid, in multi-vitamin tablets. Other nutritional supplements have been shown to contain heavy metals and pesticides. Laboratory analyses found trace amounts of one or more potentially hazardous contaminants in 37 of the 40 herbal supplements that were tested. All 37 tested positive for trace amounts of lead; of those, 32 also contained mercury, 28 cadmium, 21 arsenic and 18 residues from at least one pesticide.

There are two likely reasons why a high percentage of nutritional supplements are tainted. First, it could be the result of cross-contamination. This occurs when the same machines are used to process different types of products without proper cleaning of the equipment. In other words, it's due to poor quality control. Second, manufacturers may deliberately "spike" the nutritional supplement with an illegal or banned substance with the hope that it will work better. Obviously, a product that works better can lead to greater sales.

The moral of the story is that you may be consuming unknown substances that could pose a significant threat to your health. If you choose to take nutritional supplements, make sure that the products have been tested for undeclared ingredients and certified by an independent organization such as NSF International.

FOOD FOR THOUGHT

Most of the claims concerning nutritional supplements are purely speculative and anecdotal with little or no scientific or medical basis. These products offer more hype than hope.

As long as you consume a variety of foods that provide adequate calories and nutrients, there's no need for you to take nutritional supplements. And it makes more sense to invest your money in high-quality foods than spend it on expensive nutritional supplements. Remember, there are no shortcuts on the road to proper nutrition.

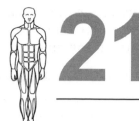

21 Nutritional Quackery

The health and fitness industry continues to be overrun by hordes of unscrupulous and unsavory entrepreneurs who seek to make quick and easy profits on the naiveté of consumers. Many individuals are easily tempted by seductive promises that nutritional supplements can help them to decrease fat, increase muscle, lose weight, get fit, improve appearance and enhance performance.

When nutritional supplements are promoted that are unproven and/or ineffective, it constitutes nutritional quackery. Each year, millions of Americans spend billions of dollars on nutritional supplements that are worthless and sometimes dangerous. But nutritional quackery isn't anything new.

SNAKE OIL SALESMEN

No other product is more closely associated with nutritional quackery than snake oil. In China, snake oil has been used for centuries as a medicinal product. In the United States, its use dates back more than 150 years. Legend has it that in the mid-1860s, Chinese laborers gave snake oil to co-workers who suffered from aches and pains while building the First Transcontinental Railroad. Over time, the term snake oil was used to describe a health product that was fraudulent. And anyone who sold such a product was subsequently referred to as a snake oil salesman.

During the late 1800s, snake oil salesmen thrived in the Midwest and rural areas of the South. This early form of consumer rip-off combined free amusement with the sale of "secret" goods that supposedly had curative powers. Traveling by horse and wagon, these "medicine shows" began innocently enough with complimentary entertainment – ranging from musical acts to magical tricks – that was given by various performers to entice an unsuspecting audience. Soon afterward, a "doctor" (or "medicine man") peddled his elixirs and tonics in colorful glass bottles as remedies for a wide assortment of ills, aches and pains to the gullible and all-to-eager masses using a spellbinding sales pitch.

A shill was often planted among the spectators who offered convincing – and scripted – testimony about how the product cured his condition. To get things moving, it wasn't unusual for the shill or another accomplice to purchase the first bottle. Thereafter, the performers circulated throughout the crowd to sell the "doctor's" product. Once money and "medicine" exchanged hands, it was only a matter of time until the showmen decided to load up their wagon and "git outta Dodge" before people realized that they had been swindled.

The products that were sold in those days – many of which were advertised as "cure-alls" – included salves, liver pads, hair growers, electric belts, powdered herbs, common forms of liniment or laxative, bunion and corn remedies and, of course, snake oil. Few could resist the alluring names and assorted purposes. For instance, Dr. Kilmer's Swamp-Root was touted as a "kidney, liver and bladder remedy"; Renne's Magic Oil was promoted for "pain killing"; Dr. McClintock's Dyspeptic Elixir was advertised as "effectual for combating dyspepsia" and a cure for "heartburn, nervousness, indigestion and all other symptoms arising from want of tone in the stomach"; McDonald's Cough Annihilator was sold to remove "the most fearful cold in a few hours"; Hamlin's Wizard Oil was said to treat "pneumonia, cancer, diphtheria, earache, toothache, headache and hydrophobia" using the marketing motto of "there is no sore it will not heal, no pain it will not subdue"; and Clark

Stanley's Snake Oil Liniment was billed as a cure for bruises, frost bite, sore throat, lumbago and sciatica and "good for man or beast." Who could refuse?

Some of the best showmen of that era were actually women: Madame DuBois had a brass band, sold medicine and pulled teeth; Princess Lotus Blossom – who was portrayed as an immigrant from China but was really Violet McNeal, a farm girl from Minnesota – sold Vital Sparks which she described as a "rejuvenator for lost manhood" that was made from male turtles and could restore "health, virility and happiness." Alas, Vital Sparks was actually aloe-coated candy.

Fast forward to the present day and only a few things have changed. The promises of combating dyspepsia and curing heartburn have shifted to "burning" fat and building muscle; the touring medicine shows and ubiquitous newspaper advertisements that were used to hawk products have been replaced by infomercials, websites and e-mails (spams); and, of course, there's considerably more money to be made. But today, as in the past, snake oil salesmen still prey on naïve consumers, targeting them with products that pledge miracles.

THE ART OF THE SEDUCTION

Make no mistake about it: The sale of nutritional supplements is a big business. The

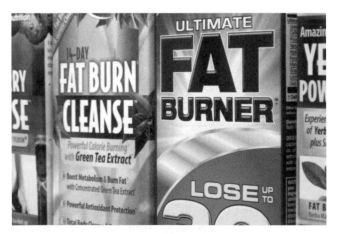

Today, as in the past, snake oil salesmen still prey on naïve consumers, targeting them with products that pledge miracles.

highly sophisticated marketing tactics used to seduce consumers are very appealing and cunning while the advertisements for products are often misleading, if not pure fabrication. Here are 10 characteristics that are common to the sales pitch for nutritional supplements:

Alluring Names

Most nutritional supplements have catchy brand names to bait consumers. Consider this random sampling of real-life products: Mega Mass, Monster Mass, Serious Mass, Elite Mass, True-Mass, Re-Built Mass, Carnivor Mass, H.U.G.E. Mass, Amplified Mass XXX, Iso Mass Extreme Gainer, Hyperbolic Mass Gainer, Mass-Tadon, Bulk Up Weight Gainer, Russian Bear 5000 Weight Gainer, CytoGainer, N-Large[2], Muscle Juice, Black All Natural Testosterone Booster, TestostroGROW, TestoJack 100, TestoRipped, Test Freak, T-Bomb, T-Up, Anabolic Freak, Anabolic Pump, Anabolic Prescription, Animal Pak, PowerFULL, Bullet Proof, Androbolix, MyoBuild, Platinum Hydro Builder, D4 Thermal Shock, Amplified Muscle Igniter 4X, Physio-Burn, Beta Burn, MethylBurn Extreme, Thermo Burst Hardcore, Thermo Detonator, Arson, Nuke, Jet Fuel, Ripped Fuel, Ripped Abs, Ripped Fast, Meltdown Fat Assault, UltraLean, AdrenaLean, Sculpted Abs, Monster Amino, Amino Burst 3000, Amino Freak and Amino Fuel. Again, this is just a sample; the list is practically endless.

Many of the names employ terms or their derivatives that connote aggressive action (amplify, grow, boost, build, bomb, shock, ignite, detonate, nuke, assault) with bodybuilding lingo (mass, ripped, pump, burn, sculpted) and scientific – or pseudoscientific – terminology (anabolic, hyperbolic, physio). The idea is to make the product sound unique, irresistible and absolutely essential for your nutritional needs.

Bodybuilding Magazines

For the most part, "muscle mags" are essentially catalogs for nutritional supplements that are neatly packaged with some articles on training. Advertisements for nutritional supplements are often strategically placed

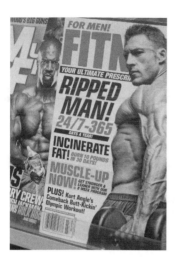

For the most part, "muscle mags" are essentially catalogs for nutritional supplements that are neatly packaged with some articles on training.

adjacent to articles that promote the very same nutritional supplements. Plus, having photographs of bodybuilders with heavily muscled physiques throughout the magazine – and usually accompanying the advertisements – implies that you can achieve the same results.

Meaningless Credentials

Support for nutritional supplements often comes from individuals with degrees or titles that aren't nationally recognized such as a certified nutritionist, nutritional consultant, nutritional counselor, nutritional specialist, nutritional therapist and doctor of nutramedicine. These credentials are meaningless, frequently having been self-conferred or received through some type of diploma mill or dubious organization. In the early 1980s, a physician famously obtained a "professional membership" for his dog in the American Association of Nutrition and Dietary Consultants and his cat in the International Academy of Nutritional Consultants merely by submitting the animal's name, address and 50 dollars.

The most reputable and recognized individual for dispensing nutritional information is a registered dietician (RD). These professionals must earn a four-year degree from an accredited college or university, complete an internship of at least six months in a supervised setting and pass a national exam. And to maintain their credentials, RDs must update their accreditation on an annual basis.

Remember, not even an MD or a PhD guarantees that a person is qualified as an authority on nutrition (or exercise). For example, a PhD who dispenses information on nutrition (or exercise) may have a degree in an unrelated field such as sport sociology or endocrinology.

Natural Products

Many nutritional supplements claim to be natural (or even legal). One study found that there's no scientific evidence to support the promotional claims for 42% of the natural products that were reviewed. Another 32% of the products had some scientific evidence to support their claims but were judged to be marketed in a misleading manner. In other words, 74% of the natural products either had no scientific evidence to support their claims or were marketed in a misleading manner.

Keep in mind, too, that because a product has natural ingredients doesn't mean that it's necessarily safe. Few things are more natural than dirt but you wouldn't want to consume it with your breakfast cereal. And, in fact, a number of natural substances can cause serious harm, including high doses of certain vitamins, minerals and herbs. (Chapter 20 discusses the safety aspect of nutritional supplements in more detail.)

Nebulous Terminology

Scientific-sounding names can be confusing and, at the same time, appealing. This is particularly true for those who seek quick and easy results. Many advertisements contain ambiguous language and rely upon the inability of consumers to understand complex terms. For instance, one product is said to contain adaptogens, metabolic intermediates, exogenous anabolic activators and energetics. Try to find those terms in any nutrition textbook.

Patent Numbers

Stating that a nutritional supplement is patented or "patent pending" can give the false impression that the US Patent and Trademark Office (USPTO) has approved the effectiveness of the product. A patent is a way to protect an inventor so that no one else makes, uses or sells the same product. Moreover, a patented product indicates that it's new and useful. New means that it's not identical to anything done before; useful means that it has a use (not that it works). The USPTO is tasked with distinguishing one product from another, not in evaluating or guaranteeing the effectiveness of a product.

Personal Testimonials

The use of personal testimonials from seemingly ordinary people is highly effective. Maybe even more effective is the use of celebrity testimonials from actors and athletes. For the right price, some individuals can be pretty eager to offer testimonials to promote practically any product.

It's fairly standard practice for testimonials to employ what's become known as before-and-after photographs. These photographs can be easily faked or "photoshopped," especially nowadays. Also, there's no evidence that the "after" photograph is truly the result of using the product.

Testimonials also come from those whom consumers trust or hold in high regard such as scientists and physicians. But reputable scientists and physicians aren't in the business of selling nutritional supplements; their testimonials should immediately raise skepticism.

Phony Endorsements

Some manufacturers make claims about their products by implying or falsely stating endorsement by professional groups. For instance, some products are said to be "university tested" which may actually mean that someone at a university was merely involved. In other cases, university testing may not have even occurred.

Since the mid-1980s or earlier, there have been commercials in which actors have said, "I'm not a doctor but I play one on TV." Then, the actors endorsed some type of product but at least they gave full disclosure. Many endorsements come from individuals who wear a white lab coat and stethoscope. Naturally, consumers assume that these people are physicians. However, if they're not referred to as physicians, they probably aren't. That's because it's illegal to impersonate a physician.

Product Labels

The label of a nutritional supplement rarely contains false claims. Untruthful or misleading information could trigger federal action since only factual data is allowed on labels. As a way around this, some manufacturers place misleading information in their advertisements – rather than on their labels – where it may be overlooked by regulators.

While on the subject, the exact content of many nutritional supplements is unknown and may not be represented accurately on the list of ingredients. In one study, for example, researchers bought 12 brands of nutritional supplements from various stores in Los Angeles. Only one of the 12 brands contained 90 to 110% of the amount of ingredients that were declared on the label; the others had significantly more or less.

Some products may even contain small amounts of banned substances such as anabolic steroids or may actually be anabolic steroids but not labeled as such. Researchers bought 58 nutritional supplements from retail outlets and Internet sites. Of the 54 nutritional supplements that were successfully analyzed, 13 (25%) had low levels of steroids and six (11%) had banned stimulants.

Questionable Research

In their advertisements, many manufacturers claim to have made a "breakthrough," conducted "scientific research" or had "secret research results." Oftentimes, though, the "research" that's noted by manufacturers is so unscientific that it's basically useless. Many of the studies, for example, were never published in a scientific journal and/or were poorly designed.

EVALUATING THE RESEARCH

As just noted, one way that manufacturers seduce consumers is to cite research. For instance, an advertisement might say "in a university study, subjects increased their muscular strength by 20%" or "more than 50 studies have proven the effectiveness of the key ingredients."

The mere mention of studies makes it sound as if there's credible evidence that a nutritional supplement is effective. But the studies may be poorly designed, irrelevant, outdated or taken out of context. And that's why it's imperative for you to "study the study" whenever possible so that you can educate yourself and separate *science fact* from *science fiction*. But once you get your hands on a study – an entire study, not just an abstract or a media report – how do you evaluate it?

Questions to Ask

Here are eight questions that should be asked to determine if a study on a nutritional supplement has any merit:

1. Was the study published in a scientific journal?

Some of the studies that are mentioned in advertisements for nutritional supplements haven't been published anywhere; others appear in non-scholarly publications. In either case, it means that the study didn't go through a rigorous peer-review process in which experts in a related field (aka referees) do an impartial review of the manuscript to determine whether or not it should be published.

With very few exceptions, magazines that are found in bookstores and on newsstands are non-scholarly publications. Any claims about the effectiveness of nutritional supplements in these types of publications are largely based on anecdotal evidence, meaning that the support is rooted entirely in personal experience, not scientific research.

This isn't much better than someone in a fitness center who says that after he took a certain nutritional supplement, his arm circumference increased by 1.5 inches, his sprint time in the 40-yard dash decreased by 0.2 seconds and his bench press improved by 50 pounds. Basically, his "success story" is anecdotal evidence. The individual may have gotten bigger, faster and stronger but there's no concrete proof that the changes were caused by the nutritional supplement.

Also be wary about information that's available on the Internet where nutritional quackery abounds. Although the emergence of the Internet has given people access to an unbelievable amount of information that's literally at their fingertips, not all of it is credible. Remember, any crackpot with a keyboard can post information on the Internet.

2. Was the study properly designed?

Because a study is published in a peer-reviewed journal doesn't guarantee that it's well designed. The gold standard for researching the effectiveness of a nutritional supplement is a randomized, double-blind, placebo-controlled study. What does this mean?

In a randomized study, subjects are randomly assigned to groups – rather than selected or chosen for a certain group – in such a way that the physical/physiological profile and size of each group are roughly the same. In a double-blind study, the researchers who are distributing the treatments and the subjects who are receiving the treatments are unaware – or "blinded" – as to who is getting what. And in a placebo-controlled study, one group of subjects receives a nutritional supplement and another group – a control group – receives the placebo.

Note: A placebo is a substance that contains no active ingredients; it's usually a sugar tablet and should be similar in appearance, taste and smell to the nutritional supplement being studied so that the subjects can't distinguish between the nutritional supplement and a placebo.

Also keep in mind that studies of short duration or with too few subjects aren't scientifically meaningful. Additionally, the results should be corroborated in other studies by other researchers at other laboratories.

3. Who were the participants/subjects in the study?

In evaluating studies, it's important to consider the population that was examined. Obviously, for a study to be relevant, the subjects in the study should be somewhat similar to you.

Here's an example: Fucoxanthin, a compound that's found in brown seaweed, has been promoted as a nutritional supplement for losing weight/fat. In a study that's often used to support this belief, subjects who were fed brown seaweed had a 5 to 10% reduction in weight. However, the subjects in the study were rats and mice. (By the way, this particular study wasn't published.)

Responses that are experienced by animals can't always be generalized to humans. A classic example of this is resveratrol, a chemical found in red grapes and wine that has been touted as a "fat-burning" supplement. One study that involved mice found positive benefits from resveratrol. But in order to get the same relative amount of resveratrol as the mice did in the study, two scientists estimated that a human would have to consume *about 333 glasses of red wine each day*.

Even if a study does involve humans, they may be much different than you. Boron is a nutritional supplement that's promoted for increasing muscular size and strength. The initial claims were triggered less than three months after the publication of a study showing that 12 subjects who received boron increased their testosterone. What the advertisements didn't mention was that these subjects were postmenopausal women, aged 48 to 82, whose testosterone was normally low. (Also not mentioned was the fact that prior to taking the nutritional supplements, the women had been deprived of an adequate intake of boron for 119 days.) Of course, this population may be considerably different than you or another individual who might be seduced by an advertisement for boron in a bodybuilding magazine.

4. Did the study find significant improvements?

A term that appears frequently in research studies is significant (or a derivative of the term such as significantly). In normal dialogue, significant means important; in statistical dialogue, significant means probably true. The term significant is used to describe the amount of change that was made by a group as well as the difference between two or more groups. When the amount of change is said to be significant, it means that it's probably true that the amount of change was the result of the treatments rather than pure chance; when the difference between two or more groups is said to be significant, it means that it's probably true that the difference was the result of the treatments rather than pure chance.

Consider, for example, a study in which subjects are randomly assigned to two different groups: One group receives a nutritional supplement and the other group receives a placebo. Both the nutritional supplement and placebo could produce a significant increase in some variable – such as size or strength – without there being a significant difference between the two substances. So the group that received the nutritional supplement might experience a greater amount of change than the group that received the placebo but the difference might not be large enough to conclude that the nutritional supplement is superior to the placebo. Rather, the difference may be due to pure chance.

5. Were the results of a study replicated by other researchers at other laboratories?

Oftentimes, a number of studies show impressive results about a nutritional supplement but are conducted by the same group of researchers. For there to be compelling evidence about the effectiveness of a nutritional supplement, similar results need to be found by different groups of researchers at different laboratories.

Similar results produced by different researchers also reduce the chance that the studies were biased toward a specific result. Otherwise, we're left to wonder, "Did the doctor 'doctor' the data?"

6. Was there a selective reporting of results from the study?

There's an old saying that if you torture the data long enough, you can make it confess to anything. This is often true when it comes to the marketing of nutritional supplements.

Advertisements for one nutritional supplement note that a study found increases in lean-body mass and maximum strength in the bench press. However, these results were selected from a handful of other findings. In the study, the researchers randomly assigned 36 men to three groups: One group received whey protein, another group received whey protein plus creatine monohydrate and the third group received a placebo. All groups used the same strength program. After six weeks, those who received whey protein plus creatine had significantly greater increases than the other groups in lean-body mass, maximum strength in the bench press and knee extension peak torque. But there were no significant differences between the groups in maximum strength in the squat and knee flexion peak torque.

7. Did the study find any adverse effects?

A study might show that a nutritional supplement lives up to the hype but it's important to know whether or not there are adverse effects. Sodium citrate is a nutritional supplement that's promoted for improving endurance. In a study, nine elite athletes ran 3,000 meters on two separate occasions, one after receiving sodium citrate and another after receiving sodium (table salt). The athletes ran the 3,000 meters significantly faster – by an average of about 10 seconds – after consuming sodium citrate than after consuming sodium. However, when using sodium citrate, eight of nine athletes experienced gastrointestinal distress.

Even if a study didn't find any adverse effects, the duration might have been too short; long-term studies are needed to assess safety. Remember, individuals might use a certain nutritional supplement for months or years, not days or weeks.

Also take into account that some studies don't investigate adverse effects. In other cases, adverse effects aren't reported.

Finally, individuals often take more than one nutritional supplement. Adverse effects can be produced when one nutritional supplement is combined with another.

8. Was the study funded and, if so, by whom?

Many scientific journals require researchers to disclose all sources of their funding and professional relationships with any company or organization that may benefit from favorable outcomes. And for good reason.

Studies on nutritional supplements are often funded or sponsored by manufacturers of those same nutritional supplements. When a manufacturer pays to have its own product investigated, it increases the possibility that the study could be biased in some way. Needless to say, studies that are funded by manufacturers that have a direct financial interest in the results should be viewed with suspicion.

There's strong evidence that the results of a study tend to favor the funder. An analysis of 206 studies found that studies with industry funding were about four to eight times more likely "to be favorable to the financial interests of the sponsoring company" than studies without industry funding. That's nothing: Another analysis of 398 studies found that researchers who had a conflict of interest were 10 to 20 times more likely to present favorable findings than those without a conflict of interest.

Therefore, you should try to determine if one or more researchers have any financial ties to the sponsor of the study. This includes being a paid employee or consultant, receiving honoraria, owning stocks and having a patent agreement. If there's a conflict of interest, you must decide whether it could have influenced (biased) the outcome of the study. (Note: Just because there's a conflict of interest doesn't mean that the study is biased.)

CONSUMER PROTECTION

Fortunately, consumers aren't alone in confronting nutritional quackery. The two main federal agencies that are tasked with protecting consumers are the Federal Trade Commission (FTC) and the Food and Drug Administration (FDA). Both organizations have been safeguarding the public for more than a century.

In 1903, the Bureau of Corporations was created by Congress. The bureau became the FTC in 1914 when President Woodrow Wilson signed the Federal Trade Commission Act into law. The primary duty of the FTC is to protect the public against unfair methods of competition (such as monopolies) but the agency is also sanctioned to move against false and deceptive advertising, mislabeling and misrepresentation of quality, guarantee and terms of sale.

In 1906, President Theodore Roosevelt signed the Pure Food and Drug Act into law which authorized the federal government to oversee the safety and quality of food. The responsibility for enforcing this act was given to the US Department of Agriculture and its Bureau of Chemistry. The bureau was renamed the Food, Drug and Insecticide Administration in 1927 and shortened to its present name in 1930. In 1938, the Federal Food, Drug and Cosmetic Act replaced the 1906 Pure Food and Drug Act. This new act was signed into law a little more than six months after Elixir Sulfanilamide, an untested "wonder drug," killed 107 people in 15 states. The act extended the range of commodities that came under federal control – to include cosmetics and medical devices – and increased penalties for violators. It also prohibited statements in food labeling that were false or misleading.

The Dietary Supplement Health and Education Act of 1994 amended the Federal Food, Drug and Cosmetic Act of 1938. This act – co-authored by Senator Orrin Hatch of Utah, a state that's home to many manufacturers of nutritional

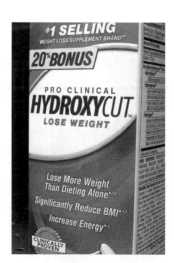

In 2009, the FDA questioned the safety of Hydroxycut after 23 cases of liver toxicity were reported in a seven-year period.

supplements – has had a drastic impact on the way that the FDA does business. Essentially, it shifted the role of the FDA from pre-market approver to post-market enforcer. Under this act, manufacturers can send a nutritional supplement directly to the market without submitting any proof about its safety or effectiveness to the FDA. Essentially, the FDA can take action against a nutritional supplement only after it's proven to be unsafe. The lone exception is when a nutritional supplement contains a "new dietary ingredient" (which is defined as one that wasn't marketed in the United States in a nutritional supplement prior to October 15, 1994 when the act became law).

Manufacturers of nutritional supplements are allowed to make specific claims of health benefits – referred to as structure/function claims – on the label of a product. However, a claim that's made on the label that a specific nutrient or ingredient has an effect on the structure or function of the body requires this disclaimer: "This statement has not been evaluated by the Food and Drug Administration. This product is not intended to diagnose, treat, cure or prevent any disease."

The FTC and FDA in Action

Besides protecting the public against nutritional quackery, the FTC and FDA have a myriad of other responsibilities as well as limited resources to review the vast amount of nutritional supplements that proliferates on the market. Nonetheless, the FTC and FDA have flexed their regulatory muscles for decades.

In 1927, the FTC filed its first weight-loss case against McGowan's Reducine, a cream that was said to "dissolve" excess fat and "slenderize" body parts. Since 1990, the FTC has been particularly active in investigating weight-loss products. In 2011, the agency settled charges against three individuals and two companies for making false and deceptive claims that their product, derived from the plant Hoodia gordonii (or, simply, Hoodia), would lead to weight loss and curb appetite.

In 2004, the FDA banned the sale of products that contained ephedra (aka ma huang) because research showed that it was associated with an increased risk of hypertension, stroke, heart palpitations and psychiatric symptoms. And in 2009, the FDA questioned the safety of Hydroxycut, a product that was touted as a weight-loss supplement, after 23 cases of liver toxicity were reported in a seven-year period. The FDA ordered the manufacturer to cease distribution and recall the product from the marketplace. (Note: The product has been reformulated and is back on store shelves.)

CAVEAT EMPTOR

Although the source of the quote is the subject of debate, a very bright person once said, "There's a sucker born every minute." Then the person added, "And two to take his money." Unfortunately, this is probably an underestimate on both counts.

Translated from Latin, caveat emptor means "Let (or may) the buyer beware." This advice certainly holds true for nutritional supplements. Don't fall prey to nutritional quackery.

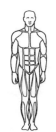

22 Weight Management

Weight management refers to gaining, losing or maintaining bodyweight. Managing your weight boils down to the mathematical interplay of two variables: caloric consumption and caloric expenditure. If you consume (eat) more calories than you expend (use), you'll gain weight. If you expend (use) more calories than you consume (eat), you'll lose weight. And if you consume (eat) the same number of calories as you expend (use), you'll maintain the same weight. The dynamics of weight management can be summarized below.

weight gain: calories in > calories out

weight loss: calories in < calories out

weight maintenance: calories in = calories out

A CLOSER LOOK

While the end result of caloric consumption and caloric expenditure boils down to simple arithmetic, there's a right way and a wrong way to manage your weight. Here's a closer look at the proper approach to weight management, especially as it pertains to gaining and losing weight.

Gaining Weight

Some people will look, feel and perform better if they gained weight. Technically, the main goal of weight gain isn't merely to gain weight; rather, it's to gain muscle.

A mistake that's often made is gaining weight too quickly. There's a limit as to how much muscle an individual can gain in a given amount of time. And it's not as much as many people think.

In order to gain weight, a caloric surplus must be produced. The daily caloric surplus shouldn't be more than about 350 calories above the amount that's necessary for weight maintenance. If the weight gain is more than about 0.5% (one-

half percent) of your bodyweight per week, it's likely that at least some of the increase was in the form of fat, not muscle. In practical terms, this means that the weight gain shouldn't exceed about one pound per week. For most people, an increase of about one-half pound per week is probably more realistic. If the weight gain isn't too great and the result of a demanding fitness program in conjunction with a moderate increase in caloric consumption, then it will probably be in the form of increased muscle.

One pound of muscle has about 2,500 calories. Therefore, if you consume 250 calories per day (cal/day) above the amount that you need to maintain your weight – a 250-calorie surplus – it will take you 10 days to gain one pound of muscle [2,500 cal ÷ 250 cal/day]. So if a 200-pound man who's very active requires 5,200 cal/day to maintain his bodyweight [200 lb x 26 cal/lb], he must consume 5,450 cal/day – 250 calories above his need – to gain one pound of muscle in 10 days. This estimate must be recalculated on a regular basis to account for changes in bodyweight. After increasing his bodyweight to 201 pounds, for example, he'll now require 5,226 cal/day to meet his energy needs [201 lb x 26 cal/lb]. In order to gain another pound of muscle in 10 days, he must increase his caloric consumption to 5,476 cal/day – 250 calories above his need.

Specific Tips

There are many tactics that you can employ to gain weight. What follows are 10 tips for gaining weight in a manner that's safe, practical and effective.

1. Eat at least three meals per day.

In order to gain weight, you need to consume more calories. It's that simple. To get enough calories, you'll need to eat at least three meals per day on a regular basis.

Your body doesn't absorb one or two large meals very well; most of these calories are jammed through your digestive system. As a matter of fact, if you consume a large number of calories at one time, the sudden and severe rush of food will wreak havoc on the digestive process and cause some of those calories to be stored as fat. A better approach, then, is to spread the calories over three or more regular-sized meals.

2. Eat at least three nutritious snacks per day.

Besides getting at least three meals per day, you'll need to get at least three snacks per day. But it shouldn't be any kind of snacks just for the sake of getting more calories; the snacks should have some nutritional value. Examples are low-fat yogurt, whole-grain crackers and certain energy/snack bars.

If you have a hectic or an unpredictable schedule, you'll probably find this tough to accomplish without good planning. For instance, you can pre-package nutritious snacks that you could eat at work or school.

Note: Consuming three meals intermingled with three snacks essentially amounts to eating every three hours or so.

3. Consume foods that are high in calories (but not too high in fat).

You can "get more bang for your buck" by choosing foods with a high caloric density. These

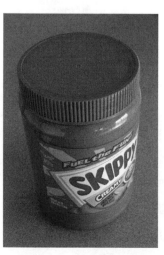

To gain weight, you can "get more bang for your buck" by choosing foods with a high caloric density.

foods have a relatively large number of calories in small portions. A bagel with peanut butter, a peanut butter and jelly sandwich and nuts (such as almonds, peanuts and walnuts) are good examples of calorie-dense foods.

4. Eat calorie-dense fruits and vegetables.

Not to belabor a point but to gain weight, you need to consume more calories. This means eating calorie-dense fruits (such as bananas, pineapples and raisins) and vegetables (such as peas, corn and carrots). An added bonus is that fruits and vegetables are rich sources of vitamins and minerals.

5. Drink calorie-dense beverages.

A great way to gain weight is by drinking calorie-dense beverages such as low-fat milk and fruit juice. These beverages contain more calories – and more nutrients – than water or unsweetened beverages.

6. Eat a healthy breakfast.

If you're the type of person who frequently skips meals, then it will be all the more difficult for you to get the amount of calories that you need to gain weight. Perhaps no other meal is skipped more than breakfast. Pass on breakfast and you'll spend a good part of the day trying to compensate for the hundreds of calories that you didn't get earlier.

7. Increase the size of your portions.

One of the easiest and most effective ways to get more calories is to increase the size of your portions. Naturally, this assumes that you're already eating a balanced inventory of foods and not merely cramming calories down your digestive tract just for the sake of getting more calories.

Increasing portion sizes is fairly easy to do: You can simply use a larger plate for your food and a larger glass/cup for your beverage.

8. Make a dedicated effort.

Gaining weight requires total dedication for seven days each week. Additional calories must be consumed on a regular basis until you achieve the desired increase in weight. You won't gain weight by making a half-hearted attempt or applying these tips every now and then.

9. Do strength training on a regular basis.

Most people who try to gain weight also engage in a strength program. However, some people overemphasize the muscles of their torso and arms and underemphasize the muscles of their hips and legs (or they ignore these muscles altogether). Neglecting your hips and legs means that an enormous amount of muscle mass isn't receiving any stimulus for growth.

10. Get adequate recovery.

Doing any type of physical training with a high level of intensity requires an adequate amount of recovery. This has even greater importance when trying to gain weight.

Make sure that you get enough recovery between your workouts. And make sure that you get enough sleep, preferably around eight hours each night.

Losing Weight

Some people will look, feel and perform better if they lost weight. Technically, the main goal of weight loss isn't merely to lose weight; rather, it's to lose fat.

A mistake that's often made is losing weight too quickly. There's a limit as to how much fat an individual can lose in a given amount of time.

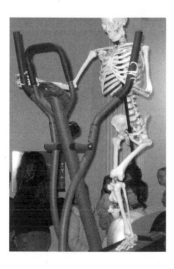

When losing weight too quickly, a significant amount of the loss can be in the form of muscle.

And similar to gaining weight, it's not as much as many people think.

In order to lose weight, a caloric deficit must be produced. The daily caloric deficit shouldn't be more than about 1,000 calories below the amount that's necessary for weight maintenance. If the weight loss is more than about 1% of your bodyweight per week, it's likely that at least some of the decrease was in the form of water and/or muscle, not fat. In practical terms, this means that the weight loss shouldn't exceed about two pounds per week. For most people, a decrease of about one pound per week is probably more realistic. If the weight loss isn't too great and the result of a demanding fitness program in conjunction with a moderate decrease in caloric consumption, then it will probably be in the form of decreased fat.

One pound of fat has about 3,500 calories. Therefore, if you consume 250 cal/day below the amount that you need to maintain your weight – a 250-calorie deficit – it will take you 14 days to lose one pound of fat [3,500 cal ÷ 250 cal/day]. So if a 200-pound man who's very active requires 5,200 cal/day to maintain his bodyweight, he must consume 4,950 cal/day – 250 calories below his need – to lose one pound of fat in 14 days. Remember, this estimate must be recalculated on a regular basis to account for changes in bodyweight. After decreasing his bodyweight to 199 pounds, for example, he'll now require 5,174 cal/day to meet his energy needs [199 lb x 26 cal/lb]. In order to lose another pound of fat in 14 days, he must decrease his caloric consumption to 4,924 cal/day – 250 calories below his need.

Actually, there are three ways to lose weight: You can (1) decrease the number of calories that you consume and maintain the same amount of activity that you do; (2) maintain the same number of calories that you consume and increase the amount of activity that you do; or (3) decrease the number of calories that you consume and increase the amount of activity that you do.

The third way – eating less and exercising more – is the preferred way. Why? Well, suppose that your goal is to lose 10 pounds of fat in 10 weeks. This represents a rate of one pound of fat per week. Since one pound of fat has 3,500 calories, you'd need to come up with a deficit of 500 calories per day. Eating 500 less calories per day can be quite a challenge; the same can be said about using 500 more calories per day. And don't forget, this 500-calorie deficit would need to be achieved every day for 70 consecutive days.

The best way, then, is to do a combination of the two: Eat a little less and exercise a little more. And it doesn't have to be a 50-50 split. In this example, you could achieve a deficit of 500 calories by eating 200 less calories and using 300 more calories. Same result but less overwhelming. Or, perhaps a 250-calorie deficit is more realistic for you than a 500-calorie deficit.

Several problems are associated with losing weight too quickly. For one thing, a significant amount of the weight loss can be in the form of muscle. Consider a 200-pound man with 20.00% fat. This means that he has 40 pounds of fat [200 lb x 0.20] and 160 pounds of fat-free (lean-body) mass. If he lost 10 pounds, he'd weigh 190 pounds. But if it was done too quickly, it's possible that only one pound of the weight loss was from fat. In this case, he'd have 39 pounds of fat and 151 pounds of fat-free mass . . . meaning that he's now *20.53% fat*. So, he lost weight but his percentage of body fat actually increased. A loss of muscle isn't desirable since muscle is functional tissue: Muscle produces movement of your bones which enables you to perform mechanical work (physical activity).

In addition, muscle is a metabolically active tissue. Having less muscle decreases your metabolic rate (the rate at which you use calories). In other words, you'll be less efficient at "burning" calories which will make it more difficult for you to lose weight. Remember, you want to lose *fat weight*, not *muscle weight*.

And when you lose weight too quickly, it's often temporary as your body can't sustain such extreme changes. It's not unusual for people to regain much of the weight that they lost. Look at it this way: If you're 10 pounds overweight, you probably didn't get that way in a week. So, you

shouldn't expect to lose 10 pounds in a week, either.

Final point: In general, it's rarely a good idea to pursue a "quick fix." In order to realize long-term success, you must install changes in your lifestyle. By losing weight too quickly, you won't change any bad habits. At best, you'll only experience short-term results.

It's worth mentioning that the numbers on bathroom scales and height/weight charts are poor indicators of whether or not someone should lose weight. The need for weight loss should be determined by *body composition*, not *bodyweight*. This is especially true for active individuals. For the most part, active individuals tend to be larger and have more lean-body (muscle) mass than the general population. Think about it: Two people could be same height and weight but have markedly different body compositions. For example, one might have 15% body fat and the other 30% body fat. If this was the case, then only one person might need to lose weight: the one with the higher percentage of body fat.

A variety of methods can be used to measure body composition such as air displacement plethysmography, bioelectrical impedance analysis, computerized tomography, dual energy x-ray absorptiometry, hydrostatic (underwater) weighing and near infrared reactance. But perhaps the most popular method of measuring body composition is to use skinfold calipers. In general, this is considered to be the most practical and least expensive method of assessment without sacrificing much in the way of accuracy (assuming that the person who takes the measurements is reasonably skilled and the equation that's used is valid).

Note: In most sports, a low percentage of body fat is desirable; in some sports, however, a high percentage of body fat is actually advantageous. For instance, long-distance swimmers obtain increased buoyancy and thermal insulation from higher levels of body fat.

Specific Tips

There are many tactics that you can employ to lose weight. What follows are 20 tips for losing

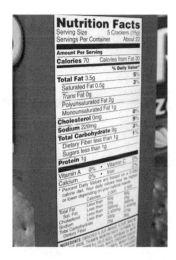

With respect to weight loss, pay particular attention to the serving size, servings per container, total calories, calories from fat and total fat.

weight in a manner that's safe, effective and practical.

1. Read food labels.

Whenever you purchase food in a supermarket or convenience store, examine the food label. Based on federal law, food labeling is required for most packaged foods including breads, cereals, canned/frozen foods, snacks, desserts and beverages.

An important part of the food label is the Nutrition Facts panel. With respect to weight loss, pay particular attention to the serving size, servings per container, total calories, calories from fat and total fat.

Also be wary of the fine print. For example, a container of food that has 100 calories per serving means that the container has 100 calories if – and only if – it has one serving. If a container of food has 100 calories per serving but has four servings per container, eating the entire contents will give you 400 calories.

2. Become more knowledgeable.

Most full-service and fast-food (aka quick-service) restaurants don't readily disclose the nutritional information of their foods . . . and for good reason. An Extra Value Meal at McDonald's® that consists of a Quarter Pounder® with cheese, small fries and 16-ounce soda has 890 calories with 37 grams of fat. "Supersize" to medium fries and 21-ounce soda and the meal balloons to 1,100 calories with 45 grams of fat. Get a McFlurry® with M&M's®

and wash it down with a refill of soda and this adds another 790 calories and 23 grams of fat to your tab. The grand total for this meal is a staggering 1,950 calories of which 68 grams are from fat, meaning that it's about 31.4% fat. For many people, that's about a day's worth of calories and fat . . . all in one meal.

Value meals are tempting but understand that the "value" is *economical*, not *nutritional*. Although you get a lot of food for your money, it's usually a lot of bad food for your money: more calories and more fat.

Needless to say, the gory nutritional details aren't made too obvious at the majority of full-service and fast-food restaurants. More knowledge is only a few clicks away, though, since most of these establishments have websites that list their nutritional information.

3. Eat more frequently.

The notion that eating more meals can help you lose weight seems counterintuitive. Indeed, how is it possible to eat more and weigh less? Well, the number of meals should be higher but the size of those meals – in terms of calories – should be smaller. In spreading calories over more meals – rather than cramming calories into less meals – you're better able to keep your hunger at bay.

In one study, subjects ate all of their calories in either three meals per day for eight weeks or two meals per day for two weeks and one meal per day for six weeks. After an 11-week washout period, the subjects were switched to the other diet for eight weeks. The researchers found that eating three meals per day produced lower ratings of hunger and higher ratings of satiety (fullness) compared to eating one meal per day. And as time went on, those ratings became more pronounced.

One of the worst things that you can do is skip a meal. In this case, you'll be ravenous and the next time that you have a meal, you'll probably satisfy your appetite by eating anything that doesn't move.

4. Decrease the size of your portions.

If you're already eating a balanced array of foods, a highly effective tactic for weight loss is to reduce the size of your portions. Decreasing portion sizes is fairly easy to do: You can simply use a smaller plate for your food and a smaller glass/cup for your beverage. Essentially, doing this helps you to limit the size of your portions and, as a result, lower the number of calories that you consume. And it certainly makes sense that if you decide to eat an entire bowl of potato chips, for example, a smaller bowl would yield fewer calories than a larger bowl.

In one classic study, 85 people were invited to attend an ice cream social. Unbeknownst to the individuals, they were randomly given either a small (17 ounces) or large (34 ounces) bowl as well as either a small (two ounces) or large (three ounces) spoon with which they scooped their serving. Those who used a larger spoon and a larger bowl consumed 56.8% more ice cream than those who used a smaller spoon and a smaller bowl. Perhaps even more startling is the fact that the participants in this study were faculty, graduate students and staff members of a nutrition and food science department at the University of Illinois.

Along these lines, here's something else that's interesting: People tend to pour more fluids into short, wide glasses than tall, narrow ones. For instance, researchers discovered that 86 experienced bartenders in Philadelphia unknowingly poured 20.5% more alcohol into short tumblers than tall "highball" glasses of the same volume.

You can use larger plates, bowls and glasses/cups to your advantage. With these items, you can give yourself bigger servings of healthier foods such as fruits and vegetables.

5. Sit away from the serving area.

When you sit near a serving area – whether it's at home or a buffet-style restaurant – the food is readily available and easily accessible, tempting you to eat more than you should. It doesn't require much effort to reach across the table or get up and take a few steps to grab second – or third – helpings. And don't forget something else

about sitting away from food: Out of sight, out of mind, out of mouth.

6. Avoid doing activities while eating.

Certain activities are associated with eating. This includes watching television, playing a board game and reading a book. When engaged in such activities, people focus on what they're doing rather than what they're eating. Therefore, it's a good idea to refrain from eating while doing these and other activities.

If you do get caught in these or other situations, use your non-dominant hand to pick up food. It sounds strange but the added effort makes it less likely that you'll overeat.

7. Confine eating to a designated area.

People tend to eat more when they're distracted. And as just mentioned, eating is triggered by some activities such as watching television. A great way to keep you from doing this is to restrict your eating to a designated place or room (and not in front of something with a screen).

8. Chew your food slowly.

At first glance, this tip might seem odd. If you chew your food slowly, however, you're less likely to mindlessly inhale it as if you're the defending champion in an eating contest.

In one study, subjects were given a plate of food and told to eat as much as they wanted. When they ate quickly, they consumed 646 calories in 8.6 minutes or about 75.1 calories per minute; when they chewed their food slowly, they consumed 579 calories in 29.2 minutes or about 19.8 calories per minute. Besides eating fewer calories when they chewed their food slowly, the subjects reported greater feelings of satiety and lower feelings of hunger. And they enjoyed the meal more.

The fact of the matter is that by chewing your food slowly, your brain is given adequate time to receive a signal from your stomach that it's full. In addition, taking the time to chew your food facilitates the digestive process.

To help you slow down, you can place your fork or spoon on the table between bites. So, pay attention to the food that you eat and take the time to really savor the flavor.

9. Start your meals with soup and/or salad.

This is a very simple and easy tactic for you to implement. Because they're comprised mostly of water, soups and salads provide you with relatively few calories but give you a feeling of satiety. If you lead off with soup and/or a salad, then, you're less likely to consume as many calories during the remainder of your meal.

Key point: Broth-based soups usually have fewer calories (and less fat) than cream-based ones. And even though they're both salads, a garden salad usually has fewer calories (and less fat) than a Caesar salad.

10. Eat foods that are low in fat.

A food that's high in fat is loaded with calories. Packed with nine calories per gram, fats are more than twice as dense as carbohydrates and protein which have four calories per gram. Or look at it this way: A food that's high in fat has more calories for the same weight than a food that's low in fat.

In particular, you should reduce your intake of saturated fats (found in red meats, certain oils, high-fat dairy products and many processed foods) and trans fats (found in shortenings, stick margarine, cookies, crackers, snack foods, fried foods, doughnuts, pastries, baked goods and other processed foods). Limiting your consumption of fat dramatically decreases the number of calories that you eat. Plus, your food choices are much healthier.

This isn't to say that you should eliminate fat completely; fat does perform several functions that are vital to your health. In the context of losing weight, however, you must reduce your intake of calorie-dense foods.

Studies have shown that people tend to eat about the same weight of food each day; not the same calories of food, the *same weight of food*. So choosing foods with a low caloric density – those

that have the smallest number of calories in the largest portions – means that you'll consume fewer calories without sacrificing satiety.

Consider, for example, grapes and raisins. Essentially, raisins are dried grapes. In terms of weight and volume, 100 calories of grapes are more food – and more filling – than 100 calories of raisins.

11. Eat more fruits and vegetables.

Foods (and beverages) that offer very few calories along with a feeling of satiety are great choices for those who are trying to lose weight. Fruits and vegetables meet these criteria because they contain exceptionally high amounts of water.

Moreover, fruits and vegetables have an extra benefit: They're jam-packed with vitamins and minerals. Truly, nothing on the planet comes closer to being a magical food than fruits and vegetables.

Yet, many people struggle with getting enough fruits and vegetables. An effective way to meet this challenge is to keep fruits and vegetables on hand and available. Then, you can incorporate different tactics to increase your intake. For example, you can eat apples as snacks. You can add carrots to soup. Or, you can put sliced tomatoes and/or lettuce on sandwiches. In short, use your imagination.

And while on the subject, it's important for you to consume a variety of fruits and vegetables. Since fruits and vegetables come in such a wide range of colors, just follow this simple directive to ensure variety: Eat a rainbow.

12. Get more fiber.

Fiber is a type of carbohydrate that can't be digested. Foods that are high in fiber tend to have fewer calories, an obvious advantage for weight loss. Also, fiber slows the rate at which food passes through your digestive system thereby increasing satiety. You can boost your intake of fiber by eating fruits, vegetables and whole-grain products (such as breads and cereals).

13. Eat spicy foods.

Spicy foods can increase your metabolic rate by raising your body temperature. The greatest increase in body temperature is triggered by capsaicin, an ingredient that's found in chili peppers; it's what makes hot peppers hot.

The effect of capsaicin on metabolic rate is temporary and small. Keep in mind, too, that eating *any* food will increase your metabolic rate. The reason is that the body uses calories to digest, absorb and transport food. This thermic effect of food is roughly 10% of your caloric intake.

However, the real benefit is the fact that eating spicy foods seems to curb appetite. Research indicates that spicy foods produce an increase in satiety and a decrease in caloric intake.

A few words of caution: Some individuals may experience gastrointestinal distress from spicy foods. Therefore, spicy foods should be avoided by anyone who suffers from ulcers and chronic heartburn.

14. Decrease your intake of sweetened beverages.

Included among sweetened beverages are non-diet soda, fruit drinks, lemonade and iced tea. Essentially, sweetened beverages are liquid sugar. The problem here is twofold: Sweetened beverages provide a significant amount of calories and no nutritional value whatsoever. Also, numerous studies have found a strong association between the intake of sweetened beverages and obesity.

The average non-diet soda has about 100 calories per eight ounces. Drinking one 12-ounce can of soda on a daily basis translates into about 54,750 calories in a year . . . or *about 15.6 pounds.*

15. Drink more water.

It's a wise move for you to drink plenty of water before, during and after meals. Remember, water has weight but no calories. Therefore, drinking water creates a feeling of satiety without adding anything to your caloric budget.

Here's something of interest: In one study, subjects ate the same food for lunch but drank a different type of beverage (either regular cola, diet cola or water). Regardless of the beverage, the subjects ate the same number of calories. So, the calories from the beverage were added to the calories from the meal. This means that when water was the beverage that accompanied the meal, fewer calories were consumed.

16. Choose healthy snacks.

There's nothing inherently wrong with snacking. It becomes problematic, however, when poor choices are made. As a rule of thumb, unhealthy snacks are those that are high in calories and fat (as well as sodium and sugar) and low in nutrients.

But a food that's loaded with calories and fat without much in the way of nutrients – such as cookies, cake and ice cream – isn't necessarily bad as long as it's consumed in moderation. In other words, something like ice cream is generally okay provided that it's not eaten in large quantities and/or on a habitual basis.

Healthy snacks include fruit, raw vegetables, low-fat yogurt, popcorn (sans butter), whole-grain crackers, pretzels, cereal and certain energy/snack bars.

Note: A number of energy/snack bars are little more than glorified – and expensive – candy bars. To tell, check the facts panel on the wrapper. Remember, the ingredients are listed by weight from highest to lowest. If the first few ingredients include sugar in one or more of its many forms – usually words that end in "ose" – it's basically a

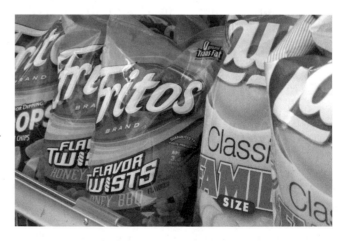

Unhealthy snacks are those that are high in calories and fat (as well as sodium and sugar) and low in nutrients.

candy bar. A healthy energy/snack bar should be low in calories and fat (and sugar) and have some nutritional value.

17. Minimize unhealthy foods in your home.

Unhealthy foods include those that are high in calories, fat and sugar and low in nutrients. When there are little or no healthy options in your home, it's virtually impossible for you to make healthy choices. To add to an earlier point: Out of house, out of sight, out of mind, out of mouth.

18. Restrict the number of meals that you eat in fast-food restaurants.

It's estimated that each day, one out of every four Americans eats fast food. Currently, there are nearly 200,000 fast-food restaurants in the United States. Sales at fast-food restaurants were projected to reach nearly 167.7 billion dollars in 2011 (compared to 194.6 billion dollars at full-service restaurants).

Fast food is inexpensive, convenient and fast. But for the most part, it's not very healthy or nutritious. Fast food tends to be high in calories and fat (and sodium). Research has shown that on the days that people eat fast food, they tend to consume more calories and fat than on other days.

19. Make activities less sedentary and more physical.

Studies have reported that an increase of sedentary activities and a decrease of physical activities are contributing factors to the steady rise of obesity. Obviously, you should do less sedentary activities and more physical activities. But whenever possible, sedentary activities should be made more physical. For example, use the steps, not the elevator; at a mall or work, park farther from the building, not closer.

20. Do strength training and aerobic training.

Like all types of physical training, strength training and aerobic training use calories. Strength training is unique, though, in that it can decrease fat and increase muscle thereby improving body composition and enhancing

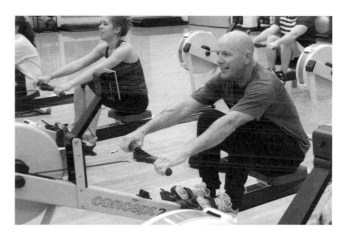

Aerobic training is important since it can produce a sustained and significant use of calories. (Photo provided by Greg Hammond.)

appearance. Muscle tissue is more metabolically active than fat tissue, meaning that it requires more calories to function. As a result, those with more muscle are more efficient at using calories. (Each pound of muscle that you gain will increase your caloric expenditure by about 10 more calories per day.) Aerobic training is also important since it can produce a sustained and significant use of calories.

Gaining and Losing Weight: General Tips

There are several tactics that you can employ to gain or lose weight. What follows are three general tips for gaining or losing weight in a manner that's safe, effective and practical.

1. Set SMART goals.

Many individuals who try to manage their weight aren't very successful. One of the main reasons why this happens is that they don't set any goals. Effective goals are SMART: Specific, Measurable, Attainable, Realistic and Timed.

Specific: One of the main reasons why people fail to achieve their goals is because they're not specific. The truth is that those who have specific goals in mind are more likely to reach them. A general goal is to get fit; this is abstract and has numerous interpretations. A specific goal is to increase the number of repetitions that you do in the leg press in your next workout; this is concrete and has one clear objective.

Measurable: If a goal can't be measured, it can't be managed. And if a goal can't be measured, it can't be assessed. Indeed, how do you know if you've achieved a goal if there's no way to measure it? So rather than have an ambiguous goal to exercise more, a measurable goal is to do strength training an average of two days per week; rather than have an ambiguous goal to eat more vegetables, a measurable goal is to consume three servings of vegetables per day. Goals that can be measured are more likely to be met.

Attainable: Although some people have goals that are specific and measurable, they're often far too difficult to achieve. A goal of losing 50 pounds of fat in three months, for example, can't be attained. An attainable goal is to lose one pound of fat per week for the next two months. Remember, too, that a successful outcome is more likely when a goal is within reach.

Realistic: Having realistic goals is closely related to having attainable goals. Don't set your sights on running a six-minute mile if the last time that you did so was 10 years and 20 pounds ago. Don't think about trimming your mid-section by a few inches if you get your three daily servings of fruit from a blueberry muffin, an apple pie and a banana split. In making realistic goals, it's important to be honest with yourself. Take into consideration things like your age, situation and motivation.

Timed: This means that you should put a time requirement on achieving your goal. A goal to gain five pounds of muscle has good intentions but when is it supposed to be attained? In two months? Six months? Whenever? The point is that it's easy to put off goals unless a deadline is attached. The deadline could be weeks or months or a specific date. For instance, a timed goal might be to gain 10 pounds of muscle by June 30. Or it might be to run a 5K by your 40th birthday.

2. Keep a food/activity diary.

Another important tactic for weight management is to keep a food/activity diary. Chronicling your efforts helps you to stay focused on your goals and progress (or lack thereof).

Essentially, using a food/activity diary holds you accountable to yourself.

One study found that people who used a food/activity diary for at least six days per week lost about twice as much weight in six months as those who didn't use such a diary. There's no reason to think that this wouldn't also work for those who are interested in gaining weight.

You should record the specific foods that you eat as well as a rough idea of the quantity. By documenting this information, you may discover that you actually eat a different amount of food – either less or more – than you thought. You should track good choices (such as the servings of fruits and unsweetened beverages) and bad ones (such as the number of cookies and sweetened beverages). Although calories count, there's no need to literally count calories. You do need to be mindful of calories, however, without it being obsessive.

Since engaging in a fitness program is also an integral aspect of weight management, it's a good idea to maintain a record of your activities as well. Note the types of activities that you do along with the duration of the activities and, if applicable, the distances that you complete. Participation in formal activities (such as strength training and aerobic training), informal activities (such as walking, skiing and playing "pick-up games") and organized sports should be included.

3. Implement a few changes at a time.

There are countless changes that you can employ to manage your weight. Although they have the best intentions, many people are often unsuccessful in their attempts for two reasons: One is trying to make major changes; another is trying to make too many changes.

Dr. James Hill, the Director of the Center for Human Nutrition at the University of Colorado Denver, is an advocate of what's known as the small-changes approach. He and his colleagues have calculated that 90% of the population gets a surplus of up to 50 calories per day which, of course, results in an increase in weight. Because of the metabolic costs that are associated with storing fat, 50 calories result from an excess of about 100 calories. Stated differently, reducing either caloric intake or caloric output by about 100 calories each day is enough to prevent an increase in weight in 9 out of 10 individuals.

Dr. Brian Wansink, the Director of the Cornell University Food and Brand Lab, has a similar perspective. He recommends that you limit yourself initially to three small, easy, doable changes that you can make without much sacrifice. Once these three changes become "mindless," you can add more.

The effectiveness of a small-changes approach has been demonstrated in a number of studies and is endorsed by many organizations. This includes the Academy of Nutrition and Dietetics (nee the American Dietetic Association), the American Heart Association and the American Cancer Society.

The fact of the matter is that making a few changes at a time that are small, easy and doable increases the likelihood that those changes will become habits. And that's what you need to do: Get to the point where a change becomes a habit. Clearly, small changes can lead to big results.

THE RIGHT "WEIGH"

Far more people need to lose weight than to gain weight. Statistically, it's estimated that 68% of Americans over the age of 20 are either overweight or obese; that's roughly two out of three people.

In an attempt to lose weight, many individuals resort to unhealthy and/or unsafe practices. This includes fasting and excessive exercise as well as the use of laxatives, weight-loss supplements and diet pills.

Many individuals also try fad diets. The list of fad diets seems endless, literally running from A (Atkins) to Z (Zone).

As the name suggests, fad diets are those that are trendy for a while and then fade away only to resurface at some point in the future (sometimes with a new name). Fad diets have at least four things in common. All fad diets (1) promise quick results (specifically, a rapid loss of weight); (2) offer short-term fixes, not long-term results; (3) fail to teach people the right way to eat; and (4) restrict one or more food groups or macronutrients.

Actually, there's one more thing that all fad diets have in common: Fad diets don't work. Weight loss can be achieved in a manner that's safe, practical and effective by following the approach as outlined in this chapter.

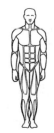

23 A Primer on Steroids

Strength training is done to increase muscular size and strength. Steroids are used as a means to accelerate these increases. As a result, strength training and steroids are inexorably linked. Therefore, any detailed discussion of strength training should include information about steroids.

A BRIEF HISTORY

In some regards, the history of steroids began thousands of years ago with the belief that certain organs and their glandular secretions had medicinal qualities. The ancient Greeks and Romans, for example, thought that the testicles had healing powers.

Scientific investigations of glandular extracts – which come from the hormone-producing glands of animals – can be traced back to the late 19th century. In June 1889, at a meeting of the Paris Biological Society, a French physician and physiologist named Charles-Edouard Brown-Sequard, then 72, announced that he had given himself 10 injections with a liquid that included a small amount of water mixed with testicular blood, seminal fluid and "juice" that was extracted from the crushed testicles of either a dog (the first five injections) or a number of guinea pigs (the second five injections). Brown-Sequard claimed that the injections, given over a three-week period, improved his strength and "intellectual labour" (and also relieved his constipation and lengthened "the jet" of his urine). Although these changes were almost certainly the result of a placebo effect, he was the first scientist to associate glandular products with physical strength.

In the late 1890s, two scientists from what was then Austria-Hungary – Oskar Zoth, a physiologist, and Fritz Pregl, a chemist and physician – injected themselves with a liquid extract of bull's testicles and concluded that it boosted the strength of their fingers. Actually, it was their middle fingers. Dr. Zoth suggested giving these injections to athletes as a way to test its effects.

The Emergence and Use of Testosterone

In 1935, within the span of about three months, three independent groups of scientists made significant contributions to the research and development of steroids. Each group was funded by a different pharmaceutical company: Organon (the Netherlands), Schering (Germany) and Ciba (Switzerland). In May, the Organon researchers isolated five milligrams of testosterone from nearly one ton of bull's testicles (and, in the process, coined the name testosterone from the words testicle, sterol and ketone). In August, the Schering researchers synthesized testosterone from cholesterol. And exactly one week later, the Ciba researchers did the same (and applied for a patent on their method).

It has been widely rumored that testosterone was given to some German athletes to prepare for the 1936 Berlin Olympics in which Germany garnered 89 medals including 33 gold, far more than any other country. (The United States was a distant second with 56 medals including 24 gold.) This was an enormous improvement for Germany in comparison to the 1932 Los Angeles Olympics where the country was ninth in the medal standings with 20 including 3 gold. (That year, the United States led the way with 103 medals including 41 gold.) Another popular rumor was that steroids were given to Nazi Schutzstaffel (SS) Troops during World War II to make them more aggressive and less fearful of violence. Even Hitler was said to have received injections of testosterone. However, none of these three reports has ever been verified. (The rumors may be attributed to the fact that much of the early research on testosterone was conducted in Germany.)

In the late 1930s, testosterone was available for purchase in the United States in drugstores without a prescription. By the early 1940s, researchers started to investigate the effects of testosterone on muscular growth. It was only natural that there was a rising interest in testosterone as a performance enhancer. In fact, the first documented case of testosterone being used to increase athletic performance was in 1941 . . . with a racehorse named Holloway. After being implanted with testosterone pellets, the horse improved its performance such that it won or placed in several races.

By the late 1940s, testosterone had muscled its way into the bodybuilding community on the west coast. From there, testosterone and its derivatives – collectively referred to as steroids – quickly infiltrated the athletic community.

As early as the 1950s, athletes of the Eastern Bloc countries were administered steroids – or steroid-like drugs – as part of a government-sponsored program. The first reported use among athletes was by the Soviet weightlifters at the 1954 World Weightlifting Championships in Vienna, Austria (where the Soviet Union and United States tied for first place, by the way, each winning seven medals). There, supposedly over "a few drinks," US team physician John Ziegler was told by the Soviet team physician that his country's weightlifters were using testosterone. In a "patriotic" response to the drug-inspired success of the Soviet athletes, Dr. Ziegler developed methandrostenolone (trade name: Dianabol) with Ciba Pharmaceutical Company . . . a move he would later regret. The steroid was given to competitive weightlifters at the legendary York Barbell Club in York, Pennsylvania, who ate the pink pills "like candy." (Note: From around 1930 to the mid-1970s, the York Barbell Club – previously known as the York Oil Burner Athletic Club – was a national power in weightlifting. As a result, the town of York was considered the Mecca of competitive weightlifting in America and nicknamed Muscletown USA. The United States,

in fact, was one of the top two or three teams in the world from the mid-1930s to the late 1950s, with many of its weightlifters coming from the York Barbell Club.)

Up until 1960, steroids were mostly used by American and Soviet weightlifters. But the rampant use of steroids – along with a new generation of growth-stimulating drugs and so-called designer steroids – has been escalating ever since.

State Plan Research Theme 14.25

In 1949, after the end of World War II, Germany was split into two countries: East Germany (the German Democratic Republic, controlled by the Soviet Union) and West Germany (the Federal Republic of Germany, allied with the United States, the United Kingdom and France). To physically separate the two countries, the Berlin Wall was built in 1961, first as a barbed-wire fence and later as a concrete barrier.

East Germany debuted at the 1968 Mexico City Olympics where the country finished fifth in the medal standings with 25 including 9 gold. In the 1972 Munich Olympics, the country improved to third in the medal standings with 66 including 20 gold. In the next three Olympics – not counting the 1984 Los Angeles Olympics which were boycotted by the Eastern Bloc countries – East Germany finished second in the medal standings each time, collecting a total of 336 including 124 gold. These were stunning accomplishments, especially considering that East Germany was roughly the size of Virginia with a population of about 17 million.

Germany remained divided – literally and figuratively – until the fall of the Berlin Wall in November 1989. Following the reunification of Germany a year later, information began to leak that would ultimately reveal the most extensive and egregious use of steroids in history. It was discovered that from 1966 to 1991, an estimated 10,000 East German athletes or more were given steroids – some of whom were 14 or younger – as part of a supervised, systematic and government-sponsored program. Code-named State Plan Research Theme 14.25, the clandestine program was controlled by the much-feared Ministry for State Security (aka the Stasi or secret police) and involved hundreds of physicians, scientists and professors. Essentially, the athletes were experimented on like guinea pigs, being told that the blue pills they received were vitamins and the injections were necessary medications. (Many of the athletes suffered long-term damage including liver disease, heart disease and cancer.)

The revelation that East German athletes had used steroids came as little surprise to most people. Suspicions had been aroused for years because of their sudden success and dominant performances accompanied by numerous accounts of East German women who sported deep voices and facial hair. One of the more memorable anecdotes occurred at the 1976 Montreal Olympics. Legend has it that Kathy Heddy, a US swimmer, ran up to her coach, Jack Nelson, and informed him that there were men in the women's locker room. Coach Nelson famously responded, "No, dear, those are the East Germans."

PREVALENCE OF STEROID USE

Up to around 1980, steroids were mainly used by athletes to improve their performance. At that point in time, many underground handbooks and guides on steroids began to surface which spawned greater use by non-athletes. Since then, the vast majority of individuals who use steroids do so to improve their *appearance*, not their *performance*. In a survey of 500 steroid users, 78.4% (392 of 500) were non-competitive bodybuilders and non-athletes.

It's estimated that as many as three million people in the United States use steroids for non-medical reasons with men having a higher prevalence of use than women. According to the 2009 Youth Risk Behavior Study, about 3.3% of the nation's high-school students took steroids without a doctor's prescription at least once in their lifetime. Studies indicate that up to 30% of those who do strength training in gyms use steroids.

Interestingly, a web-based survey of 1,955 men who used steroids for non-medical reasons determined a profile of a steroid user. The typical user was Caucasian, about 31 years old, using steroids since the age of about 26, well-educated (46% had at least a Bachelor's degree), employed as a full-time "white-collar" professional (3.9% were working in the fitness industry, by the way) and earning an above-average income (50% had an annual household income between $40,000 and $99,999). Moreover, the typical user was never involved in organized sports and took steroids to increase muscle mass, strength and physical attractiveness.

Any sport in which athletes rely on size, strength, speed and power will have a high prevalence of steroid use. For example, one study of 380 competitive bodybuilders found that 54% of the men and 10% of the women used steroids on a regular basis. Besides bodybuilding, steroids are prevalent in competitive weightlifting (Olympic-style and powerlifting), American football and track and field.

WHAT ARE STEROIDS?

Steroids are synthetic (man-made) derivatives of testosterone that have anabolic as well as androgenic properties (thus the technical term of anabolic-androgenic steroids or AAS). The anabolic (growth-promoting) effects of testosterone include increases in strength, muscle mass, bone density, protein synthesis and nitrogen retention; the androgenic (masculinizing) effects include the development of male secondary sexual characteristics such as an increase in facial and body hair, a deepening of the voice and a heightened libido. Scientists who develop steroids try to maximize the anabolic effects and minimize the androgenic effects.

Steroids can be taken by ingestion, injection, a transdermal patch or cream/gel. (By far, the most common way of self-administration is injection.) Administration of steroids typically involves "stacking" (using two or more different types of drugs at the same time); "cycling" (alternating periods in which the drugs are used with periods in which the drugs aren't used); and "pyramiding" (increasing doses of the drugs for the first half of a cycle and then decreasing doses of the drugs for the second half).

Street names for steroids include 'roids, arnolds, gym candy and "the juice." Popular steroids are methandrostenolone (Dianabol), nandrolone decanoate (Deca-Durabolin), fluoxymesterone (Halotestin), oxandrolone (Anavar) and stanozolol (Winstrol). Also of note are designer steroids that are made in such a way as to avoid detection in drug testing. An example is tetrahydrogestrinone (aka The Clear and, for short, THG) which gained considerable notoriety during the federal investigation of Victor Conte and his Bay Area Laboratory Co-Operative (BALCO) that began in 2002.

DO STEROIDS WORK?

Up to the 1980s, studies had shown that steroids weren't effective. This fact was noted regularly by the scientific and medical communities. For example, in its 1977 position stand that reviewed the existing research, the American College of Sports Medicine (ACSM) stated that steroids were ineffective for increasing size and strength. Meanwhile, government officials and scientists in East Germany must have found this research to be quite amusing since their own studies and experiments clearly showed otherwise. Not until its 1984 position stand did the ACSM acknowledge that steroids were effective for increasing size and strength.

Since the 1980s, countless studies have shown that steroids work. Research has found that steroids increase strength, especially when taken in conjunction with a strength program. Steroids also increase muscle mass. However, steroids don't decrease fat mass. As a result, body composition is enhanced but mainly through the increase in muscle mass. Upon termination of steroid use, the drug-induced improvements in size and strength gradually diminish. There's no scientific evidence that steroids increase endurance or expedite recovery between workouts.

ADVERSE EFFECTS

A multitude of adverse effects from steroids have been documented in the scientific and medical literature. It must be noted that for ethical reasons, studies often use relatively small doses of steroids and for short periods of time. In "real life," though, steroids are usually taken in much higher doses – which could be 100 times the therapeutic dose – and for longer periods of time thus presenting a much greater risk. So, if anything, research grossly underestimates the true extent of the adverse effects.

Keep in mind that what follows are potential adverse effects; there's a great deal of variability based on the type of steroid, dosing regimen and duration of use as well as individual tolerances. Also worth mentioning is that while some adverse effects are reversible with cessation of use, others are not.

These adverse effects are well-documented in the scientific and medical literature:

Liver

The second-largest organ in the body is the liver. (In case you're wondering, the largest organ is the skin.) The liver is highly vulnerable to steroid use. The most serious complications are peliosis hepatis (which results in the formation of blood-filled cysts throughout the liver) and liver tumors (both benign and malignant). These two conditions are considered life-threatening and irreversible.

Some researchers speculate that peliosis hepatis may be a pre-tumorous lesion that can become malignant with prolonged steroid use. Rupture of the blood-filled cysts or liver failure resulting from peliosis hepatis has often been fatal.

Numerous reports have been published that link the use of steroids with liver tumors. Moderate to heavy use of steroids in otherwise healthy individuals can cause liver cancer and even death over time. The period between the initial stages of liver cancer to the full-blown clinical expression may be more than five years. In other words, steroid users may have cancers growing in their livers but the symptoms have yet to reveal themselves.

The use of steroids also impairs the excretory function of the liver and results in jaundice which gives the eyes and skin a yellowish tint and occurs at relatively low doses. Finally, higher doses of steroids appear to increase the incidence of liver dysfunction.

Kidneys

Another organ of concern is the kidneys. The use of steroids increases the possibility of kidney stones, kidney dysfunction and kidney failure. Wilms' tumor – a rare kidney cancer that mostly affects children – has been associated with steroid use and can be fatal.

Cardiovascular System

There are also significant risks to the cardiovascular system. Steroids have been linked with high blood pressure (hypertension) and high cholesterol. Steroids increase low-density lipoprotein (LDL), the "bad" cholesterol, and decrease high-density lipoprotein (HDL), the "good" cholesterol. High blood pressure and high cholesterol are two major risk factors for cardiovascular disease.

A "near ideal" range for LDL is 100 to 129 milligrams per deciliter (mg/dl) with 190 mg/dl and above considered very high; a good range for HDL is 50 to 59 mg/dl with 40 mg/dl and below considered poor. One steroid user, age 22, had an LDL of 596 and HDL of 14. Within one month of discontinuing steroids, his levels improved to an LDL of 220 and HDL of 35.

Additionally, steroids are associated with several heart conditions. This includes a thickening of the left ventricular wall which makes it more difficult for the ventricular chamber to fill and pump blood. Steroids are also linked with an increased risk of acute myocardial infarction (heart attack), ventricular arrhythmia (an irregular heart beat) and sudden cardiac death.

One of the most graphic examples of the adverse effects of steroid use on the cardiovascular system was experienced by Steve Courson, a former professional football player. He encountered many adverse effects including tachycardia (an accelerated heart rate). In 1984, his resting heart rate was as high as 160 beats per minute (bpm). When Courson checked himself into a hospital in 1988, his resting heart

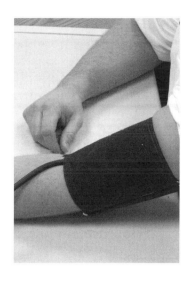

Steroids have been linked with high blood pressure (hypertension).

rate was 200 bpm. His medical problems forced him to seek a heart transplant . . . *at the age of 33.*

In 1989, Dr. Robert Malinowski, the Ashtabula County (Ohio) coroner who examined the body of Benji Ramirez, a high school football player, stated that steroids were a contributing factor in the 17-year-old's heart attack. This marked the first time that steroids had been officially linked to a death in the United States.

Reproductive System

Without question, steroids pose an enormous threat to the male and female reproductive systems. Essentially, steroids produce feminizing effects in men and masculinizing effects in women.

When a man starts to introduce exogenous testosterone into his body, his internal regulatory system reduces its own production of endogenous testosterone in order to maintain a stable internal environment (known as homeostasis). If too much foreign testosterone is added, his body will no longer produce its own supply.

This chemical balancing results in a number of chilling adverse effects. For instance, a decreased sperm count has been well-documented. One study found that the sperm count of 15 athletes was reduced by an average of 73% after two months of steroid use. Another well-documented adverse effect related to this hormonal irony is gynecomastia which is the appearance of female-like breasts on the male physique. Other male-specific effects include prostate enlargement, sterility, functional impotency, testicular atrophy, difficult or painful urination and a high-pitched voice. (Given the high potential for sterility, it's no real shocker that testosterone has been investigated as a male contraceptive.)

When a woman takes steroids, she's basically a female turning male. Women can experience physical changes that are irreversible including enlargement of the clitoris, decreased breast size, hirsutism (an increase in facial and body hair), alopecia (a loss of scalp hair) and a deepening of the voice. Other adverse effects include an increased risk of breast cancer, uterine atrophy and menstrual irregularities (such as amenorrhea).

These adverse effects and others were noted in a study that involved 10 female steroid users. In this study, all 10 women reported a lowering of the voice; nine had increased facial hair; eight experienced enlargement of the clitoris, increased libido, increased aggressiveness and irritability and acne on the face and back; and five noticed a decrease in breast size and menstrual diminution or cessation.

Women who use steroids also increase their risk of bearing children with birth defects. When taken by pregnant women, steroids can cause masculinization of the fetus. The degree of masculinization is related to the amount of steroids being taken and the age of the fetus during the steroid use.

Psyche and Behavior

Steroids have the potential to produce a wide array of adverse effects that have a profound impact on psyche and behavior. This includes anxiety, euphoria, depression, extreme mood swings, irritability, schizophrenia, paranoia, auditory hallucinations, delusions of grandeur, sleep disturbances and an increased or a decreased libido (sex drive).

In one study, researchers interviewed 41 bodybuilders and football players who had used steroids. Five of the subjects met the criteria for psychotic symptoms during periods in which they used steroids. None of the subjects had psychotic symptoms when they weren't using steroids. Of the five subjects who had psychotic symptoms, one had auditory hallucinations of voices and the other four developed various delusions. Another five subjects met the criteria for a manic episode during steroid exposure. One of these subjects bought an old car and deliberately drove it into a tree at 40 miles per hour while a friend videotaped him.

Perhaps the one psychiatric adverse effect that's most frequently documented and discussed is an increased level of unpredictable hostility, rage and aggression that's commonly referred to as 'roid rage. Because of the high potential for impaired behavior, steroids jeopardize the safety of others. A classic example of 'roid rage was demonstrated by one individual whose steroid-amplified aggression involved him in numerous brawls and created violent thoughts like "crushing people to death" and "tearing off their limbs." Another steroid user – annoyed by a traffic delay – damaged three cars (with drivers inside) using his fists and a metal bar.

Speaking of behavior, one study found an association between steroids and criminality in that the initiation of steroid use led to an increase in criminal activity. And in a study of prisoners, those who tested positive for steroids were more likely to be convicted of a weapons offense than those who tested negative.

Research has shown that about 30% of the individuals who use steroids develop a dependence on the drug. The dependency can lead to classic symptoms of withdrawal – including depression and fatigue – when steroids are discontinued.

Linked to the psychological dependency on steroids is a condition known as muscle dysmorphia, a term that was coined in 1997 and is sometimes referred to as reverse anorexia nervosa. Those with muscle dysmorphia are dissatisfied with their body, have low self-esteem and are preoccupied with their muscularity. No matter how much muscle these individuals gain, they still see themselves as too small. Muscle dysmorphia is prevalent among steroid users.

Miscellaneous Adverse Effects

There are a variety of other adverse effects, too. Steroid users are predisposed to connective tissue injuries. One theory is that steroids weaken connective tissue by inhibiting the formation of collagen, cellular proteins that provide structural support. Another theory is that connective tissue doesn't respond to steroids to the same degree that muscle tissue does. This would create a situation in which the connective tissue can't keep up with the demands from using heavier weights thereby increasing the possibility of serious tendon, ligament, fascia and meniscus injuries. This has been likened to installing a very powerful engine into a sub-compact car. Eventually, the tremendous torque generated by the new engine would overpower the original transmission and tear it to bits.

In one study, more than 14% of steroid users reported injection practices that were unsafe. This included reusing needles and sharing multi-dose vials and needles with others. Those who inject steroids run the risk of infection, blood poisoning and the spread of communicable diseases – including hepatitis and human immuno-deficiency virus (HIV) – from contaminated needles along with neural dysfunction as a result of improperly placed needles.

Adolescents who use steroids may experience a pre-mature fusing of their epiphyseal (or growth) plates that are located at each end of a long bone. A pre-mature closure of the epiphyseal plates before completion of the normal growth cycle will result in stunted growth which isn't reversible.

There's strong evidence that the use of steroids leads to the use of other drugs. This, of course, represents a big problem and manifests itself in many ways.

One study found that 77% of self-reported steroid users also took at least one other illicit or non-medical drug during the previous year. For instance, steroid users were almost 12 times more likely than non-users to take cocaine. Furthermore, studies have shown that steroid use is associated with opiate use (such as morphine and heroine) and a higher prevalence of alcohol use. In one study, 21 of 227 heroin addicts at a treatment facility were first introduced to opiates through steroid use. In fact, 17 of those 21 individuals first purchased opiates from the same drug dealer who sold them steroids.

Individuals who use steroids also tend to employ other appearance- or performance-enhancing drugs such as human growth hormone and insulin. In addition, they may use other drugs in an attempt to control the unwanted effects of steroids. For example, they may take amphetamines to combat depression; sedatives to overcome insomnia; diuretics to avoid fluid retention and reduce blood pressure; tamoxifen to prevent gynecomastia; and Human Chorionic Gonadrotropin (HCG, mainly prescribed to treat female infertility) to reverse or prevent testicular atrophy. (Diuretics and HCG are also used to mask the appearance of steroids in a drug test.)

The use of steroids can trigger an increase in oil production by the sebaceous glands of the skin and cause acne to develop anywhere on the body, usually on the back. Additional adverse effects include fluid retention, alopecia, unprovoked nose bleeds, stretch marks and peptic ulcers.

TESTING FOR STEROIDS

In 1980, Manfred Donike of West Germany developed a technique for identifying abnormal levels of testosterone in the urine. His method looks at the ratio of testosterone to epitestosterone or, for short, the T/E ratio. Since the levels of epitestosterone in the body remain stable, testosterone from an outside source will elevate the T/E ratio.

A T/E ratio of 1:1 is normal with men having a slightly higher ratio and women a slightly lower ratio. Some people have a ratio of 2:1. A ratio of 3:1 is rare. For many years, a ratio of 6:1 or greater indicated a positive test for steroids. In 2005, the threshold was lowered to a ratio of 4:1. If a test finds a T/E ratio of 4:1 or higher, a follow-up test is done using a carbon isotope ratio analysis (or other data).

Since the 1980s, laboratories have tested thousands of Olympic athletes. About 90% of them have a ratio of 1:1. More than 99% are less than 5:1. Only one in 2,000 athletes has a naturally elevated level of testosterone.

After Germany was reunified in 1990, investigators uncovered a trove of classified documents in Stasi files. One document showed the results of "in house" tests on four East German female swimmers who had won a total of 10 Olympic gold medals. The tests were done at a laboratory in East Germany on August 9, 1989, shortly before the European Swimming Championships in Bonn. (Testing of athletes had become standard practice just prior to international competitions; athletes whose test results were unacceptable weren't allowed to participate.) Testing positive (T/E ratio in parentheses) on that date were Heike Friedrich (8.8:1), Dagmar Hase (10.0:1), Daniela Hunger (12.5:1) and Kristin Otto (17.0:1). Remember, these were females.

Many East German athletes were often given a "counterinjection" of epitestosterone to normalize their T/E ratio in an attempt to avoid the detection of steroids. This practice is still done by athletes and, as a result, epitestosterone – which has no ergogenic value – is banned by the World Anti-Doping Agency as a masking agent.

OVERT SIGNS OF STEROID USE

Coaches, parents and employers may be interested in identifying the use of steroids. Although this is virtually impossible without testing, there are a few tell-tale signs.

Because steroids can be taken by injection or in tablet/pill form, users may have needles, syringes and pill bottles either hidden or in their possession. Puncture marks, bruises, scar tissue or calluses on the upper thighs and buttocks from injections are overt signs.

Many physical indicators of steroid use are related to the adverse effects. For example, users often have a bloated, puffy look to their faces and skin due to fluid retention. In addition, their eyes and skin may have a yellowish tint (from jaundice). A sudden and significant increase in size, weight and strength can also be a sign of steroid use. Other physical indicators are severe acne, alopecia, gynecomastia, unprovoked nosebleeds and stretch marks (likely due to the sudden and significant increase in size).

In terms of psychological signs, unpredictable hostility, rage and aggression are noticeable adverse effects of steroid use. Other indications of steroid use can be severe depression and a significant change in libido.

Just because one or two of these signs are present doesn't necessarily indicate steroid use. However, if there are more than a few signs, the use of steroids is likely.

LEGITIMATE USES

Steroids are prescribed by physicians for a number of medical conditions. This includes anemia, breast cancer, burn injuries, recovery from surgery, osteoporosis and HIV infection.

Another legitimate use of steroids is in testosterone replacement therapy for hypogonadism, a condition in which the gonads (testicles) produce levels of testosterone that are below the normal range of healthy men. The vast majority of testosterone prescriptions are written for men who are 46 and older. To ensure that testosterone is prescribed by a physician for the treatment of hypogonadism – and not something else like the improvement of size and/or strength – individuals who are required to be drug tested may be asked to provide medical documentation that their level of testosterone is consistent with that of a hypogonadal man.

A MATTER OF ETHICS

As just noted, steroids do have some legitimate medical applications. But the use of steroids in an attempt to improve physical capacity or athletic performance is contrary to the ethical principles and regulations of competitions as established and set down by various athletic foundations and sports-governing bodies. These organizations include the International Association of Athletics Federations, the International Olympic Committee and the National Collegiate Athletic

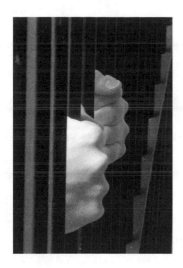

Federal law makes simple possession of steroids without a prescription punishable by up to one year in prison and/or a minimum fine of $1,000.

Association. Strong anti-steroid statements have also been issued by the National Strength and Conditioning Association, the American College of Sports Medicine and all major sports organizations, most notably the National Football League and Major League Baseball.

STEROIDS AND THE LAW

Steroids are legal in some countries but not in the United States without a prescription. Because of the potential for widespread abuse, Congress enacted the Anabolic Steroids Control Act of 1990. This amended the Controlled Substances Act of 1970, classifying 27 steroids as Schedule III controlled substances. The Anabolic Steroids Control Act of 2004 also amended the Controlled Substances Act, adding more steroids to the list of Schedule III controlled substances. (Note: Schedule III controlled substances are those that may lead to moderate or low physical dependence or high psychological dependence. Besides steroids, the list of Schedule III controlled substances includes stimulants and depressants.)

Federal law makes simple possession of steroids without a prescription punishable by up to one year in prison and/or a minimum fine of $1,000. The penalties increase for those with previous convictions for certain offenses. For first-time offenders, selling steroids or possessing them with the intent to sell is punishable by up to five years in prison and/or a $250,000 fine. Those penalties double for second-time offenders.

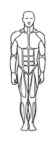

24 Strength and Fitness Q&A

There are a number of topics that don't fit neatly into the content of the previous chapters but still merit discussion. This final chapter contains 50 topics in a Q&A format that pertain to various aspects of strength and fitness.

1. How strong should the hamstrings be in comparison to the quadriceps?

It has long been suspected that an imbalance of strength between the hamstrings and quadriceps increases the potential for injury. Specifically, strong quadriceps could overpower weak hamstrings. We're told that hamstring strength should be at least 60% of quadricep strength but there's no scientific evidence for this particular number.

The exercises that provide direct work for the hamstrings and quadriceps are the leg curl and leg extension, respectively. The resistance that's used with these two exercises differs from one machine to another. The reason is because all machines are designed differently which affects leverage and, therefore, the amount of resistance that can be lifted. As a result, it's virtually impossible to make accurate comparisons of strength between the hamstrings and quadriceps (at least with conventional equipment).

Here's an example: When using a leg curl that's made by Company A, you might be able to do 15 repetitions with 100 pounds; when using a leg curl that's made by Company B, you might be able to do 15 repetitions with 120 pounds. If this is the case, which resistance is used for comparison with the leg extension?

Also keep in mind that there are two different types of leg curls – seated and prone – which also have different designs that affect the amount of resistance that you can lift. This is true even for machines that are manufactured by the same company.

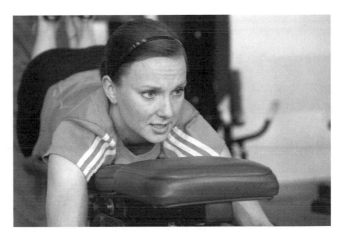

It has long been suspected that an imbalance of strength between the hamstrings and quadriceps increases the potential for injury. (Photo provided by Luke Carlson.)

So, don't worry about percentages. The important thing is to make sure that your hamstrings are as strong as possible.

2. Does the position of the feet affect which part of the gastrocnemius is used during the calf raise?

Changing the position of the limbs during the performance of an exercise is believed to target different parts of a muscle. In the calf raise, for instance, some individuals change the position of their feet thinking that this will influence different parts of their calves.

Researchers randomly assigned 20 subjects to perform the calf raise with their feet in three different positions: neutral, internally rotated (toes pointed in) and externally rotated (toes pointed out). The subjects performed one set of 12 repetitions in each of the three positions without wearing any footwear. The calf raise was done with their forefeet elevated on a 1.5-inch block while holding a barbell across their shoulders that was loaded with 30 to 35% of their bodyweight.

When their feet were externally rotated, there was significantly greater activation of the medial (inner) gastrocnemius; when their feet were internally rotated, there was significantly greater activation of the lateral (outer) gastrocnemius.

It would seem that during the calf raise, then, the position of the feet *does* target different parts of the gastrocnemius. Be that as it may, some individuals may find it uncomfortable to do the calf raise with their feet rotated excessively in one direction or the other.

3. What's the best grip width to use when doing the bench press with a barbell?

In a study that involved 24 subjects, researchers compared performance in the bench press with six different grip widths: two "narrow," two "moderate" and two "wide." The researchers found that the subjects lifted significantly more weight with a moderate-width grip. In this study, a moderate-width grip was about 26 to 32 inches or 165 to 200% of biacromial breadth. (Biacromial breadth is the distance between the most lateral points on the acromion processes. The acromion process is essentially the tip of the shoulder.)

You don't have to collect this anthropometric data and calculate your ideal grip width for the bench press. Simply use a grip that's slightly wider than shoulder-width apart.

4. Why is it easier to do a chin-up than it is to do a pull-up?

Regardless of how you position your hands, just about any type of multiple-joint movement for your torso that involves a pulling motion targets the same muscles, namely your upper back, biceps and forearms. However, there are differences in your biomechanical leverage based on the grip that you use. For example, doing a chin-up with an underhand grip (palms facing toward the body) is more biomechanically efficient than doing a pull-up with an overhand grip (palms facing away from the body). With an underhand grip, the radius and ulna – the

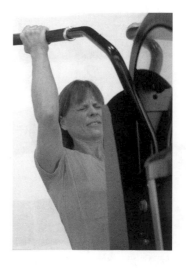

Doing a chin-up with an underhand grip is more biomechanically efficient than doing a pull-up with an overhand grip. (Photo provided by Luke Carlson.)

bones in the lower arms – run parallel to one another; with an overhand grip, the radius crosses over the ulna forming an X. In this position, the bicep tendon gets wrapped around the lower portion of the radius, creating a biomechanical disadvantage and a loss in leverage. As a result, it's more difficult to do a pull-up.

This is also true when comparing underhand and overhand grips during other pulling and rowing movements; the same muscles are used but with varying degrees of biomechanical leverage. (With a parallel grip – in which the palms face each other – the bones in the lower arms don't cross, either. Therefore, this grip is also more efficient than an overhand one.)

5. Is rotating the torso while holding a stick across the shoulders an effective exercise?

Many individuals sit on a bench, place a wooden stick (or sometimes a barbell) across their shoulders and rotate their torso from one side to another. Or, they hold a medicine ball with their arms straight and parallel to the floor and rotate their torso in the same manner. But these exercises do little, if anything, for the obliques.

In order for an exercise to be as effective as possible, you must apply a force that opposes the resistance by 180 degrees. In other words, the applied force must be *exactly opposite* the direction of the resistance. If the resistance is from the south, the force must be applied to the north;

if the resistance is from the east, the force must be applied to the west.

Gravity is a force that always pulls straight down. Because of the effects of gravity, the force that's applied to any "dead weight" – such as a barbell or dumbbell – must be straight up. When you push or pull a barbell or dumbbell (or something similar) straight up while gravity acts straight down, the application of force is absolutely perfect: It's 180 degrees out of sync with the resistance.

From this, it can be seen that rotating the torso with a stick or similar object held across the shoulders is an incorrect – and ineffective – application of force. No matter how much the object weighs, the resistance is always straight down. Therefore, the force needs to be applied straight up or *perpendicular* to the floor, not *parallel* to it.

The most effective way to do torso rotation is on a machine. Here, the direction of the applied force is congruent with the direction of the resistance.

6. Are free weights better than machines for increasing strength?

Studies have shown that there are no significant differences in the development of strength when comparing groups that used free weights and groups that used machines. The fact is that the use of *any* equipment in which a load is progressively applied on your muscles will stimulate improvements in strength (and size, for that matter).

In one study, 22 subjects were randomly assigned to two groups: One group did the bench press and shoulder press with free weights; the other group did similar exercises with machines. Both groups used the same training protocol (three sets of six repetitions done three times per week). After five weeks, the subjects in the free-weight group increased the strength of their elbow extensors by about 22% and shoulder flexors by about 12%; the subjects in the machine group increased the strength of their elbow extensors by about 24% and shoulder flexors by

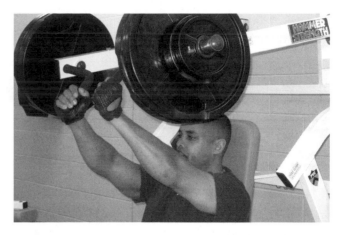

Studies have shown that there are no significant differences in the development of strength when comparing groups that used free weights and groups that used machines.

about 13%. There were no significant differences between the two groups.

Since a muscle doesn't have the ability to think or see, it cannot possibly "know" whether the source of resistance is a barbell, a machine or a cinder block. The sole factors that determine your response from strength training are your genetics and effort, not the equipment that you employ. To quote Dan Riley, who served as a strength coach in the National Football League for 27 years and at the collegiate level for eight years: "The equipment used is not the key to maximum gains. It's how you use the equipment."

7. To avoid injury, don't warm-up sets have to be done prior to a set that's taken to the point of muscular fatigue?

Warm-up sets aren't necessarily needed for your muscles to receive a proper warm-up. If you do a relatively high number of repetitions and lift the weight in a smooth, controlled manner without any explosive or jerking movements, then you'll actually warm up as you perform the set. Think about it: If you do a set of 10 repetitions with a speed of movement that's roughly six seconds per repetition, you'll have exercised your muscles for about one minute before you reach the point of muscular fatigue. After one minute of exercising, there's little doubt that you'll be adequately warmed up and prepared – both physiologically and psychologically – to reach muscular fatigue in a safe manner.

An exception to this would be individuals who do low-repetition sets such as competitive weightlifters. In this case, they should perform warm-up sets prior to their low-repetition efforts to reduce their risk of injury.

8. Do high repetitions tone muscles and low repetitions bulk them?

There's no scientific evidence that doing high repetitions will increase muscular definition ("tone") and low repetitions will increase muscular size ("bulk"). Researchers randomly assigned 24 subjects to two groups: One group did multiple sets of four repetitions and the other group did multiple sets of 10 repetitions. (A third group acted as a control and didn't train.) After 10 weeks of training, both repetition protocols produced significant and similar improvements in strength, muscle cross-sectional area, muscle girth and skinfold measurements.

In another study, 38 subjects were randomly assigned to three groups: One group did four sets of 3 to 5 repetitions, the second group did four sets of 13 to 15 repetitions and the third group did four sets of 23 to 25 repetitions. (A fourth group acted as a control and didn't train.) After seven weeks of training, all three repetition protocols produced significant and similar improvements in hamstring and quadriceps thickness.

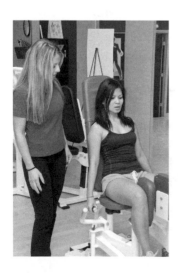

There's no scientific evidence that doing high repetitions will increase muscular definition and low repetitions will increase muscular size. (Photo by Pilar Martinez.)

Other than monozygotic (identical) twins, each person has a different genetic potential for achieving muscular definition and muscular size. Some people are predisposed toward developing highly defined physiques while others are predisposed toward developing heavily muscled physiques. Whether sets consist of high repetitions or low repetitions (or intermediate repetitions), you'll still develop according to your genetics (provided that the sets are done with similar levels of intensity).

9. Are high repetitions as effective as low repetitions for increasing muscular strength?

Muscular endurance and muscular strength are directly related. If you increase your muscular endurance, you'll also increase your muscular strength.

One way to measure muscular strength is to do one repetition with a maximum amount of weight (known as a one-repetition maximum or 1-RM); one way to measure muscular endurance is to do as many repetitions as possible with a sub-maximum amount of weight. Now, suppose that your 1-RM in the bench press is 100 pounds (your muscular strength) and you can do 10 repetitions with 75 pounds (your muscular endurance). And after several months of training with high repetitions – say, using a range of about 5 to 10 – suppose that you've progressed to the point where you can do 90 pounds for 10 repetitions. Given the fact that you increased the amount of weight that you could lift for 10 repetitions by 20% – from 75 to 90 pounds – it's likely that your 1-RM will now be greater than your previous effort of 100 pounds. So even though you trained with high repetitions, you increased your muscular strength.

By the way, it works the other way as well. If you increase your muscular strength, you'll also increase your muscular endurance. Here's why: As you get stronger, you need fewer muscle fibers to sustain a sub-maximum effort (muscular endurance). This also means that you have a greater reserve of muscle fibers available to extend the sub-maximum effort.

10. When lifting weights, should the eccentric phase of a repetition be minimized since it's associated with excessive muscular soreness?

One long-standing criticism of eccentric exercise is that it produces a large degree of muscular soreness. However, research has shown that soreness can occur if a muscle is loaded excessively in a concentric, isometric *or* eccentric manner.

Moreover, it has been shown that eccentric exercise has a protective (or repeated-bout) effect. This means that any muscular soreness that may occur as a result of eccentric exercise will be lessened after doing subsequent workouts that involve eccentric exercise.

Keep in mind, too, that when lifting weights, the duration of the eccentric phase of a repetition involves a relatively brief period of loading. If you lower a weight in about three to four seconds per repetition, for instance, then the eccentric loading that occurs during a set of 15 repetitions only lasts about 45 to 60 seconds. Even when this amount of time is extrapolated over the course of a workout, it's a far cry from the amount of eccentric loading that's used in most studies. In one study, for example, the subjects did *100 continuous eccentric repetitions* on the leg extension with their dominant leg. Two weeks later, they ran five intervals on a treadmill at a 10% decline for eight minutes per interval – *a total of 40 minutes of eccentric activity* – at a speed that corresponded to 80% of their predicted maximum heart rate. (Two minutes of recovery were given between each of the five intervals.) The subjects had no prior experience with eccentric training or intermittent downhill running. Is it any wonder that this eccentric exercise/activity produced a significant amount of "muscle tenderness"?

The eccentric phase of a repetition – and eccentric exercise/activity, for that matter – is safe and productive as long as it isn't performed to an extreme. As your muscles become more familiar with eccentric loading, any amount of muscular soreness that you may experience will be reduced.

11. What's the correct way to breathe when lifting weights?

It doesn't seem to matter too much whether you inhale as you raise the weight and exhale as you lower it or do the opposite. As it turns out, inhaling and exhaling naturally usually results in correct breathing. This is fortunate since it may be difficult for some individuals to maintain a set pattern of breathing when lifting weights.

One thing that must be avoided while strength training, however, is breath holding. When the breath is held during exertion, it creates an elevated pressure in the abdominal and thoracic cavities which is referred to as the Valsalva maneuver. The elevated pressure interferes with the return of blood to the heart. This may deprive the brain of blood and trigger a loss of consciousness.

12. What's the bilateral deficit?

The term bilateral deficit refers to the fact that the sum of the force produced by two limbs separately (unilaterally) is greater than the force produced by the same two limbs simultaneously (bilaterally). Consider the leg extension, for example. If you produce 50 pounds of force with one leg and 50 pounds of force with the other, it adds up to 100 pounds of force. It seems logical to think that you should be able to produce at least 100 pounds of force when you do the exercise with both legs at the same time. But you can't because of the bilateral deficit.

There's no consensus among researchers as to why this phenomenon occurs. Theories include neural inhibition and a reduced utilization of fast-twitch fibers. In any event, studies have shown that the bilateral deficit is about 85%. So in the aforementioned example, if you produced 50 pounds of force with each leg separately – a sum of 100 pounds – you'd be able to produce about 85 pounds of force with both legs simultaneously. Strange but true.

13. What's the best way to stimulate fast-twitch fibers in the fitness center or weight room?

It's important to first understand how muscle fibers are recruited. Under normal circumstances, the nervous system innervates muscle fibers in an orderly fashion according to the intensity or force requirements, not the speed of movement. Demands of low muscular intensity are met by slow-twitch fibers. Intermediate (hybrid) fibers are recruited when the slow-twitch fibers are no longer able to continue the task. Fast-twitch fibers are recruited only when the other fibers are fatigued to the point that they can't meet the force requirements. All fibers are working when the fast-twitch fibers are being used. The orderly recruitment pattern remains the same regardless of whether the repetition speed was fast or slow.

This pattern is consistent with the size principle of recruitment that was proposed by Dr. Elwood Henneman in the 1950s. He described the experimental basis of his principle in 18 related articles that were published in the *Journal of Neurophysiology* over the course of 25 years. According to this principle – which is widely regarded as one of the most important advances *ever* in the field of motor control – motoneurons are recruited based on increasing size: The motor unit with the smallest motoneuron is recruited first and the motor unit with the largest motoneuron is recruited last. (A motor unit

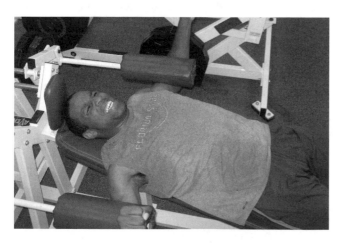

In order to engage as many fast-twitch fibers as possible, it's critical to train to the point of muscular fatigue. (Photo by Michael Bradley.)

consists of a motoneuron and all the muscle fibers that it innervates.) In general, the smallest motoneurons innervate slow-twitch fibers and the largest motoneurons innervate fast-twitch fibers. Therefore, slow-twitch fibers are recruited first and fast-twitch fibers are recruited last. (Note: An exception to the size principle is when a muscle is made to contract by electrical stimulation. In this case, the order of recruitment is reversed.)

What's the implication of this? In order to engage as many fast-twitch fibers as possible, it's critical to train to the point of muscular fatigue.

14. Can isometrics increase strength?

Basically, isometrics are exercises in which an individual pushes or pulls against an immovable resistance. The popularity of isometrics increased enormously in the middle of the 20th century primarily because of two events: First, in the 1950s, Erich Müeller and Theodor Hettinger of Germany released their research findings that showed the benefits of isometrics. Second, in 1961, Bob Hoffman – who was the president of the York Barbell Company and coach of the US Olympic Weightlifting Team – authored an article in which he claimed that isometrics were largely responsible for the outstanding performances that were made by two of his weightlifters, Bill March and Louis Riecke. Hoffman declared that isometrics were "the greatest system of strength and muscle building the world has ever seen." (His claims were later discredited when it was discovered that the two weightlifters had also taken steroids while performing isometrics.)

Can isometrics increase strength? Absolutely. But isometrics have several disadvantages. For one thing, isometrics increase blood pressure beyond what would normally be encountered when strength training with conventional methods. In addition, isometrics don't involve full-range repetitions. As a result, any increases in strength are specific to the joint angle being worked plus or minus a relatively small number of degrees. And since isometrics don't involve full-range repetitions, the muscles don't receive any stretch whatsoever. So after a while of doing a program of isometrics, an individual will likely lose flexibility.

15. What's a good equation for estimating a one-repetition maximum?

Over the years, a number of prediction equations have been developed and used to estimate a one-repetition maximum (1-RM) based on the relationship between muscular strength and muscular endurance. By using a prediction equation, a 1-RM can be estimated in a safe and practical manner without having to "max out." The following equation can be used to predict a 1-RM based on repetitions-to-fatigue (where X equals the number of repetitions performed):

$$\text{predicted 1-RM} = \text{weight lifted} \div (1.0278 - 0.0278X)$$

As an example, suppose that you were able to do 8 repetitions to the point of muscular fatigue with 150 pounds. Inserting these values into the equation yields a predicted 1-RM of about 186 pounds [0.0278 x 8 = 0.2224; 1.0278 - 0.2224 = 0.8054; 150 ÷ 0.8054 = 186.24].

In a study that involved 48 subjects, researchers found that this equation had a high correlation for predicting a 1-RM in the bench press and squat; in a study that involved 67 subjects, researchers found that this equation had a high correlation for predicting a 1-RM in all three of the competitive powerlifts: the bench press, squat and deadlift. It should be noted that this equation is most accurate for predicting a 1-RM when the number of repetitions-to-fatigue is 10 or less.

Because genetic factors – particularly muscle fiber types – play a major role in muscular endurance, prediction equations aren't accurate for everyone. However, they're still very practical for much of the population.

16. How effective is it to do exercises on a stability ball?

Despite the core-training craze, people have trained their cores (essentially, their mid-sections) for years. Nowadays, one of the most popular items to use for core training is the stability ball.

Researchers randomly assigned 10 subjects to perform the bench press in two conditions: stable (on a bench) and unstable (on a Swiss ball). The study found that the force exerted during the unstable condition was *59.6% less* than during the stable condition. In other words, when exercising in an unstable condition, the subjects couldn't produce as much force. This is consistent with other studies that showed decreased force output with decreased stability. In this particular study, there were no significant differences in muscle activation between the stable and unstable conditions. However, a number of other studies have shown that exercising in an unstable condition results in much less muscle activation. Needless to say, producing less force and generating less muscle activity aren't desirable when it comes to strength training.

On a related note, the use of stability balls has been shown to improve performance in arbitrary tests of core stability but not athletic performance. A study that involved collegiate swimmers found that training on a stability ball improved performance in tests of core stability but not performance in swimming; a study that involved high-school athletes found that training on a stability ball improved performance in tests of core stability but not maximum oxygen intake, running economy or running posture. (Core stability, in itself, is an ambiguous term that's subject to different interpretations.) According to Dr. Jeffrey Willardson, an assistant professor in the Physical Education Department at Eastern Illinois University, ". . . research has failed to demonstrate a significant relationship or improvement in sports performance consequent to performing exercises on unstable surfaces."

And to date, there's no scientific evidence to support the contention that instability training – on balls or other unstable objects (such as balance discs and wobble boards) – improves neuromuscular coordination or balance in another activity that requires some degree of balance. What about certain practices such as squatting while balancing on a stability ball or jumping from one stability ball to another? To quote the researchers in one study: "Whether some of these circus-type maneuvers provide specific crossover training adaptations to sport is still under debate and demands further investigation."

Not to be ignored is the potential for injury when exercising on a stability ball while holding weights. In September 2005, Peter Royal broke both wrists and one forearm and injured both shoulders when an "anti-burst" stability ball burst as he was about to do the bench press with a pair of 75-pound dumbbells. He incurred five surgeries and more than $100,000 in medical bills. About two years after the accident, he and his wife filed a lawsuit, contending that the gym, a YMCA, failed to maintain safe conditions. In 2009, Francisco Garcia, a guard-forward for the Sacramento Kings, broke his right forearm when a "burst resistant" stability ball burst while he was doing the bench press with a pair of 90-pound dumbbells. He missed 57 games that year and 24 the next. Garcia and the Kings filed lawsuits against the manufacturer of the stability ball. These aren't isolated cases; the Federal Trade Commission's Bureau of Consumer Protection estimates that more than 870 individuals have been injured using stability balls since 2004. Key point: Anything that's inflatable has the potential to burst.

Done safely, exercising on a stability ball can provide variety to workouts. But when outlandish claims are made or unsafe activities are advocated, the use of stability balls is getting just a bit unstable.

17. What's blood flow occlusion training?

Restricting the flow of blood to exercising muscles is known as blood flow occlusion training. This type of training has its roots in Japan, where it's referred as KAATSU Training. Credit for its development has been given to Yoshiaki Sato who received the "inspiration" for KAATSU Training in 1966 and went public with the idea in 1983.

Blood flow is occluded via pressurized cuffs with sensors or restrictive straps. For the most part, the application of pressure is limited to the proximal areas of the arms, thighs and calves.

Research has shown that blood flow occlusion, using as little as 20% of a one-repetition maximum, can improve strength and size. Anecdotal reports have been made that are nothing short of miraculous, including an older wheelchair-bound man who supposedly regained the use of his legs.

But is it safe? In a survey of 12,642 individuals in Japan who had received KAATSU Training, 1,651 (13.1%) sustained a subcutaneous hemorrhage. That's a pretty significant number of people. Another 164 (1.3%) experienced numbness and 35 (0.3%) cerebral anemia. There's also the potential for blood clots, muscle cell damage and necrosis. Sato, himself, was hospitalized with severe numbness in his leg due to, in his words, "reckless KAATSU Training."

Restricting your blood flow isn't normally a good thing. And it can be even more problematic when done while exercising.

18. Is vibration training effective?

A relatively new method of training is whole-body vibration (WBV). The use of WBV is becoming increasingly popular among a wide range of populations from the athletic to the elderly.

WBV has two main elements. One is the vibration that comes from a vibration device or platform. The other is the exercise/activity. WBV can be done using a single leg or both legs; static or dynamic contractions; or unloaded or loaded conditions (with additional weight).

It's touted as an effective way to prevent and treat osteoporosis and muscle atrophy as well as improve "muscle performance," "athletic power" and "body balance." As with most methods of training, however, anecdotal reports are one thing and scientific studies are another.

Most of the long-term studies (12 to 24 weeks) that used one or more comparison groups found that WBV wasn't significantly better than strength training in improving strength, vertical jump, speed of movement and fat-free mass. The acute (immediate) effects from WBV – most notably increases in vertical jump and flexibility – have led some to view WBV as a potential warm-up procedure rather than a recommended training protocol.

When administered for up to 24 weeks at 26 to 45 Hertz, WBV appears to be safe with very few adverse effects reported in the scientific literature. Nevertheless, the effects of long-term exposure to vibration are unknown.

19. Do lifting belts reduce the risk of injury or improve performance?

The use of lifting belts is fairly widespread. According to one survey, lifting belts were worn by 27% of the members of a fitness center. Moreover, 90% of the individuals who wore lifting belts said that they did so to prevent injury; 22% wore lifting belts to improve performance.

To date, no studies have looked at the effect of lifting belts on the incidence of injuries during strength/fitness applications. However, several studies have shown that doing the barbell squat and deadlift while wearing a lifting belt increases inter-abdominal pressure (IAP). An increased IAP is thought to stabilize the spine and decrease compressive forces. In addition, one study found that the use of lifting belts produced less spinal shrinkage when performing the deadlift (although the study used a protocol of eight sets of 20 repetitions with 22 pounds which is totally unrealistic).

Interestingly, no studies have looked at the effect of lifting belts on performance during strength/fitness applications. As a result, there's no scientific evidence to support the notion that the use of lifting belts improves performance.

20. Does grunting help someone lift more weight?

Walk into most gyms and you'll hear a cacophony of sounds including an assortment of grunts. In 2006, reports quickly spread across the country about a man who was escorted from Planet Fitness (a commercial gym) by local police for grunting, a violation of the gym's policy. In fact, the story was deemed so newsworthy that it made the front page of *The New York Times*.

Among other things, the incident triggered intense debate about whether or not a gym should have a no-grunting rule. Lost in the shuffle, though, was whether or not there's any merit to grunting while lifting weights.

In one study, 31 subjects did three maximal grunts. The researchers measured the maximum decibel level and averaged the three grunts. On a later day, the subjects made three grunt and three non-grunt efforts while performing an isometric deadlift. In order to be characterized as a grunt, the decibel level had to be more than 90% of maximum; a non-grunt was less than 25% of maximum.

The study found that grunting produced an improvement in peak force but not significantly more than non-grunting. So it seems as if grunting does help but not too much.

21. What's exertional rhabdomyolysis?

Rhabdomyolysis is a condition in which muscle fibers are broken down in such an extreme manner that the cell membranes are destroyed. This releases or "leaks" intracellular contents into the bloodstream in concentrations so high that it can have dire consequences. Complications include cardiac arrhythmia (an irregular heartbeat), cardiac arrest (a sudden loss of heart function), compartment syndrome and renal (kidney) failure.

The most common risk factors for rhabdomyolysis are drug abuse, alcohol abuse, bacterial and viral infections, blunt trauma and crush injuries. But in many instances, it results from severe exertion. Here, it's referred to as exertional rhabdomyolysis or exercise-induced rhabdomyolysis. Most cases of exertional rhabdomyolysis involve military and law-enforcement personnel, often recruits/trainees. During 2011, for example, there were 435 cases of exertional rhabdomyolysis in the US military (of which 207 required hospitalization). However, there are numerous and growing reports of exertional rhabdomyolysis sustained by individuals who were pushed too hard by their coaches or trainers.

Factors that increase the risk of rhabdomyolysis are a sudden increase in physical activity; exercises that are severe, repetitive and unfamiliar; workouts that overemphasize one or two muscles; and a hot, humid environment, especially when coupled with inadequate hydration.

Rhabdomyolysis is a medical emergency. As a result, early recognition is extremely critical. Local signs and symptoms include muscle pain, tenderness, swelling, bruising and weakness. Systemic signs and symptoms include fever, nausea, confusion, agitation and tea-colored urine (which is often the first and perhaps most tell-tale sign of rhabdomyolysis; the dark color is due to the high urinary concentration of myoglobin, a muscle protein).

22. What can be done to avoid headaches that are caused by lifting weights?

Exercise-related headaches are somewhat common. These headaches are triggered by many activities including running and weightlifting. Since most of the headaches are benign and relate to exertion, they're referred to as benign exertional headaches.

During a six-month period, a group of physicians reported that their emergency department diagnosed four patients with headaches that were related to lifting weights. The headaches were described as persistent and severe: One patient said that the pain was so severe that he felt as if he was "going to pass

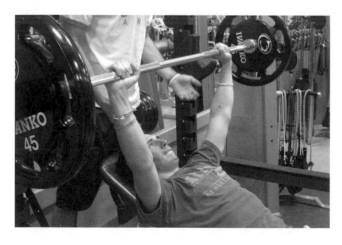

To avoid exertional headaches, it's important for you to employ proper breathing and good technique. (Photo by Stevie Harrison.)

out"; another said that it was "the worst headache" of his life. In all four patients, the onset of the pain was sudden. The location of the headache varied, although most were in the occipital (posterior and lower) area of the head.

To avoid this type of headache, it's important for you to employ proper breathing (no breath holding) and good technique (no excessive straining). Any activity that aggravates the condition should be avoided.

Keep in mind that headaches could be indicative of something more serious. It's a good idea, then, for those who experience this condition to seek medical attention.

23. How many calories are used in the recovery period after strength training?

One study had 15 women do one set of nine exercises to muscular fatigue in an average of 21.3 minutes. Researchers determined that in the two hours post-exercise, the women used about 22.4 calories above their baseline values. Or look at it this way: During the two hours post-exercise, the "afterburn" was about 1.05 calories per minute of activity.

Interestingly, the study also had the same 15 women do three sets of nine exercises to muscular fatigue in an average of 63.1 minutes. Researchers determined that in the two hours post-exercise, the women used about 22.6 calories above their baseline values. So during the two hours post-exercise, the afterburn was about 0.36 calories per minute of activity.

Another study had seven men do six sets of 10 exercises to muscular fatigue in 90 minutes. It was estimated that in the two hours post-exercise, the men used 34.0 calories above their baseline values. During the two hours post-exercise, then, the afterburn was about 0.38 calories per minute of activity which is strikingly similar to the afterburn that was produced by the multiple-set protocol in the study of 15 women.

So after strength training, there's an increased expenditure of calories above baseline values. Nonetheless, it isn't as much as might be thought.

24. What's the best way to trim fat from the abdominal area?

The abdominal area probably gets more attention than any other body part. Many people perform countless repetitions of abdominal crunches, knee-ups and other abdominal exercises – sometimes more than once per day – with the belief that this will give them a highly prized set of "washboard abs."

In exercise science, the belief that exercise can produce a localized loss of body fat is known as spot reduction. A litmus test for evaluating spot reduction is to determine whether a significantly greater change occurs in an active (or exercised) muscle compared to an inactive (or unexercised) muscle. Spot reduction has been investigated since at least 1962. The research shows that spot reduction isn't possible.

In a classic study, 19 subjects were assigned to two groups. One group performed a sit-up program for 27 days, amounting to 5,004 sit-ups per subject (with their legs bent at a 90-degree angle and no foot support). The other group served as a control and did no sit-ups. Those who did sit-ups significantly decreased the diameter of the fat cells in their abdominals, subscapular and gluteals to a similar degree. In other words, exercising their abdominals didn't preferentially affect the fat in their abdominal area more than their subscapular or gluteal areas. There were no significant differences in the rate of change in the fat-cell diameter between the three sites.

In a more recent study, 24 subjects were randomly assigned to two groups. One group performed seven abdominal exercises for two sets of 10 repetitions five days per week for six weeks, amounting to 4,200 repetitions per subject. The other group served as a control and did no abdominal training. Those who did abdominal exercises increased their abdominal endurance more than those who did no abdominal exercises. However, there were no significant differences between the two groups in decreasing abdominal fat, abdominal skinfold and waist circumference.

Why isn't spot reduction possible? Well, when you exercise, fat (and carbohydrates) is drawn from throughout your body as a source of energy,

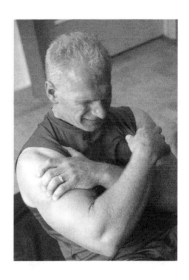

Abdominal exercises have no preferential effect on the subcutaneous fat that resides over your abdominal muscles. (Photo provided by Luke Carlson.)

not just from one specific area. Abdominal exercises certainly involve the abdominal muscles. But abdominal exercises have no preferential effect on the subcutaneous fat that resides over your abdominal muscles (and beneath your skin). For that reason, you can do abdominal exercises until you pass out but these Olympian efforts will not automatically trim your abdomen.

By the way, there's no scientific evidence that spot reduction can occur in other areas of the body, either. One study involved a group of 20 male and female tennis players. These athletes had used one side of their body much more than the other for at least six hours per week for at least two years. As expected, their upper and lower arms on their preferred side were larger than on their non-preferred side. Among men, for example, the difference in the circumference of their lower arms was about 0.89 inches; with their upper arms, the difference was 0.37 inches. But there was no significant difference in the thickness of the subcutaneous fat over the muscles of the arm. So, exposing one arm to considerably more activity over a fairly lengthy period of time resulted in an increase in size . . . without any preferential loss of fat.

25. Does electrical muscle stimulation increase size and strength?

Electrical muscle stimulation (EMS) has been used for years to rehabilitate muscles after injury or surgery. Because of its success in those applications, EMS has been proposed as an alternative or adjunct for healthy individuals who want to increase their size and strength.

Understand that EMS devices aren't anything new. Introduced in 1949, the Relaxacisor was perhaps the first EMS device peddled to the general public. More than 400,000 units were sold before the Food and Drug Administration stepped in and pulled the proverbial plug on the device in 1970 for being "ineffective and dangerous." Since then, not much has changed.

In one study, researchers examined an EMS device that was marketed to the public and could be purchased over the counter. In the study, 27 subjects were randomly assigned to two groups. One group received stimulation from the device according to the manufacturer's recommendations. The second group received sham stimulation from a device that looked identical to the other but was modified by the researchers so that it didn't transmit any electrical current. (The subjects in the latter group were told that they'd receive a lower current that "should be less noticeable.") After eight weeks, there were no significant differences between the two groups in terms of size and strength (or in skinfold measurements). And here's a real shocker: When piloting the procedure, the researchers received a small superficial burn from the electrode.

While previous research found that EMS is effective for increasing size and strength, the studies used high-quality, medical-grade devices which, of course, aren't available for general use. Plus, the studies typically examined one or two muscles which is much different from a comprehensive strength program.

Be advised that over-the-counter EMS devices have several drawbacks. For one thing, the devices may be wildly inaccurate and of very poor quality. Also, the electrical current may be too uncomfortable for many individuals.

26. Does a sauna belt help someone lose weight and melt fat?

A product that has been popularized in a number of infomercials is the so-called sauna belt. And like EMS devices, it's not a new idea. Sauna belts were introduced as early as the 1960s. Back then, it was simply a rubber wrap that secured around the waist. Today's high-tech version plugs into a wall socket and produces heat.

Promoters claim that the sauna belt melts fat. Can fat melt? Yes. But in order to do so, your body temperature would be so high that your brain would boil and your blood would probably coagulate. Other claims with no scientific basis are that the sauna belt can "flush out and eliminate toxins" and "enhance metabolism." But perhaps the most outrageous claim is that a belt uses "600 calories in 30 minutes." To get the same caloric expenditure, a 165-pound individual would have to run about 4.65 miles in 30 minutes, a pace of about 9.3 miles per hour. Since the only physical effort is to put on the belt and plug it in, a caloric expenditure that high is simply impossible.

A sauna belt will make you sweat and, theoretically, this could produce a small amount of weight loss. But the weight loss is from water and water has no calories. And when people are instructed to set the belt to as much as 176 degrees to supposedly promote fat loss, is anyone surprised that there are countless reports from consumers who burned their skin?

A sauna belt is basically a glorified heating pad. And an overpriced one at that.

27. Can wearing certain bracelets enhance balance and strength?

Nowadays, many individuals wear bracelets that supposedly improve a wide range of physical abilities. However, these products and other "performance jewelry" don't live up to their hype.

In one study, 42 collegiate athletes were randomly assigned to do tests of flexibility, balance, strength and power. The athletes did these four tests twice, once while wearing a bracelet that's marketed as performance jewelry and another while wearing a placebo bracelet. Neither the athletes nor the examiners knew which bracelet was being worn during which trial.

The researchers found no significant differences between the performance jewelry and the placebo jewelry in any of the measures. Interestingly, the athletes always did significantly better in the second trial regardless of which bracelet they wore. It's likely that the increased performance in the second trial was the result of what amounts to practicing the tests in the first trial.

So, there's no scientific evidence that performance jewelry enhances performance.

28. Can wearing certain shoes tone the hips and legs?

One of the latest products that supposedly tones and firms the muscles of the hips and legs is walking shoes. It's also claimed that the shoes can promote weight loss and improve posture.

The basic premise of the shoes is to provide instability through various designs – such as rocker-like soles and air pockets built into the soles – which make it more challenging for the wearer to maintain balance. Conceptually, this is similar to the difficulty that's encountered when trying to maintain balance on an unstable object such as a wobble board.

Promoters often point to a study in which five women walked for five minutes on a treadmill three different ways: wearing the toning shoes, wearing regular walking shoes and barefoot. It was found that the toning shoes produced significantly greater muscle activity in the gluteals, hamstrings and calves.

However, the study had severe limitations that cast a shadow of doubt on its findings: The study was short duration (involving only 500 steps), had a small number of subjects (five) and wasn't published in a peer-reviewed journal. Also raising an eyebrow is the fact that the study was funded by a manufacturer of the shoes.

Your best bet is to walk away from footwear that purports to tone your muscles.

29. Why does the resistance on some cable columns feel lighter than what's shown on the weight stack?

The force that's required to lift the weight on a cable column is dependent on the mechanical efficiency of the pulley arrangement. All cable columns have a fixed pulley directly above the weight which doesn't move when the weight is lifted. But some cable columns also have a "traveling" or moveable pulley directly above the weight which does move.

If the machine only has a fixed pulley, it offers no mechanical advantage. In this case, 100 pounds on the weight stack feels like 100 pounds. If the machine has two pulleys – one fixed and one traveling – the mechanical advantage is 2. In this case, 100 pounds on the weight stack feels like 50 pounds. So, the extra pulley cuts the resistance in half.

Here's another point of interest in comparing one pulley versus two: With one fixed pulley, when the bar moves a distance of two feet, the weight stack moves a distance of two feet; with one fixed pulley and one traveling pulley, when the bar moves a distance of two feet, the weight stack moves a distance of one foot. So, the extra pulley also cuts the distance that the weight moves in half.

30. What are some recommendations for individuals who have exercise-induced asthma?

Exercise-induced asthma (EIA) is an acute narrowing of the airway that, as the name suggests, is triggered by exercise. Classic symptoms include chest tightness, coughing, wheezing, excess production of mucous, sore throat and shortness of breath during or after exercise.

The condition is much more prevalent than you might think. It's estimated that 12 to 15% of Americans have EIA. Moreover, the condition is found in recreational athletes as well as elite athletes. One study found that 17% of the athletes in the 1998 Winter Olympics had EIA (with cross-country skiing as high as 50%). An estimated 70 to 90% of all individuals with chronic asthma experience EIA.

The symptoms are more likely – and more severe – during efforts that are intense or prolonged. So, those who suffer from EIA should adjust the level of their intensity and duration of their effort accordingly. Cold, dry air causes more symptoms. An effective tactic here is for individuals to cover their nose and mouth when exercising outdoors in cold weather. A basic, lightweight surgical mask (or dust mask) can be used as a barrier against cold air. Warm, humidified air lessens the degree of bronchospasm which suggests that swimming is an excellent activity.

Finally, anyone who suffers from EIA should seek the advice of a physician (who may prescribe medication as a preventive measure).

31. What's a "stitch in the side"?

At one time or another, many individuals have probably developed a "stitch in the side" when exercising. Technically referred to as exercise-related transient abdominal pain, its cause is subject to some debate. In the opinion of most authorities, however, it's due to a restricted supply of blood to the diaphragm – the main muscle that's used in respiration – and spasm.

The pain is localized in the abdominal area. When severe, the pain is sharp; when less severe, the pain is more like a cramp, an ache or a pull. It's related to activities that involve repetitive movements of the torso such as running and swimming. The condition is fairly common: One study reported that nearly 20% of runners experienced a stitch in the side during the previous year.

The good news is that the pain often subsides quickly. A few words of advice, though: Having a pain in the side of the abdomen doesn't automatically mean that it's a stitch in the side. The pain could be related to an abdominal strain, for example. Or it could be something that's far

worse. To be on the safe side, then, it's important to consult with a physician.

32. Is it okay to exercise when sick?

The best guide for deciding whether or not to exercise when you're sick is the location of the symptoms. More specifically, are the symptoms located above or below your neck?

When the symptoms are above your neck – such as a stuffy or runny nose, headache, sore throat or sneezing – the illness is relatively mild and probably will not worsen with exercise. Sometimes, in fact, the symptoms may temporarily improve while exercising. For example, exercise may unclog a stuffy nose.

But when the symptoms are below your neck – such as a chest cold, hacking cough, muscle aches, fever, chills, nausea or vomiting – the illness is more severe and probably will worsen with exercise. In this case, rest is needed.

If the illness is mild and you choose to exercise, you should employ a level of intensity that's below normal. Symptoms that worsen during exercise are a clear indication to stop.

A related issue that often gets ignored is whether or not the illness can spread to others in the fitness center. Something like this shouldn't be taken lightly as the health of others is now at stake.

When in doubt, hold off on exercising until you're healthy. And, of course, seek medical advice.

33. Are there differences in the energy requirements between running outdoors on a road and running indoors on a treadmill?

Assuming that "running outdoors on a road" is done in a relatively calm environment – meaning that the wind doesn't offer any substantial amount of air resistance – not really. In one study, eight subjects (who were runners) ran on a track and a treadmill at three different speeds: 6.7, 7.8 and 9.7 miles per hour. The researchers found that, statistically, there were no significant differences in the energy requirements between running on a track and treadmill.

So if inclement weather doesn't make it feasible to run outside on a road, you can still simulate your outdoor efforts – and obtain other health and fitness benefits – with a run inside on a treadmill.

34. Is it better to run with or without shoes?

Running without shoes is one of the latest movements afoot (pun clearly intended). Proponents of barefoot running point out that before the arrival of running shoes, humans had run barefoot or with minimal footwear since breaking ranks with apes millions of years ago.

Studies have compared the foot strike patterns of running with and without shoes. It has been shown that those who usually run with shoes tend to land on the back of their foot while those who usually run without shoes tend to land on the front of their foot *then* the back of their foot. In addition, barefoot runners who land on the front of their foot produce lower impact forces than shod runners who land on the back of their foot. This may reduce the risk of impact-related injuries but scientific evidence is lacking.

So don't shuck your shoes just yet. Besides, running outside without shoes is a risky venture. The odds of stepping on a sharp pebble, nail or shard of glass are high. And to prevent the spread of disease, it's not a good idea to run barefoot on a treadmill in a commercial setting.

35. Is there any significance as to how quickly the heart rate recovers after exercise?

Few would argue about the importance of the resting heart rate and exercising heart rate with respect to fitness. But often overlooked is the recovery heart rate following exercise.

Recovery heart rate is actually a fairly good indicator of fitness. Indeed, those who recover more quickly from exercise are most likely in better shape than those who recover less quickly. Here's something that has even greater significance, however: Several studies have found

that recovery heart rate is an indicator of longevity.

In one of those studies, researchers at the Cleveland Clinic Foundation followed 2,428 patients for six years. The subjects were referred to the clinic for exercise testing (which was done on a treadmill). Their recovery heart rates were taken during a cool-down period one minute after completion of the test. In this study, an abnormal recovery heart rate was considered to be a reduction of 12 beats per minute or less; a normal recovery heart rate was a reduction of 13 beats per minute or more.

Of the 639 patients who had an abnormal recovery heart rate, there were 120 deaths from all causes (18.8%); of the 1,789 patients who had a normal recovery heart rate, there were 93 deaths from all causes (5.2%). The study found that having a heart rate that takes a long time to return to resting levels following exercise is "a powerful predictor of overall mortality."

36. Is the Body-Mass Index a valid indicator of being overweight or obese?

The Body-Mass Index (BMI) is simply a ratio of someone's weight to height. It's used as a quick and handy way to estimate if a person is underweight or overweight.

To calculate your BMI, follow these three steps:

- Take your height in inches and square it (multiply it by itself).

- Divide that number into your bodyweight in pounds.

- Multiply that number by 703.

If you're 6'0" and weigh 180 pounds, for example, your BMI is about 24.4 [72 x 72 = 5,184; 180 ÷ 5,184 = 0.0347; 0.0347 x 703 = 24.39]. For adults, a normal BMI is considered 18.5 to 25.0, overweight is 25.0 to 30.0 and obese is 30.0 or more.

Remember, the BMI is *an estimate*. A potential pitfall of relying on the BMI is that it doesn't distinguish fat mass from muscle/bone mass. Two people of the same height and weight would have the same BMI but it's quite conceivable that they could have markedly different levels of body fat. So even though their BMI is identical, one individual can have an excessive amount of body fat while the other can have an acceptable amount. The fact of the matter is that people who are muscular and/or have "big bones" could be mistakenly categorized as overweight or even obese.

Case in point: An individual who is 6'2" and weighs 240 pounds has a BMI of about 30.8 which is considered obese. But this happens to be the listed height and "competitive weight" of Arnold Schwarzenegger when he was a professional bodybuilder. Obviously, he wasn't anywhere near being obese. In reality, his percentage of body fat was certainly in the single digits.

Therefore, the BMI must be interpreted with caution. If anything, the BMI should be supplemented with another measure such as body composition.

37. Does caffeine improve performance when exercising?

Caffeine – a stimulant of the central nervous system – is perhaps the most widely used drug in the world. It's a component of tea, coffee, chocolate and soda as well as pills to lose weight and combat drowsiness. It has no significant nutritional value.

Interest in the use of caffeine as an ergogenic aid (or performance enhancer) was mainly inspired by two studies that were published in the late 1970s. In those studies, caffeine produced significant improvements in endurance (in cycling). To date, numerous studies done in a laboratory have shown that caffeine increases performance in cycling and running for durations of roughly 5 to 20 minutes. But studies done outside a laboratory have found mixed results. At this time, for example, it doesn't appear as if caffeine improves sprint performance (inside or outside a laboratory).

The use of caffeine doesn't seem to improve strength or muscular endurance, either. In a recent study, 14 men were randomly assigned to groups that received either caffeine or a placebo

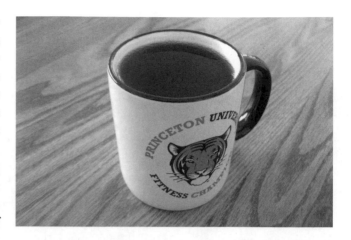

The use of caffeine doesn't seem to improve strength or muscular endurance.

one hour prior to strength training (four sets of four exercises to muscular fatigue with 70 to 80% of their 1-RM). Compared to the placebo, caffeine produced a small improvement in the number of repetitions that were done on the leg press but no improvement on the three exercises for the torso. There were no significant differences between caffeine and the placebo in the amount of weight that was lifted in any of the exercises.

In low doses, caffeine doesn't pose any serious risks for healthy individuals; when consumed in high doses, caffeine has the potential for many adverse effects such as anxiety, jitters, tremors, inability to focus, gastrointestinal distress, diarrhea, insomnia, irritability and "withdrawal headache." Since caffeine is a potent diuretic – which increases the production of urine – there has been some concern that it can increase the risk of dehydration, a major fear during physical activity, especially in a hot, humid environment.

38. Do people really need to drink eight glasses of water per day to be healthy?

One of the most oft-repeated bits of health advice is that you should drink at least eight eight-ounce glasses of water – one-half gallon of water – on a daily basis. Moreover, proponents of the so-called 8x8 Rule state that other fluids don't count toward this goal.

A high intake of water appears to be beneficial in reducing the risk of several conditions including bladder cancer, colorectal cancer and heart disease. And, of course, water has several physiological functions such as regulating body temperature (which helps to keep you from overheating).

Be that as it may, there's no scientific evidence that people need to drink eight eight-ounce glasses of water each day (or any other specific amount, for that matter). The volume of water that's needed can vary greatly from one person to another based on such factors as age, size, level of fitness and the duration and intensity of the activity as well as the environment. (Cold, heat, humidity and altitude all increase the need for water.)

And don't forget that many foods and beverages – most notably fruits, fruit juices, vegetables, vegetable juices, milk and soup – are very high in water and, thus, can be counted toward your daily total. Clearly, it's important to consume adequate amounts of fluids but this medical maxim doesn't hold any water.

39. Should water intake be limited when exercising?

In 2005, a front-page article in *The New York Times* ("Study Cautions Runners to Limit Intake of Water") quickly sparked nationwide concern about the intake of water when exercising. Much of the article was based on a study that appeared in *The New England Journal of Medicine*. The study examined 488 runners who provided blood samples at the finish line of the 2002 Boston Marathon. The researchers found that 13% of the runners had hyponatremia, a condition that's characterized by a low concentration of sodium in the blood. Three of the runners had critical hyponatremia.

The primary risk factor for hyponatremia is thought to be an excessive intake of fluids (which is why hyponatremia is sometimes referred to as water intoxication). This dilutes the level of sodium in the blood and creates an electrolyte imbalance. In the study, 35% of the runners drank so much fluid that they actually *gained weight during the marathon*. One individual was *nine pounds heavier* at the end of the race. (It's important to note that the study had several

shortcomings that weren't mentioned by the writer of the newspaper article, including a small sample size and reliance on self-reported data. Plus, imagine being asked to fill out a questionnaire immediately after running 26.2 miles.)

While overhydration during exercise is certainly a concern, the take-home message of the article was that people should restrict their intake of water when exercising. No doubt, many individuals were frightened into the extreme, thinking that they should refrain from drinking fluids altogether.

Certainly, endurance athletes should be aware of the potential for overhydration. But for the average person, overhydration is extremely rare. In hot, humid weather, proper hydration is absolutely critical. It's recommended that you weigh yourself before and after activity and adjust your fluid intake as needed.

40. Is bottled water significantly better than tap water?

Everyone assumes that bottled water is more pure than tap water. After all, it costs much more. But is it really much better?

One study compared the fluoride levels and bacterial content of commercially bottled water to that of tap water in Cleveland. The researchers examined 57 samples of five categories of bottled water that were purchased from local stores. (The five categories were spring, artesian, purified, distilled and drinking.) They also examined 16 samples of tap water that were collected from four local water processing plants. (Four samples were taken from each plant on unannounced visits.)

Only three samples (5%) of bottled water contained fluoride levels that were in the recommended range for drinking water as required by the state of Ohio. Meanwhile, 100% of the samples of tap water were in the recommended range. In terms of bacterial count, 15 samples (26%) of bottled water had significantly more bacteria than tap water. Compared to the average bacterial count of the tap water, six samples (11%) of bottled water had at least 1,000 times the bacteria of tap water. One sample of bottled water contained *nearly 2,000 times that of the most contaminated sample of tap water.*

But what about taste? Surely bottled water must taste better. In a survey of 2,800 people in England, 60% couldn't tell the difference between bottled water and tap water. It's also interesting to note that the Natural Resources Defense Council tested more than 1,000 samples of 103 brands of bottled water and found that "an estimated 25 percent or more of bottled water is really just tap water in a bottle."

41. Is there anything wrong with eating energy bars in place of a meal?

First, keep in mind that the use of the term energy can be misleading. Numerous products use the word energy in their names. This suggests that the product will improve your stamina or make you more energetic. In truth, calories provide you with energy and three nutrients provide you with calories: carbohydrates, protein and fat. In short, people get energy from food. Technically, then, a can of non-diet soda is an energy drink, a hot dog is an energy roll, a pad of butter is an energy square, a slice of bacon is an energy strip, a chocolate-chip cookie is an energy disc and an ice-cream sandwich is an energy bar.

That being said, there's nothing inherently wrong with most of the products that have been dubbed energy bars. So you can eat an energy bar, especially when it's more convenient because of time constraints. But you shouldn't make a habit of eating energy bars in lieu of regular foods and meals. Remember, there's nothing wrong with energy bars . . . but there's nothing magical about them, either.

While on the subject, some energy bars are made to taste like candy bars. As they say, if something smells like a fish it's probably a fish. So if an energy bar tastes like a candy bar, it's probably a candy bar. Or at best, it's a glorified and an expensive one. When considering an energy bar, it's always a good idea to check the Nutrition Facts panel and the ingredients on the food label.

42. Do energy drinks give you energy?

Countless numbers of beverages have been marketed as energy drinks. These beverages have fueled a multi-billion dollar industry with annual sales of more than three billion dollars in the United States alone.

The implication is that energy drinks will give you energy. As just noted, it's important to realize that energy is derived from calories. Any drink that has calories gives you energy so, technically speaking, orange juice, iced tea, non-diet soda and wine are energy drinks.

Of course, what's being marketed to consumers as energy drinks is a completely different story altogether. Standard ingredients of these beverages usually include sugar as well as various vitamins, amino acids (such as taurine) and herbs (such as ginseng). But the real buzz often comes from a hefty dose of caffeine.

In cola-type beverages, the Food and Drug Administration considers that caffeine is "generally recognized as safe" when the amount is less than about 70 milligrams per 12 ounces. As a point of reference, a 12-ounce can of Coca-Cola® has about 35 milligrams of caffeine. Since caffeine isn't a nutrient, products aren't required to show the exact amount on the Nutrition Facts panel and, in fact, energy drinks rarely offer this information. One beverage, though, claims 170 milligrams of caffeine in a one-ounce "shot," a concentration that's *nearly 30 times more* than what's generally recognized as safe for a cola-type beverage.

Energy is derived from calories so any drink that has calories gives you energy.

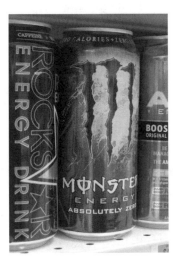

320

Concerns about the consumption of too much caffeine via energy drinks shouldn't be taken lightly. In a three-year period, 265 cases of "caffeine abuse" were reported to the Illinois Poison Center (Chicago) of which 37 were from dietary supplements and 41 were from "caffeine-enhanced beverages." In nearly 12% of the 265 cases, the patients were hospitalized for medical complications from caffeine.

43. Do thermogenic products really increase metabolism?

In an effort to lose weight, many individuals take thermogenic products. It's thought that these pills and drinks increase resting energy expenditure (REE).

Researchers randomly assigned 18 subjects to receive either three capsules of a commercially available thermogenic product or a placebo. Those who consumed the thermogenic product increased their REE by 17.3%, 19.6% and 15.3% after one, two and three hours post ingestion, respectively. Meanwhile, those who consumed the placebo decreased their REE at the same time points.

But how many more calories were used as a result of the product? Well, the REE increased by an average of about 11.46 calories during the first hour, 13.54 calories during the second hour and 10.42 calories during the third hour. This amounts to about 35.42 calories over the course of three hours. That's right, *a little more than 35 calories in three hours.*

Losing one pound of fat (3,500 calories), then, requires roughly 300 capsules of this particular product. At $39.99 for 90 capsules, that's an investment of *about $133.30 per pound of fat.*

Moreover, taking these products does absolutely nothing to improve your health and fitness or teach you good nutritional habits. It would be far better – and much cheaper – for you to lose weight by consuming less calories (eat less) and expending more calories (exercise more).

44. Does fortified water offer any advantages or benefits?

Fortified (or "enhanced") water contains vitamins but each bottle costs more than a dollar. For less than a dime, you can get pretty much the same thing by washing down a multi-vitamin/mineral supplement with a glass of water. Also of note is that fortified water usually contains more sugar – and more calories – than might be expected. An eight-ounce serving of one popular "water beverage," for example, has 13 grams of sugar. So, someone who drinks a 20-ounce bottle gets 32.5 grams of sugar (130 calories). For those who are trying to maintain or lose weight, these calories only add to their caloric budget.

Individuals who eat a balanced diet have no need to drink water that's fortified with vitamins. Remember, the best way to get vitamins (and minerals) is by eating fruits, vegetables and other wholesome foods. And the best way to get fluids is by drinking plain, old-fashioned water.

Additional "water beverages" offer an alluring array of other enhancements including amino acids, antioxidants, herbs and minerals. None of the products live up to their advance billing.

Speaking of fortified beverages, several companies have introduced soda that has been fortified with vitamins (such as Vitamins B_3, B_6, B_{12} and E) and minerals (such as chromium, magnesium and zinc). This is largely in response to consumer outcry that's directed at soda as being a major factor in the obesity epidemic along with the hope of reversing the trend of dwindling soda sales as consumers gobble up bottled water, teas, juices and sports drinks.

Yes, fortified soda is *healthier* than regular soda but that doesn't mean that it's *healthy* (or, in the words of one company's chief executive, a "health and wellness brand"). Promoting soda as "sparkling" rather than "carbonated" may be a good public relations ploy but, as they say, "A

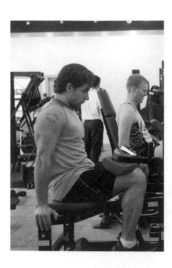

You don't have to exercise for 20 minutes before using fat as a source of energy. (Photo by Luke Carlson.)

horse by any other name is still a horse." So, let's not be fooled: Candy that's fortified with vitamins and minerals is still candy. And soda – liquid candy – that's fortified with vitamins and minerals is still soda.

45. Is it true that a person doesn't start using fat as an energy source until after 20 minutes of exercise?

The main source of energy that's used during an activity depends on the *level* of effort, not the *length* of effort. At rest, your body primarily uses fat as an energy source. As your level of effort increases, there's a greater reliance on carbohydrates to provide energy.

Therefore, you don't have to exercise for 20 minutes before using fat as a source of energy. In fact, as you read this book, your body is primarily using fat as an energy source. Besides, it's absurd to think that your body automatically switches to fat as an energy source at exactly the 20-minute mark.

46. Does eating after 6:00pm cause someone to gain weight?

Simply because you consume calories after a certain time doesn't mean that it will result in weight gain. The most important thing that determines whether or not you gain (or lose) weight is the number of calories that you consume and expend, not the time of day.

Does it makes sense that it would be okay to eat up until 6:00pm but doing so one minute later

would result in weight gain? And think about this: Suppose that you're in Georgia a few feet from its border with Alabama. Georgia is in the Eastern Time Zone and Alabama is in the Central Time Zone. So if you're in Georgia and it's 6:00pm, you're not supposed to eat or you'll gain weight. But if you quickly step across the border into Alabama where it's 5:00pm, is it now suddenly okay for you to eat without fear of gaining weight?

47. Are organic foods more nutritious than conventional foods?

Even though organic foods are more expensive than conventional foods, many people don't seem to mind paying a higher price for foods that they feel are healthier and more nutritious. But organic foods aren't really better than conventional foods when it comes to nutritional value.

British researchers examined 55 studies that were deemed to be of satisfactory quality. The studies analyzed 100 different foods and presented data on 455 nutrients and relevant substances that the researchers grouped into 98 nutrient categories. It was found that organic and conventional foods are comparable in their nutrient content. In other words, conventional foods are just as nutritious as organic foods.

Not to be overlooked, however, is the fact that organic foods control the use of chemicals in crop production (such as herbicides and pesticides)

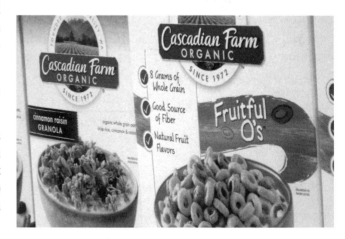

Research has found that conventional foods are just as nutritious as organic foods.

and medicines in animal production (such as antibiotics and growth hormones).

48. Is weight gain associated with high fructose corn syrup?

High fructose corn syrup (HFCS) is a synthetic sweetener that was created in the late 1960s. The manufacturing process starts out with kernels of corn and ends up with a concoction of fructose and glucose. It's found in numerous foods and beverages, ranging from the fairly obvious (yogurt and sweetened beverages) to the totally unexpected (bread and tomato soup).

One study looked at the short- and long-term effects of consuming HFCS. The study consisted of two experiments. In Experiment 1, male subjects who were fed HFCS with their meals gained more weight than those who were fed sucrose (a sugar) with their meals and those who were just fed their meals for eight weeks. In Experiment 2, male and female subjects who were fed HFCS with their meals gained more weight and abdominal fat than those who were just fed their meals for six months (males) and seven months (females).

However, the study was met with heavy criticism. Some described the study as "flawed" with "inconsistent results." It was noted that the subjects were fed enormous amounts of HFCS and even then, the weight gain was extremely small ("statistically indistinguishable"). A final point is that the subjects in this study were rats. And any data collected on rodents can't always be extrapolated to humans.

What's more, it's totally unreasonable to think that weight gain can be narrowed down to one single food or ingredient. The cause of weight gain is a function of two variables: eating too much and exercising too little.

49. Does vinegar "burn" fat?

In 2008, an article was published in *Sports Illustrated* about Jesse Chatman, who was a running back in the National Football League. The article reported on Chatman's efforts to maintain his bodyweight at an appropriate level. According to the article, the player got down to 223 pounds and then arranged a weigh-in with the trainer for the San Diego Chargers. He weighed 221 pounds "after chugging pickle juice en route to the team's facility (vinegar burns fat)."

Is this even possible? For the sake of argument, let's assume that the two-pound loss of weight came entirely from fat (especially since it's pointed out that "vinegar burns fat"). At rest – or nearly at rest such as driving a car – an individual who weighs 223 pounds uses about 1.77 calories a minute. One pound of fat has 3,500 calories. Under resting conditions, then, a 223-pound individual would "burn" two pounds of fat in roughly 3,946 minutes or about two days, 17 hours and 46 minutes. So unless the player drove to San Diego non-stop at an average speed of 60 miles per hour from somewhere like Fairbanks, Alaska, or another place that's about 3,642 miles away, it's simply impossible to "burn" two pounds of fat while driving a car.

For the record, there's absolutely nothing in vinegar that could "burn" fat. Nor is there any other substance currently known that can "burn" fat.

50. Do carbohydrates make people fat?

Contrary to what some may believe, *eating too much and exercising too little* make people fat. If anything, it's important for active individuals to consume carbohydrates to fuel their lifestyles. The primary function of carbohydrates is to supply energy, especially during intense exertions. The other two macronutrients that are sources of energy – fat and protein – have major

It's important for active individuals to consume carbohydrates to fuel their lifestyles.

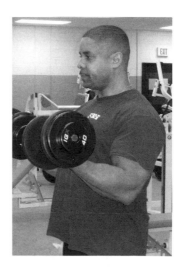

limitations for active individuals. Fat is an inefficient source of energy so it's preferred during low-intensity efforts when there's no need to be efficient; protein is generally a last resort since it resides in the muscles and if you're in a situation where you must depend on it as an energy source, then you're literally cannibalizing yourself.

There's no doubt that eliminating carbohydrates from your diet will inhibit your stamina and endurance. In addition, it's important to note that consuming too much fat and protein is associated with a greater risk of heart disease. And if you avoid carbohydrates, you also avoid foods with highly valuable nutrients such as fruits, vegetables and whole grains. This may lead to vitamin and mineral deficiencies. Clearly, carbohydrates are miscast villains.

APPENDIX A: SUMMARY OF FREE-WEIGHT EXERCISES

EXERCISE	EQUIPMENT	MUSCLE(S) STRENGTHENED	REPS
Deadlift	BB DB TB	gluteus maximus, hamstrings, quadriceps and erector spinae	15-20
Ball Squat	BW DB	gluteus maximus, hamstrings and quadriceps	15-20
Lunge	BW DB	gluteus maximus, hamstrings and quadriceps	15-20
Step-Up	BW DB	gluteus maximus, hamstrings and quadriceps	15-20
Seated Calf Raise	DB	soleus	10-15
Standing Calf Raise	DB	gastrocnemius	10-15
Dorsi Flexion	DB	dorsi flexors	10-15
Bench Press	BB DB	chest, anterior deltoid and triceps	5-10
Incline Press	BB DB	chest (upper portion), anterior deltoid and triceps	5-10
Decline Press	BB DB	chest (lower portion), anterior deltoid and triceps	5-10
Dip	BW	chest (lower portion), anterior deltoid and triceps	5-10
Bent-Arm Fly	DB	chest and anterior deltoid	5-10
Bench Row	DB	upper back, biceps and forearms	5-10
Bent-Over Row	DB	upper back, biceps and forearms	5-10
Chin-Up	BW	upper back, biceps and forearms	5-10
Pull-Up	BW	upper back, biceps and forearms	5-10
Pullover	BB DB EZ	upper back	5-10
Shoulder Press	BB DB	anterior deltoid and triceps	5-10
Lateral Raise	DB	middle deltoid and trapezius (upper portion)	5-10
Front Raise	DB	anterior deltoid	5-10
Bent-Over Raise	DB	posterior deltoid, trapezius (middle portion) and rhomboids	5-10
Internal Rotation	DB RB	internal rotators	8-10
External Rotation	DB RB	external rotators	8-10
Upright Row	BB DB	trapezius (upper portion), biceps and forearms	5-10
Shoulder Shrug	BB DB TB	trapezius (upper portion)	8-10
Scapulae Adduction	DB	trapezius (middle portion) and rhomboids	8-10
Bicep Curl	BB DB EZ	biceps and forearms	5-10
Tricep Extension	BB DB EZ	triceps	5-10
Wrist Flexion	BB DB	wrist flexors	8-10
Wrist Extension	DB	wrist extensors	8-10
Finger Flexion	BB DB	finger flexors	8-10
Abdominal Crunch	BW	rectus abdominis	8-10
Knee-Up	BW	iliopsoas and rectus abdominis (lower portion)	8-10
Side Bend	DB	obliques and erector spinae	8-10
Back Extension	BW	erector spinae, gluteus maximus and hamstrings	10-15
Stiff-Leg Deadlift	BB DB	erector spinae, gluteus maximus and hamstrings	10-15

EQUIPMENT CODES: BB = Barbell; BW = Bodyweight; DB = Dumbbells; EZ = EZ Curl Bar; RB = Resistance Band; TB = Trap Bar

NOTE: If two or more muscles are involved in an exercise, the first one listed is the prime mover. For example, the bench press involves the chest, anterior deltoid and triceps but it's considered to be a chest exercise.

APPENDIX B: SUMMARY OF MACHINE EXERCISES

EXERCISE	EQUIPMENT	MUSCLE(S) STRENGTHENED	REPS
Leg Press	PM SM	gluteus maximus, quadriceps and hamstrings	15-20
Hip Extension	SM	gluteus maximus and hamstrings	10-15
Hip Flexion	SM	iliopsoas	10-15
Hip Abduction	PM SM	gluteus medius and gluteus minimus	10-15
Hip Adduction	PM SM	hip adductors	10-15
Prone Leg Curl	PM SM	hamstrings	10-15
Seated Leg Curl	PM SM	hamstrings	10-15
Leg Extension	PM SM	quadriceps	10-15
Seated Calf Raise	PM	soleus	10-15
Calf Extension	SM	gastrocnemius	10-15
Dorsi Flexion	PM	dorsi flexors	10-15
Chest Press	PM SM	chest, anterior deltoid and triceps	5-10
Seated Dip	PM SM	chest, anterior deltoid and triceps	5-10
Pec Fly	PM SM	chest and anterior deltoid	5-10
Seated Row	PM SM	upper back, biceps and forearms	5-10
Underhand Lat Pulldown	PM SM	upper back, biceps and forearms	5-10
Overhand Lat Pulldown	PM SM	upper back, biceps and forearms	5-10
Pullover	PM SM	upper back	5-10
Shoulder Press	PM SM	anterior deltoid and triceps	5-10
Lateral Raise	PM SM	middle deltoid and trapezius (upper portion)	5-10
Rear Deltoid	PM SM	posterior deltoid, trapezius (middle portion) and rhomboids	5-10
Internal Rotation	CC PM	internal rotators	8-10
External Rotation	CC PM	external rotators	8-10
Upright Row	CC PM	trapezius (upper portion), biceps and forearms	5-10
Scapulae Adduction	PM SM	trapezius (middle portion) and rhomboids	8-10
Bicep Curl	CC PM SM	biceps and forearms	5-10
Tricep Extension	CC SM	triceps	5-10
Wrist Flexion	CC	wrist flexors	8-10
Wrist Extension	CC	wrist extensors	8-10
Abdominal Crunch	PM SM	rectus abdominis	8-10
Side Bend	CC	obliques and erector spinae	8-10
Torso Rotation	SM	obliques and erector spinae	8-10
Back Extension	SM	erector spinae, gluteus maximus and hamstrings	10-15
Neck Flexion	PM SM	sternocleidomastoideus	8-10
Neck Extension	PM SM	neck extensors and trapezius (upper portion)	8-10
Neck Lateral Flexion	PM SM	sternocleidomastoideus	8-10

EQUIPMENT CODES: CC = Cable Column; PM = Plate-loaded Machine; SM = Selectorized Machine

NOTE: If two or more muscles are involved in an exercise, the first one listed is the prime mover. For example, the seated row involves the upper back, biceps and forearms but it's considered to be an upper-back exercise.

APPENDIX C: SUMMARY OF MANUAL-RESISTANCE EXERCISES

EXERCISE	MUSCLE(S) STRENGTHENED	REPS
Hip Abduction	gluteus medius and gluteus minimus	10-15
Hip Adduction	hip adductors	10-15
Prone Leg Curl	hamstrings	10-15
Seated Leg Curl	hamstrings	10-15
Leg Extension	quadriceps	10-15
Dorsi Flexion	dorsi flexors	10-15
Push-Up	chest, anterior deltoid and triceps	5-10
Bent-Arm Fly	chest and anterior deltoid	5-10
Bent-Over Row	upper back	5-10
Seated Row	upper back, biceps and forearms	5-10
Lat Pulldown	upper back	5-10
Shoulder Press	anterior deltoid and triceps	5-10
Lateral Raise	middle deltoid and trapezius (upper portion)	5-10
Front Raise	anterior deltoid	5-10
Bent-Over Raise	posterior deltoid, trapezius (middle portion) and rhomboids	5-10
Internal Rotation	internal rotators	8-10
External Rotation	external rotators	8-10
Bicep Curl	biceps and forearms	5-10
Tricep Extension	triceps	5-10
Wrist Pronation	wrist pronators	8-10
Wrist Supination	wrist supinators	8-10
Abdominal Crunch	rectus abdominis	8-10
Neck Flexion	sternocleidomastoideus	8-10
Neck Extension	neck extensors and trapezius (upper portion)	8-10

NOTE: If two or more muscles are involved in an exercise, the first one listed is the prime mover. For example, the bicep curl involves the biceps and forearms but it's considered to be a bicep exercise.

About the Author

Matt Brzycki, BS, has nearly 30 years of experience at the collegiate level as a coach, instructor and administrator. This includes work as a Health Fitness Supervisor at Princeton University (May 1983 to September 1984), Assistant Strength and Conditioning Coach at Rutgers University (September 1984 to July 1990) and a variety of positions at Princeton University including Strength Coach and Health Fitness Coordinator (August 1990 to December 1993); Coordinator of Health Fitness, Strength and Conditioning (December 1993 to March 2001); Coordinator of Recreational Fitness and Wellness Programs (March 2001 to June 2007); and his current role as Assistant Director of Campus Recreation, Fitness (June 2007 to present).

He served in the US Marine Corps from 1975 to 1979, earning various distinctions including the Leatherneck Award (for rifle marksmanship), meritorious promotion to the rank of sergeant, Meritorious Mast, Good Conduct Medal, Certificate of Merit, Drill Instructor Ribbon and rifle expert badge (three awards). After completing his four-year enlistment, Matt enrolled at The Pennsylvania State University where he earned his Bachelor of Science degree in Health and Physical Education in 1983. In college, he was a competitive powerlifter and bodybuilder.

Matt has authored eight books, co-authored seven books and edited two books. In addition, he has authored more than 465 articles/columns on strength and fitness that have been featured in 45 different publications. Matt has given presentations throughout the United States and Canada including the Princeton University Cross Country Camp; Princeton University Wrestling Camp; Princeton University Strength & Speed Camp; American College of Sports Medicine's Health & Fitness Summit & Exposition; Athletic Business Conference & Expo; Tampa Bay Buccaneer Strength and Conditioning Seminar; NSCA Strength & Conditioning Conference for Football; Toronto Football Clinic; FBI Law Enforcement Executive Development Seminar; and Operational Tactics National SWAT/Sniper Symposium. In addition, he has given presentations to the Central Intelligence Agency; US Customs and Border Protection; and US Secret Service Academy. He has been a guest on radio shows in Atlanta, Cincinnati and Phoenix.

Previously, Matt was a coadjutant (part-time lecturer) for the Department of Exercise Science and Sport Studies at Rutgers University from March 1990 to July 2000, teaching a course in Strength Training Theory and Applications. In January 2012, he returned to Rutgers as a coadjutant, teaching a course in Principles of Weight Training. He taught a similar course for the Department of Health and Physical Education at The College of New Jersey from 1996 to 1999. Matt has co-developed two certification courses, the SWAT (Special Weapons and Tactics) Fitness Specialist certification (in 2003) and the Youth Fitness Instructor/Trainer (YouthFIT™) certification (in 2010).

Matt served on the Alumni Society Board of Directors for the College of Health and Human Development at Penn State from 2001 to 2007, chairing its Awards Committee during his final two years. He was appointed by the governor to serve on the New Jersey Council on Physical Fitness and Sports as well as the New Jersey Obesity Prevention Task Force.

He finished third in the 200 (29.89) and the 400 (1:04.33) in his age group (50-54) at the 2010 Mid-Atlantic Open and Masters Outdoor Track and Field Championships. His time in the 400 was below the qualifying standard of 1:06.20 for the 2011 Summer National Senior Games.